DATE DUE

FEB 2 8 2008		
DEC 2 7 2007		
MAR 1 1 2008		
JUN 2 2 2012		

GAYLORD   #3523PI   Printed ir

DISEASE SURVEILLANCE

THE WILEY BICENTENNIAL–KNOWLEDGE FOR GENERATIONS

*E*ach generation has its unique needs and aspirations. When Charles Wiley first opened his small printing shop in lower Manhattan in 1807, it was a generation of boundless potential searching for an identity. And we were there, helping to define a new American literary tradition. Over half a century later, in the midst of the Second Industrial Revolution, it was a generation focused on building the future. Once again, we were there, supplying the critical scientific, technical, and engineering knowledge that helped frame the world. Throughout the 20th Century, and into the new millennium, nations began to reach out beyond their own borders and a new international community was born. Wiley was there, expanding its operations around the world to enable a global exchange of ideas, opinions, and know-how.

For 200 years, Wiley has been an integral part of each generation's journey, enabling the flow of information and understanding necessary to meet their needs and fulfill their aspirations. Today, bold new technologies are changing the way we live and learn. Wiley will be there, providing you the must-have knowledge you need to imagine new worlds, new possibilities, and new opportunities.

Generations come and go, but you can always count on Wiley to provide you the knowledge you need, when and where you need it!

WILLIAM J. PESCE
PRESIDENT AND CHIEF EXECUTIVE OFFICER

PETER BOOTH WILEY
CHAIRMAN OF THE BOARD

DISEASE SURVEILLANCE

A Public Health Informatics Approach

Edited by

Joseph S. Lombardo

The Johns Hopkins University
Applied Physics Laboratory
Laurel, Maryland

David L. Buckeridge

McGill University
Montreal, Quebec
Canada

BICENTENNIAL
1807
WILEY
2007
BICENTENNIAL

WILEY-
INTERSCIENCE

A JOHN WILEY & SONS, INC., PUBLICATION

Copyright © 2007 by John Wiley & Sons, Inc. All rights reserved.

Published by John Wiley & Sons, Inc., Hoboken, New Jersey.
Published simultaneously in Canada.

For general information on our other products and services or for technical support, please contact our Customer Care Department within the United States at (800) 762-2974, outside the United States at (317) 572-3993 or fax (317) 572-4002.

Wiley also publishes its books in a variety of electronic formats. Some content that appears in print may not be available in electronic format. For information about Wiley products, visit our web site at www.wiley.com.

Wiley Bicentennial Logo: Richard J. Pacifico

Library of Congress Cataloging-in-Publication Data:

Disease surveillance : a public health informatics approach / [edited by] Joseph S.
    Lombardo, David Buckeridge.
        p.; cm.
    Includes bibliographical references and index.
    ISBN 978-0-470-06812-0 (cloth : alk. paper)
    1. Public health surveillance.   2. Medical informatics.   I. Lombardo, Joseph S., 1946–
II. Buckeridge, David, 1970–
    [DNLM: 1. Population Surveillance—methods.   2. Public Health Informatics. WA 105
    D6117 2007]
    RA652.2.P82D57 2007
    362.1—dc 22   2006053118

Printed in the United States of America.

10 9 8 7 6 5 4 3 2 1

*To those public health workers who get the call at 5 P.M.
on Friday afternoon and give freely of their own time
to protect the health of the populations they serve.
It is hoped that the advance disease surveillance methods
described in this book will help them to use their time
and talents more efficiently to accomplish their mission.*

Contents

Contributors

JEFF ARAMINI, DVM, PHD, Public Health Agency of Canada, Guelph, Ontario, Canada

RAJ ASHAR, MA, The Johns Hopkins University Applied Physics Laboratory (JHU/APL), Laurel, Maryland, USA

STEVEN BABIN, MD, PHD, The Johns Hopkins University Applied Physics Laboratory (JHU/APL), Laurel, Maryland, USA

DAVID BLAZES, MD, MPH, U.S. Naval Medical Research Center Detachment, Lima, Peru

DAVID L. BUCKERIDGE, MD, PHD, McGill University, Montreal, Quebec, Canada

HOWARD BURKOM, PHD, The Johns Hopkins University Applied Physics Laboratory (JHU/APL), Laurel, Maryland, USA

JEAN-PAUL CHRETIEN, MD, PHD, Walter Reed Army Institute of Research, Silver Spring, Maryland, USA

JACQUELINE COBERLY, PHD, The Johns Hopkins University Applied Physics Laboratory (JHU/APL), Laurel, Maryland, USA

DUNCAN COOPER, BSC, MRES, Health Protection Agency, West Midlands, United Kingdom

R. LOREN ERICKSON, MD, DRPH, Walter Reed Army Institute of Research, Silver Spring, Maryland, USA

JONATHAN GLASS, MD, U.S. Naval Medical Research Center Detachment, Jakarta, Indonesia

SHILPA HAKRE, MPH, DRPH, Walter Reed Army Institute of Research, Silver Spring, Maryland, USA

SHERI HAPPEL LEWIS, MPH, The Johns Hopkins University Applied Physics Laboratory (JHU/APL), Laurel, Maryland, USA

LOGAN HAUENSTEIN, MS, The Johns Hopkins University Applied Physics Laboratory (JHU/APL), Laurel, Maryland, USA

REKHA HOLTRY, MPH, The Johns Hopkins University Applied Physics Laboratory (JHU/APL), Laurel, Maryland, USA

HAROLD LEHMANN, MD, PHD, The Johns Hopkins University School of Medicine Baltimore, Maryland, USA

KATHY HURT-MULLEN, MPH, Montgomery County (Maryland) Department of Health and Human Services Rockville, Maryland, USA

JOSEPH S. LOMBARDO, MS, The Johns Hopkins University Applied Physics Laboratory (JHU/APL), Laurel, Maryland, USA

WAYNE LOSCHEN, MS, The Johns Hopkins University Applied Physics Laboratory (JHU/APL), Laurel, Maryland, USA

HAOBO MA, MD, MS, Science Applications International Corporation, Atlanta, Georgia, USA

STEVEN MAGRUDER, PHD, The Johns Hopkins University Applied Physics Laboratory (JHU/APL), Laurel, Maryland, USA

COLLEEN MARTIN, MSPH, Science Applications International Corporation, Atlanta, Georgia, USA

SHAMIR NIZAR MUKHI, MSC, Public Health Agency of Canada, Guelph, Ontario, Canada

CECILIA MUNDACA, MD, U.S. Naval Medical Research Center Detachment, Lima, Peru

DAVID ROSS, SCD, Public Health Informatics Institute (PHII), Decatur, Georgia, USA

MARVIN SIKES, MHA, The Johns Hopkins University Applied Physics Laboratory (JHU/APL), Laurel, Maryland, USA

CAROL SNIEGOSKI, MS, The Johns Hopkins University Applied Physics Laboratory (JHU/APL), Laurel, Maryland, USA

NATHANIEL TABERNERO, MS, The Johns Hopkins University Applied Physics Laboratory (JHU/APL), Laurel, Maryland, USA

MICHAEL W. THOMPSON, PHD, The Johns Hopkins University Applied Physics Laboratory (JHU/APL), Laurel, Maryland, USA

JEROME I. TOKARS, MD, MPH, Centers for Disease Control and Prevention (CDC), Atlanta, Georgia, USA

RICHARD WOJCIK, MS, The Johns Hopkins University Applied Physics Laboratory (JHU/APL), Laurel, Maryland, USA

Preface

During the last quarter of the twentieth century, countries with advanced healthcare systems felt comfortable in their ability to manage the spread of diseases that would have had high morbidity and mortality in earlier years. Smallpox had been eradicated and the memory of the Spanish Influenza outbreak of 1918 had faded. Toward the end of the twentieth and into the twenty-first century, the overuse of antibiotics, resulting in disease resistance, the rapid spread of HIV, and the increasing threat of bioterrorism were examples of public health issues that were beginning to increase pressure to enhance existing disease surveillance processes.

Among these concerns, the clandestine release of a deadly pathogen on an unsuspecting population maybe the most insidious public health threat. Most pathogens available as bioweapons can cause high mortality and could lead to the collapse of the healthcare delivery and emergency response systems in an area under attack. The contamination and the possible closure of major medical centers, even if only temporary, would have a serious impact on the health of the population. To mitigate the consequences of this type of public health event, an effective detection and treatment campaign must be launched early in the course of the outbreak.

Because of the threat of bioterrorism and the emergence of new infectious diseases, disease surveillance systems that utilize modern technology are becoming commonplace in public health agencies. The objective of this book is to present the components of an effective disease surveillance program that utilize modern technology. These components include the research, development, implementation, and operational strategies that are finding their way into successful practice.

Advanced disease surveillance systems automatically acquire, archive, process, and present data to the user. The development and maintenance of the systems require skilled personnel from the fields of medicine, epidemiology, biostatistics, and information technology. In addition, for the surveillance systems to be useful, they must adapt to the changing environment in which they operate and accommodate emerging public health requirements that were not conceived previously.

Research and innovation have led to the implementation of surveillance methods that would have been considered impossible or radical only a few years ago. For example, the case definitions or events under surveillance, which traditionally rely on diagnosis, have been altered in many systems to rely on less specific pre-diagonstic health indicators of syndromes. Correctly filtering data into syndromes or other categories for analysis requires knowledge of the underlying diseases and health-seeking behaviors of the population. Additionally, for analytical tools to have high specificity, they must take into account the normal range of all of the variables that comprise the background for the health indicators. Tools that fuse data and information from inhomogeneous indicators are necessary to provide decision-maker with comprehendable output. Similarly, information technologists must automate data ingestion and cleansing, optimize system architecture, and create user-friendly interfaces while meeting the challenge of using and customizing commercial, off-the-shelf products.

Users' requirements must have a higher priority than solutions that are technologically exciting. Continuing dialogue must exist among the users and the multidisciplinary development team to establish an effective surveillance capability that fits within the environment where it will be deployed. Without close interaction between these groups, effective advanced disease surveillance will be compromised. Changes to traditional thinking have resulted in the implementation of improved methods that are more suited to meeting the current challenges facing health departments. Because it is difficult to anticipate future public health emergencies, a continuing adaptation is required to maintain satisfactory system performance.

The field of public health informatics is growing rapidly as applications of technology are being applied to permit health departments to recognize and manage disease in the populations they serve. This book is intended for use (1) as a textbook for public health informatics students, (2) as a reference for health departments that are exploring modern information technology to support their surveillance activities, and (3) as training material for workshops that are components of disease surveillance and public health conferences.

The contents of this book provide insight into not only the technology but also into the difficulties and the successes that the public health community has had with the implementation and operational use of advanced disease surveillance systems. Hence, chapter authors provide not only the views of academics and developers of the technology, but also of users from health departments in the United States, Canada, United Kingdom, South America, and Asia. This wide variety of perspectives will hopefully provide a broad and balanced treatment of issues related to developing and operating advanced surveillance systems.

The book is divided into three parts. Following an introductory chapter (Chapter 1), the first part (Chapters 2 through 5) presents the methods and technologies needed to implement a modern disease surveillance system, including the data sources currently being used in syndromic surveillance systems (Chapter 2); the mechanisms for the acquisition of data for surveillance systems (Chapter 3); an overview of analytical methods for the recognition of abnormal trends within the data captured for surveillance (Chapter 4); and some basics of systems architectures, text parsing, and data visualization techniques (Chapter 5).

The second part of the book (Chapters 6 through 9) is devoted to case studies of modern disease surveillance systems and provides examples of several implementations in the United States, Canada, Europe, and Asia. These chapters indicate the breadth of the techniques used across the globe in applications of modern technology to disease surveillance.

The third and last part of this book (Chapters 10 through 12) addresses practical questions regarding the evaluation of disease surveillance systems, education of future public health informatics personnel and disease surveillance practitioners, and a look to the future to consider how technology will continue to influence the practice of disease surveillance.

Joseph S. Lombardo
The Johns Hopkins University
Applied Physics Laboratory
Laurel, Maryland, USA

David L. Buckeridge
McGill University
Montreal, Quebec
Canada

Acknowledgments

The chapter authors drew upon their extensive knowledge and experience to make this book a reality. Their contributions have made it possible for this book to include a depth of information on the wide variety of topics needed to implement, operate, and evaluate advanced disease surveillance applications.

In addition to the chapter authors, the talents of several individuals made this book possible. They took time from their busy lives to help assemble and review the materials from the authors. We are indebted to Steve Babin in particular for his knowledge of LaTEX and for the enthusiasm he brought to the project. The book could not have been assembled without the organizational skills of Sue Pagan who converted the diverse materials received from authors into chapters. Evelyn Harshbarger should also be recognized for the conversion of draft figures into high-quality images. Christian Jauvin's help was instrumental in creating the index. Finally, we would also like to thank Judy Marcus for her expert guidance in translating many flavors of jargon into readable material.

1 Disease Surveillance, a Public Health Priority

Joseph S. Lombardo, David Ross

Pandemic influenza, West Nile virus, severe acute respiratory syndrome (SARS), and bioterrorism are a few of the current challenges facing public health officials. The need for early notification of, and response to, an emerging health threat is gaining increasing visibility as public opinion increases the pressure to reduce the mortality and morbidity of health threats. With the greater emphasis on the early recognition and management of health threats, federal, state, and local health departments are turning to modern technology to support their disease surveillance activities. Several modern disease surveillance systems are in operational use today. This book presents the components of an effective automated disease surveillance system and is intended for use by public health informatics students, masters of public health students interested in modern disease surveillance techniques, and health departments seeking to improve their disease surveillance capacities.

This introductory chapter provides an overview of the changing requirements for disease surveillance from the perspective of past, present, and future concerns. It includes a brief history of how technology has evolved to enhance disease surveillance, as well as a cursory look at modern disease surveillance technology and activities.

1.1 INTRODUCTION

Control of infectious diseases is a cornerstone of public health. Various surveillance methods have been used over the centuries to inform health officials of the presence and spread of disease. The practice of disease surveillance began in the Middle Ages and evolved into the mandatory reporting of infectious disease cases to authorities responsible for the health of populations.

A common definition of surveillance is "the ongoing systematic collection, analysis, and interpretation of outcome-specific data for use in planning, implementation, and evaluation of public health practice" [1]. One of the more challenging aspects of public health surveillance is the early identification of infectious disease outbreaks

1

that have the potential to cause high morbidity and mortality. In recent years, concern over potential uncontrolled outbreaks due to bioterrorism or the appearance of highly virulent viruses such as avian influenza has placed increased pressure on public health officials to monitor for abnormal diseases. Public concern was heightened when at the beginning of the twenty-first century, the dissemination of a biological warfare agent through the U.S. mail system revealed weaknesses in the ability of existing public health surveillance systems to provide early detection of a biological attack.

Containment of potential outbreaks is also confounded by advances in transportation technology. Modern transportation systems permit communicable diseases to be carried around the world in hours over many public health jurisdictions. Health authorities can no longer simply be concerned only with the health status of the populations they serve; they must also cooperate and collaborate in surveillance and containment activities at regional, national, and international levels.

The Internet is an enabling technology for collaboration across wide geographic areas. Information technology in general is also playing a vital role in the timely capture and dissemination of information needed for identification and control of outbreaks. The subject of this book is the use of modern information technology to support the public health mission for early disease recognition and containment.

1.2   THE EMERGING ROLE OF INFORMATICS IN PUBLIC HEALTH PRACTICE

For more than 50 years, public health has been undergoing a change in identity that strongly affects how the public health sector envisions the use of information technologies. Public health is best viewed as an emergent industry. It has grown from a collection of single-purpose disease prevention and intervention programs to a national network of professionals linked through professional and organizational bonds. The 1988 Institute of Medicine report titled "The Future of Public Health" recognized that public health was established around three core functions and 10 essential services.

The core functions are:

- Assessment

- Assurance

- Policy development

The 10 essential services are:

1. Monitor health status to identify and solve community health problems.

2. Diagnose and investigate health problems and health hazards in the community.

3. Inform, educate, and empower people about health issues.

4. Mobilize community partnerships to identify and solve health problems.

5. Develop policies and plans that support individual and community health efforts.

6. Enforce laws and regulations that protect health and ensure safety.

7. Link people to needed personal health services and assure the provision of health care when otherwise unavailable.

8. Assure a competent public health and personal health care workforce.

9. Evaluate effectiveness, accessibility, and quality of personal and population-based health services.

10. Research for new insights and innovative solutions to health problems.

Information is one of the central products produced by public health. Protecting community health; promoting health; and preventing disease, injury and disability require vigorous monitoring and surveillance of health threats and aggressive application of information and knowledge by those able to prevent and protect the public's health. Thus, public health *informatics* supports the activities, programs, and needs of those entrusted with assessing and ensuring that the health status of entire populations is protected and improves over time.

Public health informatics has been defined as the systematic application of information and computer science and technology to public health practice [2]. The topic supports the programmatic needs of agencies, improves the quality of population-based information upon which public health policy is based, and expands the range of disease prevention, health promotion, and health threat assessment capability extant in every locale throughout the world [3]. In the future, public health informatics may change to be defined as informatics supporting the public's health, a discipline that may be practiced beyond the walls of the health department.

In 1854, John Snow conducted the first comprehensive epidemiological study by linking the locations of cholera patients' homes to a single water pump. In doing so, he established that cholera was a waterborne disease. Using visual data, Snow quickly convinced the authorities to remove the pump handle. Following that simple intervention, the number of infections and deaths fell rapidly [4].

Over the past 30–50 years, public health programs have emerged around specific diseases, behaviors, or intervention technologies (e.g., immunization for vaccine preventable diseases), each having specific data and information needs. Not surprisingly, information systems were developed to meet the specific needs of each categorical program, and a culture of program-specific information system design permeated public health thinking. By the mid-1990s, leaders in public health acknowledged the need to rethink public health information systems, conceive of systems as support tools for enterprise goals, and do so through nationally adopted standards. As noted in [3] "Public health has lagged behind health care delivery and other sectors of industry in adopting new information technologies, in part because public health is a public enterprise depending on funding action by legislative bodies (local, state, and federal).

Additionally, adoption of new technologies requires significant effort to work through government procurement processes." A 1995 Centers for Disease Control and Prevention (CDC) study reported that integrated information and surveillance systems "can join fragments of information by combining or linking the data systems that hold such information. What holds these systems together are uniform data standards, communications networks, and policy-level agreements regarding confidentiality, data access, sharing, and reduction of the burden of collecting data" [5].

In the late 1990s, it became apparent that public health should be more comprehensive in understanding disease and injury threats. Reassessing its information mission has led federal programs such as CDC and Health Resources Service Administration (HRSA), to view information system integration as the driver for future information system funding. Integration across programs and organizations requires interoperability: data from various sources being brought together, collated in a common format, analyzed, and interpreted without manual intervention. Interoperability also requires an underlying architecture for data coding, vocabularies, message formats, message transmission packets, and system security. Interoperability implies connectedness among systems, which requires agreements that cover data standards, communications protocols, and sharing or use agreements. Interconnected, interoperable information systems will allow public health to address larger aspects of the public's health. The twenty-first century will probably be seen as the enterprise era of public health informatics. Once the domain of humans alone, the process of gathering and interpretating data should now be mediated by computers. Major advances in the quality, timeliness, and use of public health data will require a degree of machine intelligence not presently embedded in public health information systems [6].

The context in which informatics can contribute to public health progress is changing. New initiatives within public health and throughout the health care industry portend changes in how data are captured, the breadth of data recorded, the speed with which data are exchanged, the number of parties involved in the exchange of data, and how results of analyses are shared. Increasing use of electronic health record systems provides an opportunity to gather more granular, discrete data from a variety of sources, including nursing, pharmacy, laboratory, radiology, and physician notes, thereby changing the specificity and timeliness of knowledge about the distribution of risk factors, preventive measures, disease, and injury within subpopulations.

As agreements are reached on the major information architectural standards (data, transmission, and security) and appropriate approaches to governance and viable business models can be demonstrated, health information exchanges will emerge to assist and transform how health care is delivered. Public health considerations must be central to this transformation, and public health informatics will be central to how public health agencies participate in this rapidly evolving environment.

1.3   EARLY USE OF TECHNOLOGY FOR PUBLIC HEALTH PRACTICE

There are historical accounts in the bible of social distancing as a control measure to stop the spread of leprosy. During the spread of plague in Europe in the fourteenth century, public health authorities searched vessels looking for signs of disease in passengers waiting to disembark. In the United States, the practice of disease surveillance by public health inspection at immigration has been highly publicized as a result of the renovation of Ellis Island. The immigration law of 1891 required a health inspection of all immigrants coming into the United States by Public Health Service physicians. Between 1892 and 1924, over 22 million immigrants seeking to become American citizens were subject to health inspections (Fig. 1.1). The law stipulated the exclusion of "all idiots, insane persons, paupers or persons likely to become public charges, persons suffering from a loathsome or dangerous contagious diseases" [7]. Technology was limited to paper-and-pencil recordkeeping for these surveillance and control activities.

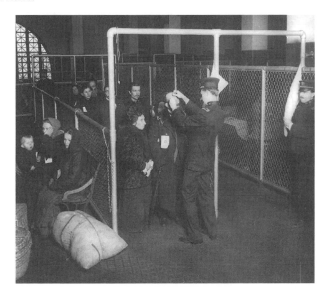

Fig. 1.1   Public health inspectors at Ellis Island looking at the eyes of immigrants for signs of trachoma. (Photo courtesy of the National Library of Medicine)

1.3.1   Early Use of Analytics, Visualization, and Communications

One of the earliest technologies used in disease surveillance was the statistical interpretation of mortality data. In 1850, William Farr analyzed the 1849 cholera outbreak in London by deriving a mathematical solution using multiple causation [8].

Florence Nightingale used statistical methods to fight for reform in the British military. She developed the polar-area diagram to demonstrate the needless deaths caused by unsanitary conditions during the Crimean War (1854–1856). Nightingale was an innovator in the collection, tabulation, interpretation, and graphical display of descriptive statistics. Figure 1.2 is Florence Nightingale's famous diagram depicting the causes of mortality for British troops during the Crimean War. The circle in the figure is divided into wedges, each representing a month of the war. The radius of each wedge is equal to the square root of the number of deaths for the month. The area of each wedge, measured from the center, is proportional to the statistic being represented. Dark gray wedges represent deaths from "preventable or mitigable zymotic" diseases (contagious diseases such as cholera and typhus), medium gray wedges represent deaths from wounds, and light gray wedges are deaths from all other causes [9].

Another example of the use of graphics to support epidemiological investigations is the 1869 chart by C.J. Minard describing Napoleon's ill-fated 1812–1813 march to Moscow and back [10]. Figure 1.3 is Minard's chart. The upper portion of the chart provides the strength of the French forces as a function of time superimposed on a map of Russia. The gray band is a measure of the size and location of the force as it advanced to Moscow; the black band represents the size and location of the retreating forces. On the lower portion of the chart is a record of the temperatures that the army encountered upon their retreat. Napoleon's army numbered 422,000 when it crossed the Polish border on the way to Russia. Only 100,000 survived to participate in the battle at Moscow. The returning army facing the Russians at the Battle of Berezina numbered only 19,000. The returning forces suffered massive casualties due to disease and hypothermia associated with the declining temperatures. Temperatures in Russia dropped to -35 degrees Celsius during the campaign.

The invention of the telegraph and Morse code in the mid nineteenth century provided a means for rapid dissemination of information over a wide geographic area. This technology had important implications for public health surveillance. During the Spanish Flu outbreak in 1918, the telegraph and the weekly *Public Health Reports* became essential tools to provide the Public Health Service with surveillance data on the progression of the pandemic.

1.3.2   Early Informatics Applications in Medicine & Public Health

Medical computing applications evolved with the development of computing technology. The very earliest applications were patient records to support diagnosis and clinical laboratory work. Bruce Blum describes the objects that are processed by computers as data, information, or knowledge [11]. A data point is a single measurement, element of demographics, or physical condition made available to the computer application or analyst. Information is a set of data with some interpretation or processing to add value. Knowledge is a set of rules, formulas, or heuristics applied to the information and data to create greater understanding.

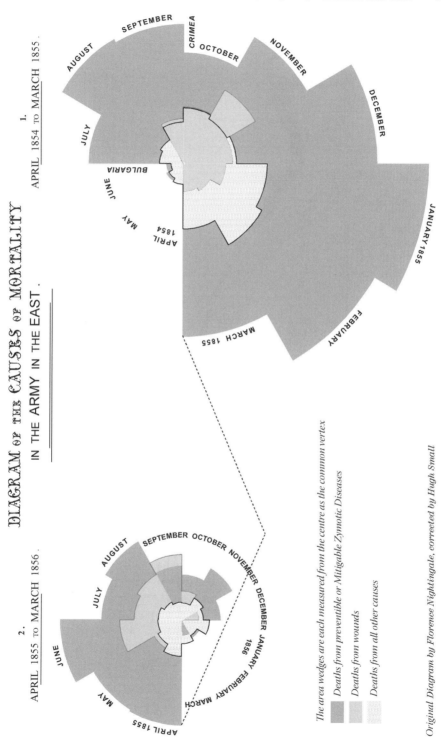

Fig. 1.2   Florence Nightingale's visualization of the causes of mortality in British troops during the Crimean War. (From Cohen [9])

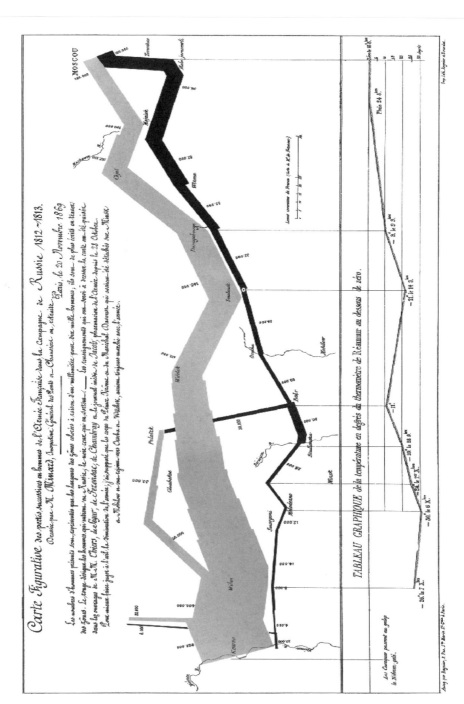
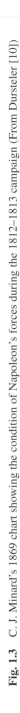

Fig. 1.3 C. J. Minard's 1869 chart showing the condition of Napoleon's forces during the 1812–1813 campaign (From Dursteler [10])

Applications using data were introduced in the 1960s when the IBM 1401 mainframe computer found use in university and research settings. In the 1970s, with the advent of low-cost minicomputers, such as the DEC PDP series or Data General Nova series, computer processing applications were developed to create information to support diagnosis in various branches of medicine. Medical imaging made great advances because images could now be acquired, stored, and processed as individual pixels, permitting multidimensional slices with high resolution. In 1970, a prototype computerized tomography system, developed by Grant [12], enabled multiaxis images to be acquired of a region under investigation. By 1973, Ledley had begun development of a whole-body CT scanner, called the automatic computerized transverse scanner (ACTA), which began clinical service early in 1974 [13].

One of the initial languages developed specifically for the organization of files in the health care industry was the **M**assachusetts General Hospital Utility **M**ulti-**P**rogramming **S**ystem (MUMPS). The language was developed by Neil Pappalardo, an MIT student working in the animal laboratory at Massachusetts General Hospital in Boston during 1966 and 1967. The original MUMPS system was built on a spare DEC minicomputer. MUMPS was designed for building database applications that help programmers develop applications that use as few computing resources as possible. The core feature of MUMPS is that database interaction is built transparently into the language [14].

The Veterans' Health Administration (VHA) adopted MUMPS as the programming language for an integrated laboratory/pharmacy/patient admission, tracking, and discharge system in the early 1980s. This system, known originally as the Decentralized Hospital Computer Program (DHCP), has been extended continuously in the years since. In March 1988, the Department of Defense launched the Composite Health Care System (CHCS), based on the VHA's DHCP software, for all of its military hospitals [15]. DHCP and CHCS form the largest medical records archiving systems in the United States. These archives are sources of indicators of emerging diseases and outbreaks.

1.3.3 Public Health Records Archiving

In the United States, state and local health departments have taken on the role of collecting and archiving vital statistics for the populations they serve. Health departments issue certified copies of birth, death, fetal death, and marriage certificates for events that occur in their population. Many departments also provide divorce verifications and registries on adoption and act as adjudicators of paternity.

The National Center for Health Statistics (NCHS) is the lead U.S. federal government agency for collecting, sharing, and developing procedures and standards for vital statistics. The NCHS is the oldest and one of the first examples of intergovernmental data sharing in public health. The data are provided through contracts between NCHS and individual record systems operated in the various jurisdictions legally responsible for the registration of vital events: births, deaths, marriages, divorces, and fetal deaths. In the United States, legal authority for maintaining registries of vital events and for issuing copies of birth, marriage, divorce, and death certificates resides with the states, some individual cities (Washington, DC, and New York City), and the territories [16, 17].

In 1916, the Illinois Department of Public Health (IDPH) assumed responsibility for collecting data on vital events such as live births, still births, and deaths. In 1938, the department acquired IBM tabulation equipment for the generation of vital statistics and other health data. A computer was first used in population monitoring to support the Census Bureau in tabulating data from the 1950 census. In 1962, the IDPH became the first state health department to convert its applications on tabulation equipment to the newly acquired IBM 1401 computer. Many applications were developed for the IDPH computers, one of the most famous for a large salmonellosis outbreak in 1985. The IDPH identified communications with local heath departments as a major weakness to the response. As a result, a minicomputer network was established that used modems and phone lines to pass information among state and local health departments. This system was known as the Public Health Information Network [18].

1.4   GUIDING PRINCIPLES FOR DEVELOPMENT OF PUBLIC HEALTH APPLICATIONS

The Public Health Informatics Institute (PHII) was formed in 1992 with a grant from the Robert Wood Johnson Foundation. The Institute helps to foster applications that provide value to public health rather than just using the latest technology for technology's sake [19]. The Institute has outlined a set of principles to assist in guiding the development and use of computer applications for public health [20]:

1. Engage all stakeholders throughout the life cycle of the project.

2. Consider the business processes and operational constraints and develop the requirements prior to system design. In other words, think logically before physically.

3. Plan for the system to be interoperable with emerging standards such as the Public Health Informatics Network.

4. Manage the project and maintain accountability through the use of detailed plans, status reports, and meetings to help focus the project on obtaining its goals.

Figure 1.4 provides a graphical representation of the PHII principles and the four major steps in the development of a public health informatics application. The first step is to determine how the new system can improve health outcomes by quantifying the health problem, developing a business case for the system, and defining the indicators for measuring success. The second step is to determine how the work will be accomplished through a series of analyses to define the workflow and business processes that will support the application. The third step is to determine the requirements for the application through performance requirements analysis and system design. Once the system is implemented, the final step is to determine how success will be measured through an evaluation and a series of metrics that measure the performance of the system. For advanced disease surveillance systems, the Centers for Disease Control and Prevention (CDC) has developed a framework for evaluating syndromic surveillance systems that contains a series of metrics [21, 22]. The framework assumes that the system has been fully developed and operational for several years; thus, a comprehensive evaluation in the early implementation stages of the system using the framework is not possible. It is one of the most comprehensive sets of metrics developed for disease surveillance systems. See Chapter 10 for a discussion of this and other frameworks.

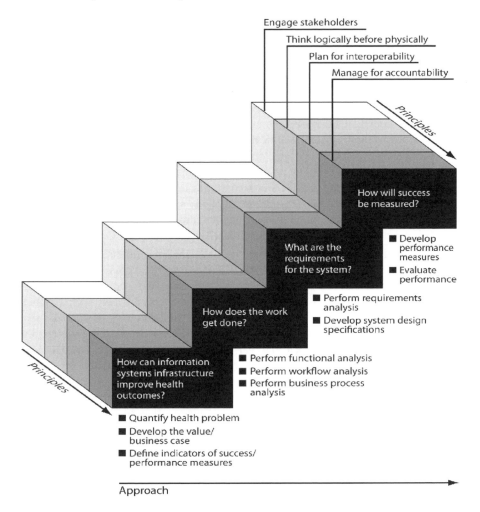

Fig. 1.4   Principles and approach for planning and design of an enterprise information system. (From Public Health Informatics Institute [20], ©PHII)

1.5 INFORMATION REQUIREMENTS FOR AUTOMATED DISEASE SURVEILLANCE

James Jekel describes surveillance as the entire process of collecting, analyzing, interpreting, and reporting data concerning the incidence of death, diseases, and injuries and the prevalence of certain conditions whose knowledge is considered important for promoting the health of the public [23]. Most surveillance systems are developed and implemented with a clear objective of the specific outcome being sought. Examples are the linkage of specific environmental risk factors to chronic diseases such as cancer or monitoring of behavioral factors associated with the transfer of sexually transmitted diseases (STDs). As mentioned earlier, a main focus of this book is surveillance systems for the early recognition of outbreaks due to highly infectious diseases that have a potential for high morbidity and mortality, such as virulent forms of influenza or disease agents of bioterrorism. A main objective of a system developed around this focus is to reduce the number of cases by enabling the administration of prophylaxis rapidly or by allowing for social distancing to reduce the spread of disease. To achieve this objective, a disease outbreak must be recognized in the very early stages for a highly contagious disease such as influenza or during the initial symptoms of a disease like anthrax so that treatment and control efforts still have a high chance of a successful outcome. Traditional disease surveillance and response can be represented by the steps shown in Fig. 1.5. Health departments have traditionally relied on reporting from health care providers or laboratories before initiating epidemiological investigations. This surveillance approach is highly specific, but neither sensitive or timely. In the case of anthrax, preventing the mortality of those infected relies on the rapid identification and treatment of the disease.

One potential approach for early identification of abnormal disease in a community is to collect and analyze data that are not used traditionally for surveillance and may contain early indicators of the outbreak. This approach relies on capturing health-seeking information when a person becomes ill. The concept of how such a system may operate is illustrated in Fig. 1.6. The concept is based on the assumption that a pathogen is released into the environment either in the air or in the water supply. If some type of sensor is present that can detect the presence of the pathogen and determine its identity, the detection phase is complete, but it is not possible for sensors to be located everywhere. Also, environmental sensors may be of little value if the health threat is due to highly contagious persons rather than pathogens released into the environment. If biological or chemical material has been released into the environment, the effect may be seen in animals, birds, and plant life, as well as in humans. Zoonotic diseases such as West Nile virus may first present with animal illness and death before presenting in humans.

Several types of data are collected routinely for purposes other than disease surveillance could contain indicators and warnings of an abnormal health event. When continual feeds are established for these data, analytical techniques can be applied to identify abnormal behavior. Signals identified through this process can fall into several different classes, where the most important is an outbreak with the potential

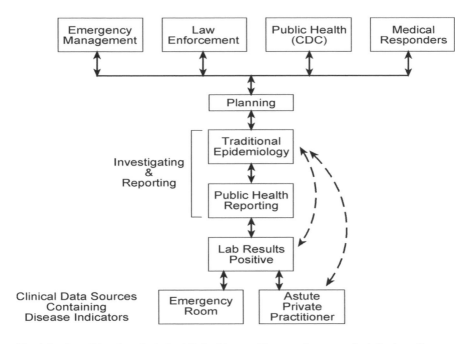

Fig. 1.5   A traditional method of public health surveillance and response for infectious diseases.

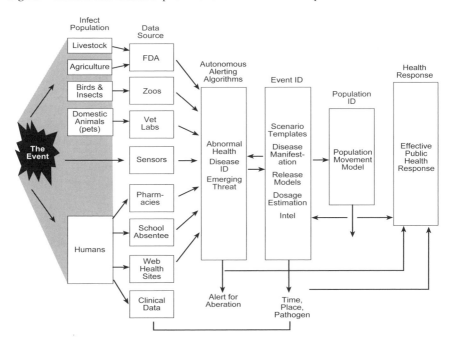

Fig. 1.6   Concept for a disease surveillance system using data sources that may contain early indicators and warnings of a health event.

for high morbidity or mortality in the population. Once it has been established that the signal is of importance, additional data are needed to understand what is occurring before a public health response can be executed.

Following the detection of a statistical aberration in surveillance data, several questions must be answered. What disease is present, and what agent is causing it? What are the characteristics of the disease and what methods are used to treat the disease? Where and when did people get infected? Was the exposure at a single point over a short duration, or was exposure over an extended time period and a large geographic area? Knowledge of the population at risk is also necessary to assess the potential public health implications of a surveillance alarm. If the disease is highly contagious, is it contagious before symptoms develop, and which persons are at risk of being infected by contact with those initially infected? Where are those who have been infected, and how can they be contacted? These are just a few of the questions for which answers would be urgently needed.

Health departments need the answers to these questions to develop and execute a response to contain an outbreak. However, surveillance systems that use non-specific data as early indicators of disease cannot provide many answers; traditional epidemiological investigations are still needed. The best modern disease surveillance systems recognize this burden and attempt to collect as much data as possible to assist investigators in pulling together as much information as possible in a timely manner.

1.6   HISTORICAL IMPACT OF INFECTIOUS DISEASE OUTBREAKS

Modern medicine has had a significant impact on the control of infectious disease outbreaks. During the majority of the past century, Western countries have had abundant supplies of vaccines and antibiotics to control emerging outbreaks. A large outbreak of an unknown strain of an infectious disease agent or a large bioterrorist event could overburden the ability of the medical communities to give high-quality care to all those infected. A review of the history of significant outbreaks provides insight into the challenges facing the public health community.

1.6.1   Smallpox

One of the most significant diseases in the history of humankind is smallpox. Early accounts of smallpox date back to 10,000 B.C., when it appeared in the agricultural settlements of northeastern Africa [24]. Egyptian merchants helped to spread the disease to India in the last millennium B.C. Lesions resembling smallpox were found on the faces of mummies, including the well-preserved mummy of Ramses V, who died in 1157 B.C.

Western civilization has been affected greatly by smallpox. The plague of Anto-nine, around A.D. 180, killed between 3.5 and 7 million persons and coincided with the beginning of the decline of the Roman Empire [25, 26]. Arab expansionism, the Crusades, and the discovery of the West Indies all contributed to the spread of smallpox. The disease was introduced into the new world by Spanish and Portuguese conquistadors and contributed to the fall of the Aztec and Inca empires. During the decade following the Spanish arrival in Mexico, the population decreased from 25 million to 1.6 million, with disease contributing significantly to the decline [27].

The diseases that ravaged Europe and Asia for centuries were for some time unknown to Native North Americans. Ultimately, infectious diseases introduced by expansionism devastated the American Indian, with the greatest number of deaths caused by smallpox — sometimes intentionally. During the Indian siege of Fort Pitt in the summer of 1763, the British sent smallpox-infected blankets and handkerchiefs to the Indians in a deliberate attempt to start an epidemic [28]. The plan to infect the Indians and quell the siege was documented in a letter written by Colonel Henry Bouquet to Sir Jeffrey Amherst, the commander-in-chief of British forces in North America.

In 1796, Edward Jenner, an English physician, observed that dairymaids who contracted cowpox, a much milder disease, were immune to smallpox. With serum taken from a dairymaid, Jenner began vaccination. When it was available, vaccination became an effective way of controlling the spread of smallpox.

In 1947, the Soviet Union established its first smallpox weapons factory in Zagorsk just northwest of Moscow. Animal tests showed that fewer than five viral particles were needed to cause infection in 50 percent of subjects. In comparison, 1500 plague cells and 10,000 anthrax spores were needed to achieve the same results. By 1970, smallpox was considered so important to the biological weapons arsenal that over 20 tons were stored annually at Zagorsk for immediate use [29].

In 1967, the World Health Organization (WHO) initiated a mass vaccination program that resulted in the eradication of smallpox by 1978 [30, 31, 32]. On May 8, 1980, WHO announced that smallpox had been eradicated from the planet. Smallpox immunization programs were discontinued, and only limited quantities of the virus were retained for research purposes at the Centers for Disease Control in Atlanta and the Ivanovsky Institute of Virology in Moscow. Coincidently, the Soviet weapons program, Biopreparat, included smallpox in the weapons improvement list in its five-year 1981–1985 plan [29].

1.6.2 Plague

Bubonic plague, or Black Death, left an indelible mark on history. In 1346, there were fearful rumors of plague in the East at major European seaports. India was depopulated; Tartary, Mesopotamia, Syria, and Armenia were covered with dead bodies. The disease traveled from the Black Sea to the Mediterranean in galleys following the trade routes to Constantinople, Messina, Sicily, Sardinia, Genoa, Venice, and Marseilles. By 1348, the Black Death had taken a firm grip on Italy. Between the years 1347 and 1352, plague accounted for the destruction of one third to one half the population of Europe, approximately 25 million victims. The disease terrified the populations of European cities because it struck so swiftly and consumed a town or city within weeks. Victims died within days in agony from fevers and infected swellings [33].

Plague had been around London since it first appeared in Britain in 1348, but in 1665, a major outbreak occurred. Two years earlier, plague ravaged Holland. Trade was restricted with the Dutch, but despite the precautions, plague broke out in London, starting in the poorer sections of the city. Initially, the authorities ignored it, but as spring turned into one of the hottest summers in recent years, the number of deaths increased dramatically. In July, over 1000 deaths per week were reported, and by August, the rate peaked at over 6000 deaths per week. A rumor that dogs and cats caused the spread resulted in a drastic reduction in their numbers, leaving the plague-carrying rats without predators.

Control measures consisted of quarantining families in their homes. When a person in a household became infected, the house was sealed until 40 days after the victim either recovered or died. Guards were posted at the door to see that no one left. The guard had to be bribed to allow any food to pass to the homes. Accounting for victims was difficult because the quarantine measures were so harsh that families were not willing to report the death of family members. Nurses went from door to door in an attempt to quantify the number dead. Estimates are that over 100,000 people (about a quarter of the population of London) perished in the outbreak. In 1666, the Great Fire of London burned down the city slums and brought the plague under control.

1.6.3   Spanish Influenza, 1918

In colonial times, laws were passed mandating the reporting of smallpox, yellow fever, and cholera [24]. By the nineteenth century, mandatory reporting at the state and federal levels became common. During the twentieth century, increasing use of vaccines and antibiotics, improvements in communication, and the dedication of individuals and organizations led to a significant decline in morbidity and mortality due to highly contagious diseases. The twentieth century also saw the pandemic or world-wide epidemic of the Spanish influenza of 1918 and the belief by government leadership that modern medicine had conquered the risk of infectious disease outbreaks by the end of the century. These beliefs led to complacency in allocating funding to improve disease surveillance activities.

There were three major pandemic influenza outbreaks in the twentieth century [34]. In 1918–1919, Spanish influenza, caused by the H1N1 subtype of the influenza A virus, infected up to one-third of the world's populations.[1] The pandemic erupted during the final stages of World War I and ultimately killed more people than the war. The number of dead is estimated at between 20 and 40 million, with the exact

---

[1]Influenza A virus subtypes are labeled by an H number and an N number. The H number represents HA antigens or hemagglutinin proteins and varies from H1 to H16. The HA antigen is responsible for binding the virus to the cell. The N number represents the NA antigen, or neuraminidase enzyme, and varies from N1 to N9. The NA antigen is responsible for releasing the virus from infected cells. H1N1 is a subtype of the of avian influenza virus species.

numbers unknown due to inadequate reporting. In the United States, the outbreak claimed 675,000 lives. It has been cited as the most devastating epidemic in recorded world history. More people died of influenza in a single year than in the four years of the Black Death from 1347 to 1351.

From analysis to determine the virulence of the H1N1 virus strain, a U.S. Armed Forces Institute of Pathology study determined that the Spanish influenza could first have appeared in a young British soldier during the Battle of the Somme in 1916 [35]. In 1916, supply lines stretching through the French town of Etaple comprised not only hundreds of thousands of troops but also piggeries and chicken coops to supply food for the forces. Etaple could have been the incubation site for the transfer of the virus from chickens and pigs to humans. The Institute of Pathology study also included the collection of virus samples from victims buried in the Alaska permafrost. Using documentary evidence and new genetic clues, researchers have been able to trace the flu's spread in three waves around the world. These studies are being used to speculate about the impact of a potential H5N1 Avian Influenza pandemic [36].

Camp Funston provides a graphic example of how the 1918 pandemic ravaged communities. The 29th Field Artillery Battalion was constituted on July 5, 1918, as part of the Army's 10th Division at Camp Funston, Kansas. There, they underwent equipment issue and tactical training and began preparations to deploy to Europe. However, during this period, Camp Funston suffered an influenza outbreak that devastated the installation. Figure 1.7 shows an emergency hospital set up at Camp Funston to care for the influenza patients. By the end of October 1918, there were 14,000 reported cases and 861 deaths in Camp Funston alone. The State of Kansas reported a total of 12,000 deaths by the time the flu had run its course and the units were healthy, the war had ended. Camp Funston was originally considered the initial site of the Spanish Influenza outbreak.

There are still several questions regarding the characteristics of the 1918–1919 pandemic. Figure 1.8 gives the mortality rate in the United Kingdom for the Spanish Flu. Three distinct waves occurred: in the spring of 1918, the fall of 1918, and the late winter of 1919. The first two waves of the pandemic occurred at a time of the year unfavorable to normal influenza virus strains. Could the virus have mutated around the world so quickly and simultaneously?

Another major difference between the pandemic strain and normal flu related to the groups affected. Mortality for influenza typically occurs among the very young or aged populations. In the 1918–1919 pandemic, disproportionate numbers of healthy young adults became victims. One theory is that earlier circulating influenza strains provided partial immunity for those exposed to a similar strain of the virus. The elderly would have been exposed to many more strains. Because most elderly could be expected to have weaker immune systems, the rates remained high. Figure 1.9 provides a comparison of the number of deaths per 100,000 persons in the United States by age group during 1911–1917 with those that occurred during 1918.

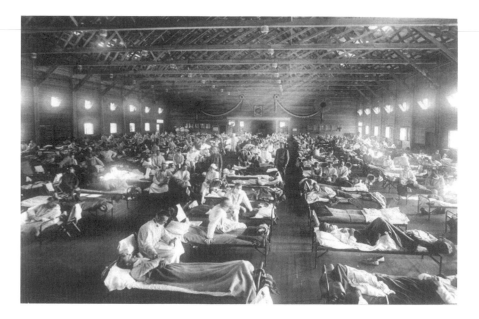

Fig. 1.7   Emergency hospital set up in Camp Funston, Kansas, during the beginning of the 1918 influenza epidemic. (Photo courtesy of the National Museum of Health and Medicine)

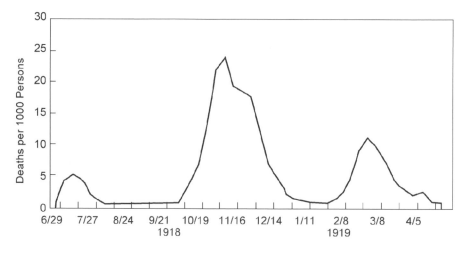

Fig. 1.8   Combined influenza and pneumonia mortality rate in the United Kingdom for 1918–1919.

1.6.4   Influenza Pandemics after 1918

Two influenza pandemics have swept the world since 1919: the Asian influenza pandemic of 1957 (H2N2) and the Hong Kong influenza pandemic of 1968 (H3N2),

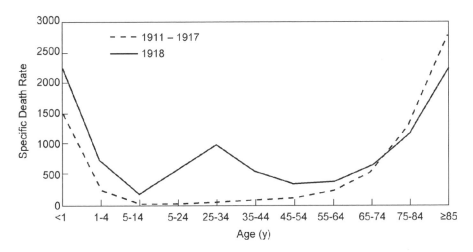

Fig. 1.9   Combined influenza and pneumonia mortality by age at death per 100,000 persons in each age group, United States, 1911–1918. Influenza- and pneumonia-specific death rates are plotted for the nonpandemic years 1911–1917 (dashed line) and for the pandemic year 1918 (solid line).

both of which were avian influenza viruses. The Asian flu pandemic probably made more people sick than the pandemic of 1918, but the availability of antibiotics to treat the secondary infections resulted in a much lower death rate. Asian flu was first identified in China in February 1957. The virus was quickly identified due to advances in scientific technology, and vaccine production began in May 1957, before the disease spread to the United States in June 1957. By August 1957, vaccine was available in limited supply in the United States. The virus claimed 1 million victims worldwide.

The Hong Kong flu pandemic strain of H3N2 evolved from H2N2 by antigenic shift. Antigenic shift is the process by which two different strains of influenza combine to form a new subtype with a mixture of the surface antigens of the two original strains. Annual flu virus mutation occurs through a process called antigenic *drift*, where the surface proteins change slowly over time. The body's immune system can react to slow changes but cannot readily adapt to a rapid antigenic shift. Because of its similarity to the 1957 Asian flu and, possibly, the subsequent accumulation of related antibodies in the affected population, the Hong Kong flu resulted in far fewer casualties than in most pandemics. Casualty estimates vary; between 750,000 and 2 million people died of the virus worldwide during the two years (1968–1969) that it was active [37].

A highly virulent form of the avian virus H5N1 is currently being spread across the world by migrating waterfowl. Domestic poultry catch the virus from contact with migratory birds. Humans have caught H5N1 from close contact with infected chickens. Originally endemic only in birds in Southeast Asia, migratory patterns threaten to infect birds everywhere. Tens of millions of birds have died of the H5N1 virus, with hundreds of millions slaughtered in an attempt to control the disease.

Figure 1.10 shows an example of the flyways currently being used by migratory bird. The flyway patterns cover most populated areas of the globe.

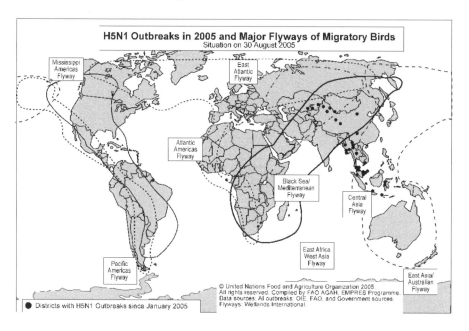

Fig. 1.10 Flyway patterns of migratory birds. (Adapted from United Nations Food and Agriculture Organization Figure [38])

The present form of the H5N1 virus does not pass efficiently between humans. However, as the virus continues to evolve, another pandemic on the order of the Spanish flu is feared. Table 1.1 presents the number of human cases of H5N1 and related deaths from 2003 until March 16, 2006. Of the 176 confirmed cases, there have been 97 fatalities, yielding a case fatality rate of 56.4%. The rate far exceeds that of previous pandemics [40].

Table 1.2 provides a list of major outbreaks considered pandemics from answers.com. There were undoubtedly many more episodes that did not make this list due to the lack of documented historical evidence prior to the eighteenth century. For the last entry, severe acute respiratory syndrome (SARS), there were fewer than 10,000 cases of the disease, but air travel spread the previously unknown contagious disease quickly.

1.7   DISEASE AS A WEAPON

Before the twentieth century, biological weapons were relatively simple. Infected materials were used to induce illness in an opponent's forces, or food or water supplies were poisoned. In the sixth century B.C., the Assyrians poisoned the drinking water of

Table 1.1   Cumulative Number of Confirmed Human Cases of Avian Influenza A/(H5N1) Reported to WHO as of March 10, 2006. Source: World Health Organization [39]

Year	Cambodia	China	Indonesia	Iraq	Thailand	Turkey	Viet Nam	Total
2003								
Cases	0	0	0	0	0	0	3	3
Deaths	0	0	0	0	0	0	3	3
2004								
Cases	0	0	0	0	17	0	29	46
Deaths	0	0	0	0	12	0	20	32
2005								
Cases	4	8	17	0	5	0	61	95
Deaths	4	5	11	0	2	0	19	41
2006								
Cases	0	7	11	2	0	12	0	32
Deaths	0	5	10	2	0	4	0	21
Total								
Cases	4	15	28	2	22	12	93	176
Deaths	4	10	21	2	14	4	42	97

their enemies; in medieval times Mongol and Turkish armies catapulted the diseased corpses of animals or humans into fortified castles; and as late as 1710, Russian armies used plague corpses as weapons. During World War I, German agents in the United States inoculated horses and cattle with glanders before they were shipped to France for use by the Allied powers.

In 1925, the first international agreement, known as the Geneva Protocol, to limit the use of chemical and biological weapons was signed. The Protocol prohibited the use in war of asphyxiating gases and of bacteriological methods of warfare. The agreement did not address production, storage, or verification mechanisms and could not be used to support disarmament. As a result, significant research was performed in the twentieth century to increase the performance of biowarfare agents and delivery methods. Biological weapons could be developed very cheaply and cause large numbers of casualties compared with conventional weapons [41].

The Soviet Union established its biological weapons program in the late 1920s after a typhus epidemic in Russia from 1918 to 1922 killed between 2 and 10 million, illustrating graphically the destructive and disruptive power of biological weapons. From the occupation of Manchuria in 1931 to the end of World War II in 1945, the Imperial Japanese Army experimented with biological weapons on thousands of Chi-

Table 1.2   Documented Pandemics

165-180	Antonine plague (smallpox)
541	Plague of Justinian (bubonic plague)
1300s	The Black Death (plague)
1732-1733	Influenza
1775-1776	Influenza
1816-1826	Cholera
1829-1851	Cholera
1847-1848	Influenza
1852-1860	Cholera
1857-1859	Influenza
1863-1875	Cholera
1899-1923	Cholera
1918-1919	Spanish flu (influenza)
1957-1958	Asian flu (influenza)
1959-present	AIDS
1960s	El Tor (cholera)
1968-1969	Hong Kong flu (influenza)
1993-1994	Plague, Gujarat. India
2002-2003	SARS

nese. These experiments were conducted in a disguised water purification plant known as Unit 731 at Pingfan, near the city of Harbin in northeastern China [42]. Japanese scientists tested plague, cholera, smallpox, botulism, and other diseases on prisoners. Their research led to the development of a defoliation bacilli bomb to destroy crops and a flea bomb to spread bubonic plague. Initial successes with this technology stimulated other developments, which enabled Japanese soldiers to launch biological attacks with anthrax, plague-carrying fleas, typhoid, dysentery, choler, and other deadly pathogens. At least 11 Chinese cities were attacked with biological weapons, resulting in an estimated 10,000 to 200,000 deaths. In addition, there are firsthand accounts of the Japanese infecting civilians through the distribution of infected food and contaminated water supplies, with estimated casualties of over 580,000 from plague and cholera. Following the war, the United States granted amnesty to the Japanese scientists in exchange for their experimentation data. Figure 1.11 shows a human vivisection experiment conducted by Unit 731 during World War II, in which a team of Japanese surgeons is removing organs while another is taking measurements on the organs.

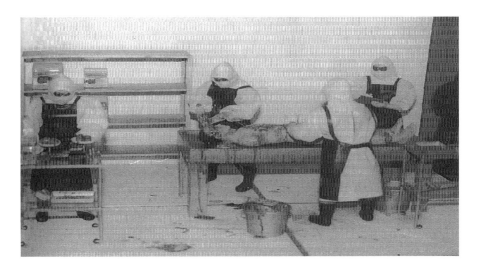

Fig. 1.11   Japanese vivisection experiment conducted on a Chinese victim infected with a biological agent. (From Hal Gold [42], p. 169)

In 1941, a biological weapons development program initiated by the United States, the United Kingdom, and Canada in response to German and Japanese weapons development activities resulted in the weaponization of anthrax, brucellosis, and botulinum toxin. During World War II, the United Kingdom developed the Allies' first anthrax bomb by experimenting with sheep on Gruinard Island in Scotland. Sheep were used because they were similar in weight to humans, are highly susceptible to anthrax, and are plentiful in the area. The research left the island contaminated with anthrax spores (Fig. 1.12).

In another World War II program, termed Operation Vegetarian, the UK manufactured and planned to drop 5 million anthrax cattle cakes on German beef and dairy herds. The plan was to wipe out the German herds and simultaneously infect the German human population. Because antibiotics were not available to the general population, the operation could have caused thousands, if not millions of human deaths. The operation was abandoned due to the success of the Normandy invasion. At the end of 1945, the British incinerated 5 million anthrax cattle cakes.

Stockpiles of biological weapons were destroyed after President Nixon unilaterally ended the United States' offensive biological warfare program. This initiative ultimately resulted in the Biological Weapons Convention in 1972. Signers of the Convention pledged to never develop, produce, stockpile, acquire, or retain biological warfare agents or the means to deliver them.

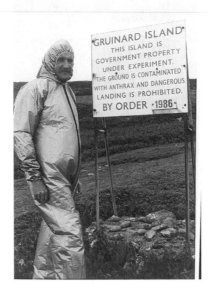

Fig. 1.12 Gruinard Island was the site of an experimental anthrax bomb (AP Photo/Press Association, used with permission.)

Following World War II, the Soviet Union formulated a doctrine on the production and use of biological weapons. Two types of biological weapons were developed: strategic weapons, consisting of such highly lethal agents as anthrax, smallpox, and plague, for use on deep targets inside the United States and other countries, and operational weapons, to be used to incapacitate vital civilian and military activities well behind the battlefront. The latter weapons contained agents causing diseases such as tularemia, glanders, and Venezuelan equine encephalomyelitis. Biological weapons were not considered for tactical targets because they were not immediately effective in stopping advancing forces [43].

Concern over the use of biological weapons against civilian populations resulted in a research effort within the United States. In June 1965, the U.S. Central Intelligence Agency released a harmless simulant into the New York City subway system during peak traffic periods to demonstrate the vulnerability of U.S. cities to a covert biological warfare attack. These experiments were performed in secret; commuters had no knowledge that they had been exposed to the simulant.

Despite signing the Biological Weapons Convention, the Soviet Union continued research and production of biological weapons in a program called Biopreparat [29]. The United States was unaware of the program until the first deputy director of Biopreparat, Dr. Kanatjan Alibekov, defected in 1992. The program employed 30,000 in the research and development of biological weapons and antidotes. Pathogens weaponized or under development included smallpox, bubonic plague, anthrax, Venezuelan equine encephalitis, tularemia, influenza, brucellosis, Marburg virus, Ebola virus, and Machupo virus.

Documented testimony indicated that the Soviets conducted aerosol attacks on Laos, Kampuchea, and, eventually, Afghanistan using "yellow rain" (trichothecene mycotoxins) and causing thousands of deaths between 1974 and 1981. In 1979, an accidental release of *Bacillus anthracis* spores from the Compound 19 production facility in the town of Sverdlovsk resulted in at least 66 fatalities. The Soviets initiated mass prophylaxis of the population, burying victims using special procedures without the attendance of family members. A massive cover-up of the incident has made it difficult to reconstruct the event to determine the actual death toll, but estimates have ranged from 200 to 1000. In 1992, President Boris Yeltsin acknowledged that the Sverdlovsk incident was an accident involving aerosol release of anthrax spores.

In 1991, the United Nations' Bioweapons Inspection Team found evidence that the Iraqis were in the early stages of developing an offensive biological warfare capability. Inspectors found several state-of-the-art facilities that could have been used for agent production, as well as evidence of the weaponization of anthrax, botulinum toxin, and aflatoxin [44]. Fortunately, these weapons were not used during Desert Shield or Desert Storm. Pressure from the United Nations resulted in the destruction of the Iraqi offensive program by 1996. Several other countries have biological warfare programs in place or under development, including Russia, Israel, China, Iran, Libya, Syria, and North Korea.

1.7.1 Bioterrorism

In 1995, the religious cult Aum Shinrikyo released sarin nerve gas in a Japanese subway system. The group was subsequently found to have been developing biological weapons, including anthrax, botulism, and Q fever. Following an Ebola outbreak in 1993, the group sent cult doctors and nurses to Zaire to bring back samples of the virus for a possible biological weapon. The group staged several unsuccessful attacks using their biological weapons before resorting to sarin for the subway attack.

In September and October 2001, letters containing anthrax spores were mailed to addressees in Florida, New York City, and Washington, DC (Fig. 1.13). The incident resulted in five fatalities, with more than a dozen victims developing full-blown infections. Tens of thousands at risk of exposure were prescribed antibiotics prophylactically. The perpetrator of the attacks has not yet been identified, but it is known that the strain of anthrax was obtained from the U.S. Army Medical Research Institute for Infectious Diseases at Fort Detrick, Maryland. The letters contained 2 to 3 grams of weaponized spores of remarkable purity, indicating use of the latest technology and a well-funded and sizable research program with possible government support. The anthrax letters revealed how unprepared the public health infrastructure in the United States was to respond to acts of bioterrorism or biowarfare.

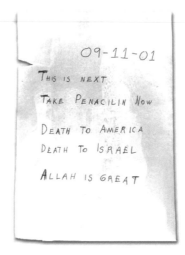

Fig. 1.13   Example of an Anthrax letter.

1.8   MODERN DISEASE SURVEILLANCE APPLICATIONS

1.8.1   Components of an Early Recognition Disease Surveillance System

In response to the need for earlier recognition of significant health events, health departments, academics, and information technologists have developed surveillance systems that use data which may provide early indications of disease, but are not specific enough to confirm the presence of any particular disease. These routinely collected data include records of over-the-counter (OTC) medication sales; school absenteeism; school nurse visits; 911 calls; calls to poison control centers; reports of illness from nursing homes; animal health data; health maintenance organization encounter data; and reports of chief complaints from emergency medical services and hospital emergency departments. These data sources have some features in common. For example, although they may provide an early indication of a health event, they do not typically provide a specific signal. OTC medication sales can increase due to sales promotions, consumers stocking-up, or just to movement of product displays in the store. Data generated by interactions with health care providers are typically more specific but arise only when symptoms become uncomfortable enough for a person to seek professional help. Figure 1.14 shows data sources that may contain indicators of health status. They are arranged from left to right, with the sources on the left more likely to provide an earlier but less specific indicator and the sources on the right likely to be more specific but less timely. Chapter 2 addresses the value of various data sources as indicators of events of interest for public health surveillance.

Since the attacks of September 11, 2001, in the United States, organizations acquiring data containing health indicators have been willing to provide data feeds to health departments for disease surveillance. Data can be acquired in a variety of

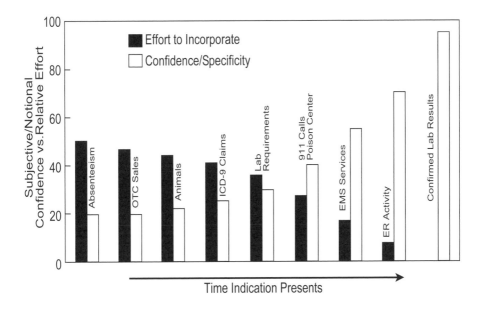

Fig. 1.14 Estimation of the value of data sources in surveillance.

modes, including real-time feeds of the data via a secure connection to the facility or batched transmission where data are aggregated over time and sent periodically to the surveillance system. Chapter 3 addresses the most common data feeds as well as data privacy issues and standards used in the formatting and transmission of data.

Once data are acquired, a variety of different analytical processes can be applied to convert them into information that can be used in surveillance. Statistical algorithms are used to find anomalies in individual data streams or in many data streams where the data elements are the same, but are coming from different facilities. Examples are sales of OTC medications from stores distributed across a region or chief complaint data from hospitals distributed across the same region. Analytic techniques may also be used to fuse data or information from several data sources to look for abnormal patterns that may not be obvious in a single data stream but become evident when data sources are used together. There are also analytic techniques for identifing clusters in time and space from single or multiple sources of data. Chapter 4 provides an introduction to some of the more popular analytical techniques used in modern disease surveillance systems.

Continued operation of a disease surveillance system is an important issue for health departments. IT resources must be allocated to operate and maintain the application, and an epidemiologist must take time to review the system's outputs. One system's architecture may fit more readily into a health department's business processes than others. Visualizing data in a specific format may fit more easily into a health department's review protocol than others. Chapter 5 presents different architectures, data processing, and visualization options available to developers of disease surveillance systems.

Because surveillance data may be nonspecific, and because algorithms detect spurious statistical anomalies as well as events of epidemiological interest, algorithms often give rise to false triggers, alarms, or alerts. The greater the number of data sources and the larger the number of algorithms applied to the data, the greater the potential for false alarms. The astute epidemiologist who is experienced in looking at local surveillance data and the alerts coming from a system can dismiss many alarms quickly. An experienced epidemiologist also can use the data and information within the system to make decisions efficiently about the health status of a population. When an epidemiologist cannot dismiss an alerts quickly, additional information may be needed to determine its importance to public health. Chapter 6 describes the business processes used by health departments to perform surveillance with nonspecific data sources.

The first place to look to for additional data to resolve a suspicious alert is the organization that provided the data causing the alert. For example, chief complaint data provided by a hospital emergency department may not contain a diagnosis or the personnel identifiers needed to contact the person or persons causing the alerts. A health department can, however, request that the hospital perform a chart review to capture the information needed to resolve the alert.

Presenting large amounts of disease surveillance data or information in a manner that is comprehensible to the users of a surveillance system is a challenge. Data can be represented as the aggregate count of patients with the same syndrome, the number of OTC medication products sold, or the number of students absent. Information can be the outputs of various detector algorithms applied to one or more data streams. Information can be presented in graphical terms, such as time-series graphs of counts over time, geographic representation of counts by zip code, or census tracks overlaid on maps, along with other information needed by the user of the system.

Figure 1.15 is an example of outbreaks indicated by a time series of counts of the number of patients presenting to military clinics in San Diego County with respiratory illness. The data in the example are simulated, but they contain many of the characteristics of previous large respiratory events in the region. The example is taken from an exercise performed to evaluate the ability of the ESSENCE surveillance system to identify the health status of the population during a simulated bioterrorism event (see Section 1.8.2). Several types of data can be shown on the same graph. As seen, the graph displays both the total count of patients seen at clinics and the number of patients who return after being seen some time during the previous 14 days. Activity decreases for two days (Saturday and Sunday), followed by an increase early in the week. Counts increase near the end of the time series, which is one indication of the beginning of a synthetic outbreak. The detector output is noted by the change in shade of the small dot representing the daily patient count. Two levels of threshold levels are provided as outputs from the algorithm. The grey shade represents a warning level and the black an alert level. Because time-series plots provide an easily interpreted overview of the data, they have become an important visualization tool in modern disease surveillance systems.

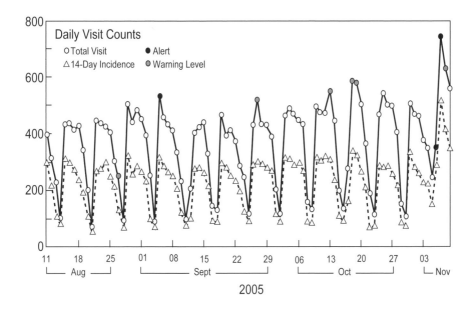

Fig. 1.15   Example of a time-series representation of respiratory syndrome counts. The solid lines represent daily counts and the dashed lines represent counts for new patients that have not been seen for at least the previous 14 days.

An example of a geographic representation of data is provided in Fig. 1.16. A map of zip codes in San Diego County is overlaid with small squares representing the sites of medical treatment facilities. The shade of the square represents the level of activity at the facility for the syndrome of interest. The intensity of the shading represents the number of patients residing in that zip code who were seen at the treatment facilities. This technique allows spatial clusters of disease to be readily identified. Another informative representation would be the number of patients seen by zip code where people spend most of their time during the day. An example would be work zip codes. The representation may identify exposure at the worksite.

The work zip codes of persons seeking treatment are also an important demographic. These data are rarely available for analysis because most disease surveillance systems do not capture them. Working adults tend to travel large distances to work, so their working zip code is probably different from their zip code of residence. School-aged and elderly persons spend more time closer to their zip code of residence.

For regions of the country where there is a large transient population due to tourism, sporting events, or other activities, the local geographic representation of data may be of limited value. Other representations for counts and detection results would be needed for patients living outside the region under surveillance.

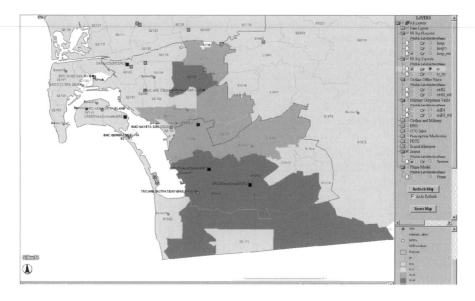

Fig. 1.16   Geographical representation of a simulated outbreak in San Diego County from an ESSENCE simulation.

Most modern disease surveillance systems provide some map graphing feature. The example shown in Fig. 1.16 is a geographic presentation of the data provided in Fig. 1.15. Different visualizations may be required for different users: epidemiologists reviewing the data would require detail, whereas higher level decision makers would require a summary view. Chapter 5 discusses approaches to the visualization of data used in modern disease surveillance applications.

The appropriate definition of regions for the aggregation and analysis of data in surveillance at a national or multinational level poses a problem. Algorithms that form clusters using all the zip codes or census tracks in the country could be a processing bottleneck if innovative analytical techniques are not employed. These concepts are explored in more detail in Chapter 4.

1.8.2   Modern Surveillance Applications for Use by State and Local Health Departments

In the mid to late 1990s, the fear of the reemergence of highly virulent forms of naturally occurring infectious diseases such as influenza and tuberculosis (TB), combined with the ever-increasing threat of bioterrorism, spurred increased development of disease surveillance systems. These systems focused on early detection rather than specificity of disease identification to reduce the risk of high mortality and morbidity.

One of the first systems in use was the Electronic System for the Early Notification of Community-based Epidemics (ESSENCE), which grew out of a pilot project for the Maryland Department of Health and Mental Hygiene and a preventive medicine project at the Walter Reed Army Institute of Research [45, 46]. The initial pilot of ESSENCE was developed for surveillance during year 2000 celebrations. Development for ESSENCE included the acquisition and evaluation of several data sources that could contain early indicators of infectious diseases. An important characteristic of ESSENCE is that it was developed in close coordination with the stakeholders in health departments, taking into consideration their business processes and operational requirements. It was the first system to integrate health indicators from both the military and civilian populations. ESSENCE became operational across the Department of Defense and was implemented by the District of Columbia, Maryland, and Virginia Health departments in a network that performs surveillance across the National Capital Region. The ESSENCE software is provided free to any health department that wants to set up its own surveillance system. ESSENCE is designed to be hosted locally by health departments so that they can keep the health indicator records within their jurisdictions [46, 47].

The Real-Time Outbreak Detection System (RODS) was developed by the University of Pittsburgh in conjunction with Carnegie Mellon University. RODS was originally developed for use by large medical centers receiving real-time data feeds from emergency departments. It was converted for use by health departments in two modes. It was the first system to provide a version of its software in open-source form on the Internet for download and installation by local users. RODS is also provided as an application service provider, connecting local hospitals to archives in the RODS Laboratory at the University of Pittsburgh and providing web access to health departments using the service [48].

The New York City Health Department has responsibility for one of the largest and most concentrated populations in the United States. The city is therefore thought to be an attractive target for terrorist activities and a favorable environment for the spread of naturally occurring diseases. Following the attack on the World Trade Center in New York in September 2001, the New York City Department of Health and Mental Hygiene initiated a fully operational syndromic surveillance project to collect data from emergency departments, pharmacy chains, and other data sources [49]. During the first year of operation, the system was able to capture data from 39 hospitals covering 2.5 million patient visits, or approximately 75% of the total visits. The system was able to provide early recognition of seasonal influenza and gastrointestinal illness shortly after it became operational.

The Early Aberration Reporting System (EARS) began as a CDC initiative to provide health departments with a set of easy-to-implement analytical tools for advanced disease surveillance applications, including bioterrorism monitoring during large-scale events. Following the terrorist attacks of September 11, 2001, the EARS tool evolved into a complete standalone application for download and use by health departments. Because it is easy to download, install, and use and is available at no cost, various city, county, and state public health officials in the United States and abroad have used or are currently using the EARS application [50].

These surveillance systems use data captured for routine business purposes in the health care industry so that little additional burden is placed on the facilities providing the data. Another model exists where data are obtained specifically for surveillance purposes. Data collected with one of these systems can be much more specific in recognizing abnormal disease occurrences. One of the first systems to exploit this feature is the Rapid Syndrome Validation Project (RSVP), developed by Los Alamos National Laboratory [51]. Physicians enter records of patient visits to a secure website. The physician is made aware of abnormal cases of disease in his or her area. The system also works with personal digital assistants (PDAs) to facilitate data entry in mobile environments. This form of data capture permits easy entry of animal health data by veterinarians and handlers on farms and ranches. This system is available commercially under the name SYRIS.

1.8.3   National Disease Surveillance Initiatives

Historically, advances in disease surveillance have been made first at the national level by federal agencies with resources and requirement sufficient to respond to political pressures regarding health matters. In the United States, the National Centers for Disease Control and Prevention (CDC) has the clearest mandate at the federal level for disease surveillance and control. The Centers have several programs for conducting advanced surveillance at the national level and supporting state and local health departments in performing their responsibilities within their jurisdictions. Support comes in the form of personnel assigned to health departments through the Epidemic Intelligence Service (EIS), which is a two-year postgraduate program of service and on-the-job training for health professionals interested in the practice of epidemiology. At least 25% of all EIS trainees are assigned to local health departments. Funding has also been provided to health departments of states and large cities through CDC cooperative agreements on public health preparedness and response for bioterrorism. These funds are intended to upgrade the preparedness of state and local public health jurisdictions for responding to bioterrorism, outbreaks of infectious disease, and other public health threats and emergencies. Many of the states have used these funds to upgrade their surveillance systems.

1.8.3.1 National Electronic Telecommunications Surveillance System   The National Electronic Telecommunications System for Surveillance (NETSS) is a computerized public health surveillance information system that provides the CDC with weekly data regarding cases of nationally notifiable diseases. Through NETSS, the CDC receives reports of notifiable diseases from the 50 state health departments, New York City, the District of Columbia, and five U.S. Territories. These reports are initiated when health care providers or laboratory directors suspect or diagnose a case of disease that is notifiable in their state. When a case of disease is reported at the local level, staff members in the local or county health department conduct further investigation, implement control measures as needed, and forward the report to the state health department.

Only designated staff in state and territorial health departments or in the New York City or District of Columbia health departments may transmit data to the CDC through NETSS. In some states, city and county staff enter data that will ultimately be transmitted to the CDC, but the weekly transmission of all reported data is overseen by the appropriate state or territorial health department staff. NETSS does not require the use of a specific computer software program. However, data are transmitted in common ASCII format, which allows the NETSS system to integrate data from surveillance systems throughout the United States.

Provisional weekly reports of notifiable diseases are published in the CDC's *Morbidity and Mortality Weekly Report* (MMWR). Final, corrected data are published in the annual *MMWR Summary of Notifiable Diseases, United States* [52]. The NETSS program began in 1984 as the Epidemiologic Surveillance Project. By 1989, all 50 states were reporting to the CDC.

1.8.3.2   National Electronic Disease Surveillance System   In 1995, the CDC initiated the National Electronic Disease Surveillance System (NEDSS). The goal of NEDSS is the automated capture and analysis of data of public health significance from public and private health entities. The vision for NEDSS is a network of complementary electronic information systems that automatically gather health data from a variety of sources on a real-time basis to facilitate the monitoring of community health and to assist in the ongoing analysis of trends and detection of emerging public health problems. The foundation of NEDSS is a series of standards for the collection, archiving, and reporting of significant health events through the use of low-cost commercial off-the-shelf (COTS) products to support state and local systems for data collection and analysis. The NEDSS system architecture is intended to integrate and eventually replace several current CDC surveillance systems, including NETSS and systems for reporting HIV/AIDS, vaccine-preventable diseases, and tuberculosis and infectious diseases [52].

The NEDSS Base System is a platform to support state-notifiable disease surveillance and analysis activities in a secure environment. The Base System is a modular platform that provides a seamless view and management of cross-program data, supports the storage and maintenance of data in an integrated database, and supports data analysis and visualization activities through the use of specific COTS products [53]. States are not required to use the Base System, but funds provided under the CDC cooperative agreements require the use of NEDSS standards in the communications among NEDSS systems.

1.8.3.3   Public Health Information Network and BioSense   The CDC's Public Health Information Network (PHIN) initiative began in 2004 with the objective of implementing a multiorganizational business and technical architecture for interoperable public health information systems. PHIN includes a portfolio of standards and software solutions to build and maintain the connectivity among information systems throughout the public health sector at the local, state, and federal levels. Applications using PHIN standards include systems for disease surveillance, national health status indicators, data analysis, public health decision support, information resources and

knowledge management, alerting and communications, and the management of public health responses [54].

BioSense is a CDC initiative to perform advanced disease surveillance at the national level [55, 56]. BioSense collects and analyzes data from emergency departments in large cities, Department of Defense and Veterans Health Affairs ambulatory visits, and laboratory test orders from the Laboratory Corporation of America. The application summarizes and presents analytical results and data visualizations by source, day, and syndrome for each zip code, state, and metropolitan area through maps, graphs, and tables. BioSense data are analyzed at CDC's BioIntelligence Center and made available to local health departments via a secure website. Substantial investments in standards and common infrastructure are also being made through Biosense to collect real-time hospital data. A goal of BioSense is to permit hospital data feeds to be sent to local health department surveillance systems in parallel with the data feed to CDC for BioSense. Figure 1.17 provides an example of where the early event detection capabilities of BioSense fit into the framework of PHIN.

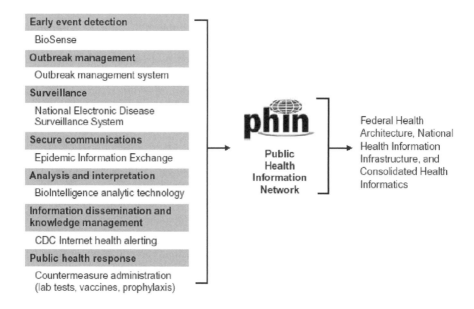

Fig. 1.17   Applications using the network standards proposed by PHIN. (From CDC [55, 56])

1.8.3.4   U.S. Department of Defense Disease Surveillance   The U.S. Department of Defense (DoD) operates its own version of ESSENCE for surveillance of all U.S. military treatment facilities worldwide. Data for the DoD instance of ESSENCE come from the TriCare system, which acquires data under the Composite Health Care System (CHCS) program. The system is operated by the Office of the Secretary of Defense for Health Affairs; users are provided with web access across the globe.

The DoD ESSENCE system currently provides service to approximately 800 users worldwide, making it the largest modern informatics program for disease surveillance.

1.9 SUMMARY

Public health organizations are facing increased challenges in rapidly identifying outbreaks in their communities. Health indicator surveillance data and modern information technology has helped to automatically collect, archive, process, and present summaries of a communities health status. Most implementations of automated surveillance systems lack the desired specificity or timeliness, but provide valuable information to monitors of disease surveillance. It is hoped that the information contained in the following chapters will provide insights to the readers to advance the technology and to better meet the challenges of the future.

REFERENCES

1. Thacker SB, Berkelman RL. Public health surveillance system in the United States. Epidemiol Rev. 1988; 10: 164-190.

2. Yasnoff WA, O'Carroll PW, Koo D, Linkins RW, Kilbourne E. Public health informatics: Improving and transforming public health in the information age. J Public Health Management Practice. 2000: 6(6): 67-75.

3. Wallace RB, ed. Maxcy Rosenau Last's Public Health and Preventive Medicine. 15th Ed. East Norwalk, CT: Appleton & Lange; 2006.

4. Smith GD. Commentary: Behind the Broad Street pump: aetiology, epidemiology and prevention of cholera in mid-19th century Britain. Int J Epidemiol. 2002; 31: 920-932.

5. Centers for Disease Control and Prevention. Integrating public health information and surveillance systems: a report and recommendations. Spring 1995. Available at http://www.cdc.gov/od/hissb/docs/Katz.htm. Accessed September 26, 2006.

6. McComb D. Semantics in business systems: the savvy manager's guide. San Francisco, CA: Morgan Kaufmann;2004:3.

7. The National Library of Medicine. Disease control and prevention. In: Images from the history of the Public Health Service: a photographic exhibit. Available at http://www.nlm.nih.gov/exhibition/phs_history/20.html.

8. Eyler JM. The changing assessments of John Snow's and William Farr's cholera studies. Soz Praventivmed. 2001; 46: 225-232.

9. Cohen IB. Florence Nightingale. Sci Amer. 1984; 250: 128-137.

10. Dürsteler JC. The golden age of visualization. The digital magazine of InfoVis.net. January 9, 2003. Available at http://www.infovis.net/ printMag.php?num=111&lang=2. Accessed September 26, 2006.

11. Blum BI, Duncan K. A History of Medical Informatics. New York: ACM Press; 1990.

12. Grant, DG. Tomosynthesis: a three dimensional radiographic imaging technique. IEEE Trans Biomed Eng. 1972; 19(1): 20-28.

13. Ledley RS, et al. Computerized transaxial x-ray tomography of the human body. Science. 1974; 186(4160): 207-212.

14. Wikipedia. MUMPS (Massachusetts General Hospital Utility Multi-Programming System). Available at http://en.wikipedia.org/wiki/MUMPS/ History. Accessed September 26, 2006.

15. Kolodner RM. Computerizing Large Integrated Health Networks: The VA Success. New York: Springer-Verlag; 1997.

16. Grove RD, Hetzel AM. Vital Statistics Rates in the United States: 1940–1960. Washington, DC: US Government Printing Office; 1968.

17. Linder FE, Grove RD. Vital Statistics Rates in the United States: 1900–1940. Washington, DC: US Government Printing Office; 1943.

18. US Public Health Service. US vital statistics system major activities and developments, 1950–1995. US Public Health Service Document 97-1003. Washington, DC:National Center for Health Statistics. 72 pp. Includes reprint of History and organization of the vital statistics system, by AM Hetzel. Washington, DC: National Center for Health Statistics; 1997. Available at http://www.cdc.gov/ nchs/products/pubs/pubd/other/miscpub/vsushist.htm. Accessed October 5, 2006.

19. Public Health Informatics Institute. Available at http://www.phii.org/. Accessed September 26, 2006.

20. Public Health Informatics Institute. Guiding principles for effective health information systems. 2004. Available at http//www.phii.org/Files/ PHII_Brochure.pdf. Accessed September 26, 2006.

21. CDC. Framework for evaluating public health surveillance systems for early detection of outbreaks: recommendations from the CDC Working Group. MMWR. 2004; 53 (RR-5): 1-13. Available at http://www.cdc.gov/mmwr/PDF/rr/ rr5305.pdf. Accessed September 26, 2006.

22. German RR. Updated guidelines for evaluating public health surveillance systems. MMWR. 2001; 50(RR13): 1-35. Available at `http://www.cdc.gov/mmwr/preview/mmwrhtml/rr5013a1.htm`. Accessed September 26, 2006.

23. Jekel JF, Katz DL, Elmo JG. Epidemiology, Biostatistics, and Preventive Medicine. 2nd Ed. St. Louis, MO: WB Saunders Company; 2001.

24. Hinman AR. Surveillance of communicable diseases. Presented at the 100th Annual Meeting of the American Public Health Association, Atlantic City, NJ, November 15, 1972.

25. Zinsser H. Rats, Lice and History. Boston: Little, Brown; 1935.

26. Littman RJ, Littman ML. Galen and the Antonine plague. Am J Philol. 1973; 94: 243-255.

27. Duffy J. Epidemics in Colonial America. Baton Rouge, LA: Louisiana State University Press; 1953.

28. Duffy J. Smallpox and the Indians in the American colonies. Bull Hist Med. 1951; 25: 324-341.

29. Alibek K. Biohazard. New York: Random House; 1999.

30. Hopkins JW. The Eradication of Smallpox: Organizational Learning and Innovation in International Health. Boulder, CO: Westview Press; 1989.

31. Brilliant LB. The Management of Smallpox Eradication in India. Ann Arbor, MI: University of Michigan Press; 1985.

32. Fenner F, Henderon DA, Arita I, Jezek Z, Ladnyi ID. Smallpox and Its Eradication. Geneva, Switzerland: World Health Organization; 1988.

33. Ziegler P. The Black Death. New York: John Day Company; 1969.

34. Kilbourne ED. Influenza pandemics of the 20th century. Emerg Infect Dis. 2006; 12(1): 9-14.

35. Taubenberger JK, Unravelling the 1918 flu mystery, US Med. 2004. Available at `http://usmedicine.com/article.cfm?articleID=917&issueID=65`. Accessed September 26, 2006.

36. Taubenberger JK, Morens DM. 1918 influenza: the mother of all pandemics. Emerg Infect Dis. 2006; 12(1): 15-22. Available at `http://www.cdc.gov/ncidod/EID/vol12no01/05-0979.htm`. Accessed September 26, 2006.

37. Jordan E. Epidemic Influenza: A Survey. Chicago: American Medical Association; 1927.

38. United Nations Food and Agriculture Organization. H5N1 outbreaks in 2005 and major flyways of migratory birds. Compiled by FAO AGAH, EMPRESS

Programme. Available at http://www.fao.org/ag/againfo/subjects/en/ health/diseases-cards/migrationmap.html. Accessed September 26, 2006.

39. World Health Organization. Epidemic and pandemic alert and response (EPR): cumulative number of confirmed human cases of avian influenza A/(H5N1) eported to WHO. Available at http://www.who.int/csr/disease/ avian_influenza/country/cases_table_2006_10_03/en/index.html. Accessed October 5, 2006.

40. World Health Organization Global Influenza Program Surveillance Network. Evolution of H5N1 avian influenza viruses in Asia. Emerg Infect Dis. 2005; 11(10): 1515-1521. Available at http://www.cdc.gov/ncidod/EID/ vol11no10/05-0644.htm. Accessed September 26, 2006.

41. Christopher GW, Cieslak TJ, Pavlin JA, Eitzen EM Jr. Biological warfare: a historical perspective. JAMA. 1997; 278: 412-417.

42. Gold H. Unit 731 Testimony. Charles E. Tuttle Company. Singapore: Yenbooks; 1996:169.

43. Alibek K. Behind the mask: biological warfare. Perspective. 1998;IX(1). Available at http://www.bu.edu/iscip/vol9/Alibek.html. Accessed October 9, 2006.

44. Zilinskas RA. Iraq's biological weapons: The past as future? JAMA. 1997;278:418-424.

45. Lewis MD, Pavlin JA, Mansfield JL, et al. Disease outbreak detection system using syndromic data in the greater Washington, DC area. Am J Prev Med. 2002; 23: 180-186.

46. Lombardo JS. The ESSENCE II disease surveillance testbed for the National Capitol Region. Johns Hopkins APL Tech Dig. 2003;24(4). Available at http://techdigest.jhuapl.edu/td2404/Lombardo.pdf. Accessed September 26, 2006.

47. Lombardo JS, et al. A systems overview of the Electronic Surveillance System for the Early Notification of Community-based Epidemics, ESSENCE II. J Urban Health 2003; 80(2 Suppl 1): i32-i42.

48. Tsui FC, et al. Technical description of RODS: a real-time public health surveillance system. JAMIA. 2003; 10(5): 399-408. Available at http://www.jamia.org/. Accessed September 26, 2006.

49. Heffernan R, et al. Syndromic surveillance in public health practice, New York City. Emerg Infect Dis. 2004;10(5). Available at http://www.cdc.gov/ ncidod/eid/vol10no5/03-0646.htm. Accessed September 26, 2006.

50. Hutwagner L, et al. Comparing aberration detection methods with simulated data. Emerg Infect Dis. 2005; 11(2): 314-316.

51. Zelicoff A, et al. The Rapid Syndrome Validation Project (RSVP). Proc AMIA Symp. 2001; 771-775. Available at `http://www.amia.org/pubs/proceedings/symposia/2001/D010001236.pdf`. Accessed September 26, 2006.

52. CDC, National Electronic Telecommunications System for Surveillance. Available at `http://www.cdc.gov/epo/dphsi/netss.htm`. Accessed September 26, 2006.

53. CDC. An overview of the NEDSS initiative. Available at `http://www.cdc.gov/nedss/About/overview.html`. Accessed September 26, 2006.

54. CDC. Public Health Information Network (PHIN). Available at `http://www.cdc.gov/phin/overview.html`. Accessed September 26, 2006.

55. Loonsk JW. BioSense: a national initiative for early detection and quantification of public health emergencies. MMWR. 2004;53(suppl):53–55. Available at `http:// www.cdc.gov/mmwr/preview/mmwrhtml/su5301a13.htm`. Accessed September 26, 2006.

56. Bradley CA, et al. BioSense: implementation of a National Early Event Detection and Situational Awareness System. MMWR. 2005;54;suppl:11–19. Available at `http://www.cdc.gov/mmwr/pdf/wk/mm54su01.pdf`. Accessed September 26, 2006.

Part I: System Design and Implementation

2 Understanding the Data: Health Indicators in Disease Surveillance

Steven Babin, Steven Magruder, Shilpa Hakre, Jacqueline Coberly, Joseph S. Lombardo

A primary goal of using modern technology to monitor infectious diseases is to obtain as early as possible an indication that a outbreak might be occurring. In any given population over a given time, many diseases are prevalent routinely or are endemic and may be considered a normal part of the human ecosystem. Therefore, particular diseases of concern must be chosen by public health authorities for routine surveillance so that appropriate monitoring and alerting methods may be developed. There are many health indicators that may be monitored for this purpose: individual, socioeconomic, environmental, and health care usage factors all reflect the health status of a population. These indicators reflect determinants of health and health outcomes. Health outcomes include morbidity and mortality. Determinants of health include genetics; socioeconomic status; drug, alcohol, and tobacco use; educational status; health care usage; air quality; environmental conditions; infrastructure quality; and health care accessibility. Health care accessibility is affected by such issues as race, ethnicity, language, disability, mobility, distance to health care, and the number of health care providers in an area. Adverse environmental conditions (including flooding, extreme heat, extreme cold, poor air quality, and inadequate water) may be more prevalent in some areas than in others. Infrastructure quality includes public utilities such as drinking water, sewage treatment, and transportation. Health care use comprises such issues as how comfortable people feel about seeking health care and how often they seek preventive care. Health determinants and outcomes are intricately related, so it can be difficult to measure accurately the influence of a single determinant on an outcome. Many determinants influence what happens when a person feels unwell, and understanding these determinants and their related outcomes is necessary for disease surveillance. For example, when people feel unwell, they may first seek remedies from their own medicine cabinet. If they have access to a local drugstore (i.e., feel well enough to shop on their own or have someone who will shop for them), they may purchase OTC remedies, depending on their needs, income, and cultural influences. These drugstore purchases are often the first place that their health-seeking behavior appears in data available for biosurveillance. Additional health indicators useful for biosurveillance include patient visits to hospital emergency departments (EDs), walk-in clinics, and physician offices; calls to 911 and nurse triage telephone hotlines; and school absenteeism. This chapter discusses how certain health indicators may be used in disease surveillance. General data issues are described first, then specific data sources, and, finally, examples of how different data sources might be evaluated and compared.

2.1   DATA SOURCE CONCEPTS

For daily disease surveillance, where the goal is the earliest possible indication of a health anomaly, the focus is on pre-diagnostic data. Not all health indicators are easily and electronically accessible for study or are strongly related to public health diseases of interest. In automated disease surveillance, the most commonly used health indicators are daily physician office visit data, hospital ED visit data, hospital admissions data, pharmacy sales, nurse-hotline data, ambulance 911 calls, and laboratory-test requests (as discussed later, test requests are used because they are considered pre-diagnostic and are more timely than test results). These indicators are likely to provide a signal at different times in the course of disease progression (see Fig. 2.1), depending on the disease and the individual patient.

Stages of Disease & Health Indicators

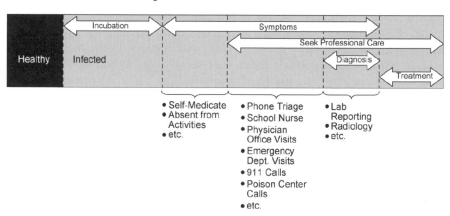

Fig. 2.1   Example of a typical progression of disease onset and health care-seeking behavior.

To facilitate analysis, these data are typically sorted into groups called *syndromes* before anomaly detection algorithms are applied. Thus, this type of disease surveillance has come to be called *syndromic surveillance*. The medical usage of the word *syndrome* must be distinguished from its usage in syndromic surveillance. The *Oxford Concise Medical Dictionary* defines a syndrome as "a combination of signs and/or symptoms that forms a distinct clinical picture indicative of a particular disorder."

A *sign* is a disease feature that is objectively determined by the physician during the physical examination, while a *symptom* is a disease feature that is subjectively reported to the physician by the patient. Therefore, a medically defined syndrome is a recognizable pattern of symptoms, signs, or other abnormalities that indicate specific traits with a single underlying cause, a specific disease, or an increased chance of developing a specific disease. In medical practice, this pattern is identified as a particular syndrome while the cause is unknown, thereby giving other physicians a tool for more easily detecting similar patterns and, ultimately, discovering the underlying cause or causes. When the cause is discovered and confirmed, the medical community typically replaces the syndrome by the disease or diseases if the syndrome results from more than one disease. However, syndromic surveillance doesn't necessarily use the term syndrome in the same way.

In syndromic surveillance, a syndrome may be a set of pre-diagnostic data that indicate the likelihood of a specific disease or that relate to a particular organ system or region of the body. Those data that relate to an organ system or part of the body are less specific than those for a particular disease, but they may be more sensitive for outbreak detection. Syndromic classifications are used to group pre-diagnostic data, which differ by source. For example, physicians' office visit data are typically in the form of International Classification of Diseases, Ninth revision (ICD-9) codes, while many hospital ED data are chief complaints in free or nonstandardized text. Chief complaints and ICD-9 codes are described in more detail in Sections 2.6 and 2.7, respectively. Figure 2.2 shows an example of such a mapping for the fever syndrome group. The table on the left lists ICD-9 codes and their corresponding descriptions that map into the fever syndrome, while the table on the right lists the chief complaints that map into the same syndrome. More details on performing syndrome grouping may be found in Chapter 5.

Some syndromic categories are much broader than specific disease patterns. For example, the gastrointestinal (GI) syndrome may be defined to include signs and symptoms that can be related to the either the abdomen or pelvis and may actually have nothing to do with the gastrointestinal system (e.g., genitourinary, musculoskeletal). Figure 2.3 shows how a respiratory syndromic category might be defined. Each of the disease descriptions listed comprises a group categorized as the respiratory syndrome. It is important to note also that syndromic categories don't have to be mutually exclusive, although the potential for "double-counting" of events should be accounted for when analyzing the data.

Important properties of pre-diagnostic data include sensitivity, specificity, latency, and completeness. *Sensitivity* is the probability that a public health event of interest will be detected in the data given that the event really occurred. Sensitivity is influenced by many factors including the type of event, the data source, and the processing algorithms that are used. A data source is more sensitive if it captures a larger fraction of the cases of interest. For example, physician visit data covering all the physicians in a city will tend to be more sensitive than a data source that includes only a subset of the physicians. The fraction of the affected population that is sampled is called the *representativeness* or *sample density* of the data source. For example, assume that

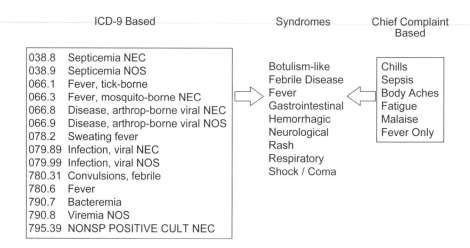

Fig. 2.2   Example of a classification system containing nine different syndromes, including fever. The ICD-9-based group on the left maps into the fever syndrome. The chief complaint-based group on the right also maps into the fever syndrome.

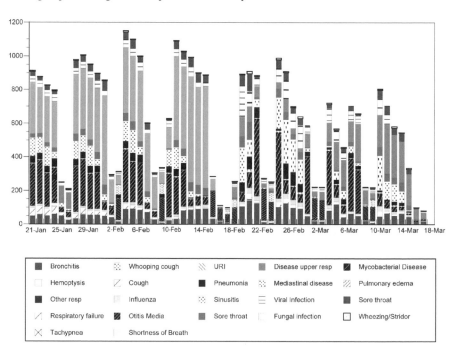

Fig. 2.3   Example of how a respiratory syndrome might be defined. This figure shows a daily decomposition of respiratory syndrome into its component disease descriptions. The vertical axis represents the number of patients seen that day with these components of the respiratory syndrome during a 3-month period.

our source of hospital ED data and our source of physicians' office visit data capture 1.9% and 64%, respectively, of the incidence of some acute condition. Figure 2.4 is a plot of the number of additional cases of this acute condition required for outbreak detection versus the number of background cases per day of this acute condition. As might be expected, the more syndromic data that occur in the background, the more additional cases are needed for outbreak detection. However, as the sample density increases, fewer additional cases above background levels are required for outbreak detection. Sample density is therefore critical for sensitive detection.

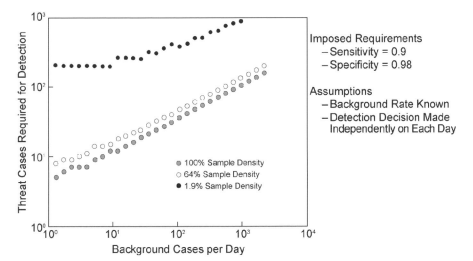

Fig. 2.4 Example of how sample density improves detection sensitivity. The number of background cases per day of an acute condition is plotted against the number of additional cases of this condition that are required for detection of an outbreak (1 standard deviation or higher than normal) of this condition. The differently shaded dots represent different sample densities plotted on a log-log scale.

A data source is also likely to be more sensitive if it carries information that can be used to group together persons potentially affected by an event while excluding those that would be unaffected. Types of information potentially useful for this purpose are the characteristics of the people sampled, such as home location, work location, or age. However, this information may be restricted by anonymity requirements. To protect patient privacy, it may be necessary to remove personal identifiers from the data that would allow identification of a specific individual or family. With spatial information, there is a trade-off between precision and privacy. The more precise the patient location information, the easier it will be to find spatial patterns in disease outbreaks. One compromise that is often used is to limit the spatial resolution to the residence zip code. Because the patient's work and school locations are often unavailable, the implicit assumption is that people go home first and then seek health care. However, working adults and college-aged children often spend considerable time away from home, so they often are not in their residence zip code when they become ill. Sensitivity is also improved when data sources carry more specific information about signs and symptoms, enabling greater focus on more probable victims of a particular event of interest.

Specificity is the probability that no health event of concern will be detected when no such event has in fact occurred. As with sensitivity, many factors influence specificity, including the type of event, the data source, and the processing algorithms that are used. Information in a data source that can distinguish different types of health events can help to enhance specificity, because the information can be used to reject health events that have a lower probability of being due to the event of interest. For example, in influenza surveillance, physician encounter data will be more specific than records of cold remedy purchases, because physician visit data include information that can better distinguish between various types of respiratory infections. Factors that may appear to have little to do with public health can reduce data specificity. For example, many data sources will be influenced by the day of week, by holidays, or by the weather. Data sources can also be affected by commercial events, such as the promotion of a new product or an arrangement with an insurance company to acquire physician visit data. It may be possible to correct for some external influences, but they still tend to reduce specificity. Information needed to correct for external factors may be obtained from ancillary sources, such as weather data or public school schedules that are not related directly to public health. Specificity can also be improved through the use of data sources that provide evidence to explain actual public health events observed in the data. For example, access to pollen count data might provide evidence that a sudden increase in headache, rhinitis, and pharyngitis was due to the pollen rather than to some more alarming cause.

Latency is the time lag between the occurrence of a health risk in the environment and the appearance of a detectable event in the data. Public health response is most effective if the health threat is observed quickly, with a short latency. The latency of a data source depends on many factors, including biological processes. For example, detection of health-seeking behavior may have longer latency than detection of a pathogen in the air or water. Latency also depends on the behavior of the victims of the health threat (e.g., how long they wait before visiting a hospital ED) and on the way the data are captured and reported. For example, physician visit data that are captured via billing to insurance companies have a latency associated with the billing process. For a given type of data (e.g., physician office visits), the latency may not be a single number but a distribution of time intervals (e.g., 5 – 7 days versus 2 days).

Another important property is data *completeness*. A data reporting problem may result in a nonrandom sampling of available data, leading to bias in the alerting algorithms. Therefore, it is important to know how much of the expected data stream has actually been received and processed. Ideally, there should be some means of including information on data completeness, although this is complicated by the fact that different data streams arrive at different times. For example, some data may be collected weekly while other data are collected daily. Different organizations may send data at different times, resulting in lags that get backfilled over time.

Multiple data streams are often used in syndromic surveillance to improve sensitivity and specificity. When multiple data streams are used, it is important to have an estimate of how these different sources might be ordered in time. Although the ordering depends both on the above-mentioned data lags and on individual health-seeking behavior, some general assumptions are often made. An example is seen in Fig. 2.1. Many people seek OTC drugs first and, if these don't work, they tend to see physicians. However, if a disease attacks suddenly and severely, telephone hotlines and ED visits may be the data through which health-seeking behavior is first revealed. All these factors may vary with location and socioeconomic status. People of low socioeconomic status may not have the resources to purchase OTC drugs and may wait until symptoms are severe before seeking help at a clinic or hospital ED. People whose residences are remote from such resources may similarly wait until symptoms are severe before seeking OTC drugs or visiting a hospital ED or clinic. For example, in urban populations, OTC drug-seeking behavior tends to precede hospital ED visits and physician office visits, but not always [1, 2].

2.2 DATA FROM PHARMACY CHAINS

Data from pharmacy chains include the date of purchase, the amount and type of drug, and the location of the store where the item was purchased. Retailers routinely collect pharmacy sales information using the manufacturer-labeled standard codes on each product. The Universal Product Code (UPC) and the National Drug Code (NDC) numbers are unique to each type of OTC remedy and prescription drug, respectively. The UPC codes are assigned and managed by the Uniform Code Council, Inc. (UCC); the NDC numbers are maintained in the Food and Drug Administration's (FDA) NDC directory (http://www.fda.gov/cder/ndc/). When a consumer purchases medications, these standard codes are scanned and the sales are electronically registered into a database. These sales are then aggregated by the retailer on an hourly, daily, or weekly basis. The resulting database may contain information on thousands of medications. If a remedy is removed from the market, the corresponding code is abandoned. Similarly, when a new medication is introduced, a new code is entered into the retailers' database. The utility of these data for surveillance therefore depends on continuous updating of the coding changes. The quantity of sales at a store is influenced by the demographic characteristics of the population, such as age group, socioeconomic status, and population size as well as that population's access to health care. For OTC sales, because the residence location or zip code of the purchaser is typically unknown, the store's location (preferably specified as the street address, or as latitude and longitude) is used for spatial reference under the implicit (though not necessarily correct) assumption that this location is spatially correlated with the residence location. In other words, it is usually assumed that a store's pharmacy sales data most likely represent only the health status of the population living or working within the vicinity of the store.

In syndromic surveillance, the type of drug may be classified both according to its target age group (children, adults) and to the symptoms it is designed to relieve (colds, sinus, headache, diarrhea, etc.). Syndromic classifications based on these criteria would tend to be as general or as specific as the product descriptions. A "flu" syndrome would include OTC drugs that have the word *flu* in their labeling. Of course, such drugs could also be used to treat colds and other respiratory infections. Similarly, some antidiarrheal OTC drugs are also used to treat nausea. Other OTC drugs, such as antifungal or antibiotic creams, have more specific indications. Drugs may also be classified by the syndrome treated (respiratory illness, gastrointestinal illness, allergy, etc.) and active ingredients in the drug (loperamide, bismuth subsalicylate, diphenhydramine, etc.) [3, 4]. For example, in a study of a waterborne *Cryptosporidiosis* outbreak in North Battleford, Saskatchewan, Canada, weekly sales of specific antidiarrheal products mirrored the epidemic curve of illness [5].

Alternatively, classification may be derived from sales data via a data-driven approach. Magruder et al. [1] began with groupings of OTC products intended primarily for adults, sorted according to the symptom indicated (e.g., cough) and the physical type of medication (e.g., pill or liquid). They considered 41 different combinations of symptom indication and physical type (Fig. 2.5). Syndrome groups were then formed out of these 41 different aggregations by comparison of the daily sales histories. If the sales histories of two different OTC groups could be fit well by a model that assumed their ratio was constant, the histories were judged similar. Otherwise, they were dissimilar. This measure of "distance" between sales histories was used to identify clusters of product groups with relatively similar sales histories. Because these clusters of products with similar sales histories were assumed to be used for similar purposes, they were aggregated into OTC syndrome groups. This empirical approach to syndrome group definitions has the advantage that it can identify flaws in assumptions about product usage. For example, in the study cited, it was discovered that usage patterns of products labeled for pain relief were similar to those for allergy products (i.e., they showed strong sales peaks during allergy season). On the other hand, sales of products advertised to treat chest congestion did not cluster well with either flu remedies or allergy remedies.

Many advantages exist in using OTC sales data for disease surveillance. First, the data may be available electronically and in near real time without the reporting delays seen in other pre-diagnostic data, such as physician office visits. Therefore, using these data may translate into earlier detection of an outbreak, although there are important exceptions [2]. Second, the data contain detailed information, such as geographic location of the store, and the date, quantity, and type of product sold. Therefore, these data offer the possibility of not only detecting spatial and temporal clustering of cases, but also disseminating preventive and control measures for the disease in a focused fashion. Third, the type of OTC medications sold reflects the symptoms experienced by the consumer and, by inference, the type of disease burdening the community. Fourth, because pharmacy sales data have been routinely collected for commercial purposes, patterns seen in current sales data may be compared to those in previous years. The availability of historical data can be used to adjust for confounding influences in the development of statistical algorithms for disease detection.

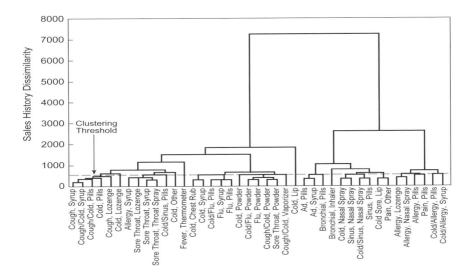

Fig. 2.5   OTC product groups clustered according to the similarity of their sales histories. Empirical syndrome groups are formed by setting a threshold on sales history dissimilarity. Products that are joined by lines falling below the threshold are aggregated into a single syndrome group.

As a result of confounding influences, fluctuations in OTC sales data may be attributable to factors other than disease. Coupons and discounts, day of the week, holidays, store hours, weather conditions, and seasonal variations affect OTC sales and may mask the impact of a disease on sales. Sales promotions affect OTC data in at least two ways. A promotion or discount on a particular drug may increase its sales as people buy it in anticipation of some indefinite future use (i.e., "stocking up"). An example of this behavior is shown in Fig. 2.6, which shows the OTC sales first reach a peak and then fall abruptly as people can now use their stocked supplies for several days without additional purchases.

Stores also use sales promotions as "loss leaders" to bring people to the store with the expectation that they will buy non-sale items while there. Such a promotion may persuade people to visit the store but does not ensure they will buy the promoted drug. They may buy a non-sale drug because it has preferred product features or is less expensive than the sale item. If they buy the on-sale item, sales of that item increase; if they don't buy the on-sale item, sales of similar items increase. Therefore, it is useful to include flags in the OTC data to indicate which products are being promoted during a particular time. However, not all promotions are chainwide. Some are managers' specials limited to a specific store or are regional specials limited to stores in a specific region that may contain as few as two or three stores. In addition, the location of the product within a store will bias the sales. For example, sales will tend to be higher for products on prominent display (e.g., near the cash register or the front of an aisle) than for other products.

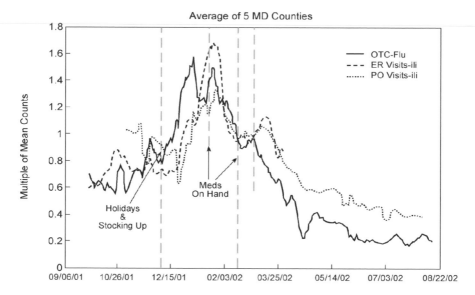

Fig. 2.6 Time-series plot of OTC flu remedy sales compared with hospital ED visits and physicians' office (PO) visits for influenza-like illnesses (ILI). The ordinate is daily sales or visits in multiples of the mean daily counts.

The other factors that affect OTC sales include day of the week and holiday effects. For example, sales may be higher on certain days and lower on following days. Adverse weather on certain days may also lower sales below what is expected. There are also seasonal effects. High pollen levels tend to occur during certain seasons, thereby affecting OTC allergy drug sales. Poor-air-quality days may affect asthma drug sales. Figure 2.7 shows various influences, such as consumer habits, marketing efforts, and the impacts of disease and environment, that may contribute to the OTC selling process and must therefore be taken into account in processing the OTC data. The electronic records are processed into a database in which the products are categorized into syndromic groups. These groups can then be evaluated for their accuracy, latency, sensitivity, etc., for detecting disease anomalies of interest. Furthermore, sales data may corroborate other surveillance data (e.g., hospital visits) and thereby increase the confidence that the detector is responding to a real disease rather than a statistical anomaly. Therefore, despite limitations that may prevent the data from being a reliable early disease outbreak detector, OTC drug sales are a useful source of data in syndromic surveillance.

Surveillance systems using OTC sales have attempted to adjust for the limitations of these data in several ways. The National Retail Data Monitor in Pittsburgh, Pennsylvania, receives health care product data daily from 10,000 stores nationwide in the United States [4]. The system addresses temporal and spatial limitations in the data by mapping sales for each OTC remedy category by store zip code and uses color coding to indicate whether the day's sales differ from what is expected based on the

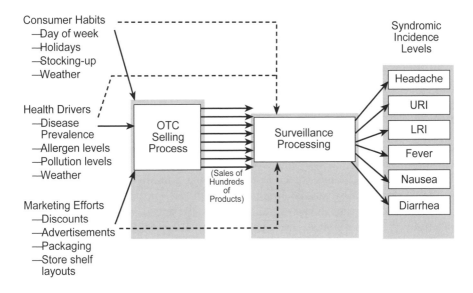

Fig. 2.7 OTC sales include other factors in addition to health indicators. These factors can cause high syndrome levels, confusing the surveillance process.

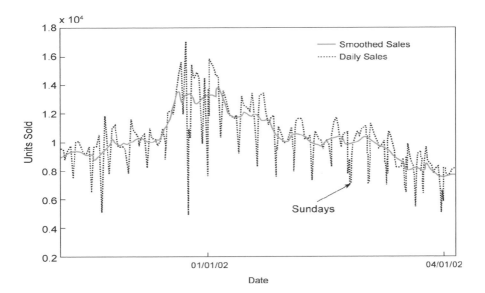

Fig. 2.8 Time series comparing daily OTC sales with those smoothed using a 7-day moving average. Note that the day-of-week effect is mitigated.

previous sales histories for that category. As shown in Fig. 2.8, using 7-day moving averages in viewing sales data is one method of addressing effects due to day of the week, holidays, and store-closing days [1]. Another way of adjusting for non-disease-related factors is to determine the percentage of change from baseline sales figures, as seen in a study conducted by Welliver et al. [6] that investigated trends in OTC cold remedy sales for signs of increased influenza in the community.

As mentioned earlier, the usefulness of a particular syndromic surveillance system and the data sources feeding it depend on how early (timeliness) and how well this system detects the presence (sensitivity) and absence (specificity) of a disease. For the data to be sensitive in detecting disease in a community, the data source would need to capture a representative sample of the affected population in the community (see Fig. 2.4). Evidence of this is seen in a 1993 outbreak in Milwaukee [7]. The public health department first became aware of the outbreak when a pharmacist noticed a 17- to 20-fold increase in sales of antidiarrheal and antispasmodic remedies at his pharmacy [8]. An outbreak investigation revealed that the public water supply to southern areas in the city was contaminated with *Cryptosporidium*. Because this outbreak was waterborne with a broad geographic distribution and affected large segments of the community, the disease was detectable in a single pharmacy's sales data. In another study conducted in New York State, Medicaid prescription data were evaluated for use in syndromic surveillance with the results that macrolide antibiotics had 50% sensitivity and 32% specificity for detecting pertussis outbreaks in a county [9]. The Medicaid program provided coverage for 4 to 20% of the county's population.

Because many people self-treat prior to, instead of, or in addition to seeking attention from the health care system, pharmacy sales data may be an earlier indicator of disease than either physicians' office visits or diagnostic data such as laboratory reports. For example, Fig. 2.9 demonstrates that OTC sales around the holidays appears to increase prior to an increase in physicians' office visits for bronchitis. Note the weekly drops in visits (related to office closures) and sales patterns. The office visits tend to peak on Mondays but this peak is lower during the last week in December because of the holidays. In contrast, OTC sales increase during this same period, possibly because of the lack of physician availability and thus an increased reliance on OTC self-medication. Once the holidays are past, physicians' office visits show a large increase that is at least partially associated with the forced deferral of visits over the holidays when offices were closed.

OTC sales data have been used for disease surveillance in several studies [1, 5, 6, 7, 8, 10]. In an investigation carried out in Los Angeles during the winter of 1976–1977, sales of cold and antipyretic OTC remedies were evaluated for detection of influenza B activity in the community. Sales of cold remedies were found to increase 3 weeks before influenza B was first isolated and 1 week before peaks in outpatient visits at a large county medical center [6]. A study conducted in the Washington, DC, area evaluated the relationship between sales of OTC influenza remedies and acute-respiratory-related physician office visits. Not only were OTC influenza remedy sales found to be strongly associated with physicians' office visits for respiratory illness, but when effects from seasonal and other non-disease factors were removed, OTC sales

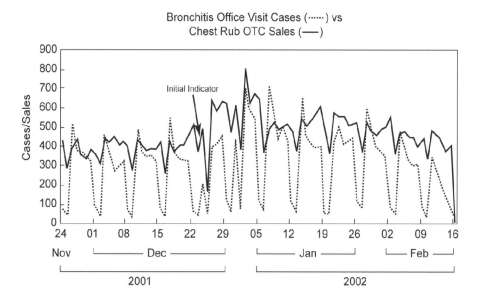

Fig. 2.9 Time series comparing daily sales of chest rub OTC products with Medicare-paid physicians' office visits by elderly patients for bronchitis.

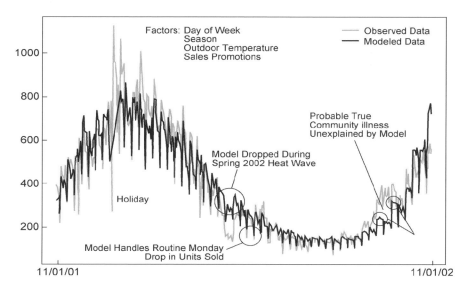

Fig. 2.10 Time series of daily OTC flu medication sales that include several confounding factors. These data were modeled in an attempt to remove the confounding factors noted in the figure.

data detected illness 2–21 days earlier than office visit data [1]. Figure 2.10 shows an example of the degree to which routine sales of OTC drugs can be fit by a simple model. The model shown here used a Poisson regression based on six parameters to describe day-of-week effects, two parameters to describe seasonal fluctuations, one parameter to describe the influence of outdoor temperature, and one parameter to describe the effects of product promotions.

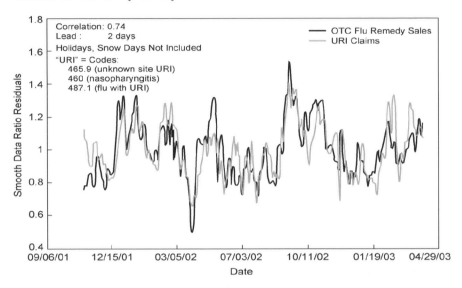

Fig. 2.11   Time series of the ratio of the actual data to the model data. Both OTC sales and physicians' office visits for URI are plotted. The effects of confounding factors in Fig. 2.10 were mitigated by the model. Note the high correlation between OTC flu remedy sales and physicians' office visits for URI, with the OTC sales leading the visits by about 2 days.

In another illustrative example, the sinusoidal seasonal variation and a linear trend were modeled separately and then subtracted from both the OTC time series in Fig. 2.10 and for a time-series of physicians' office visits. The resulting time series were then smoothed with a moving 7-day average to eliminate day-of-week fluctuations. Figure 2.11 shows the final time series of both OTC sales and physicians' office visits with only short-term fluctuations not explained by the models remaining. Transformation of the two data sources in this way, allows for a comparison of the relative latency of the short-term fluctuations in the two series without contamination from seasonal and day-of-week effects. Because these confounding effects often vary by region, it is important to know how the regional differences affect both the correlations and lead times. Aggregating data into smaller regions, as shown in Fig. 2.12, may improve the correlation between OTC sales and physicians' office visits, as is evident from a comparison of the correlation in Fig. 2.11 with the correlations shown in Table 2.1.

In a study conducted in six U.S. cities to determine if sales of electrolytes were indicative of respiratory and diarrheal disease outbreaks in children, electrolyte product sales were strongly associated with hospital diagnoses for respiratory and diarrheal

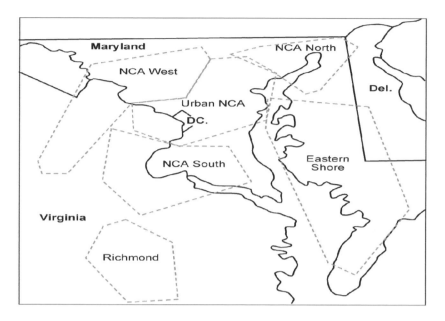

Fig. 2.12   Map of the United States in the vicinity of the NCA showing the regions used in Table 2.1.

Table 2.1   Correlation and Lag Analysis of OTC Sales vs. Physicians' Office Visits (PO) for Different Geographic Regions in the Vicinity of the National Capital Area (NCA)

Region	Mean Weekly OTC Count	Mean Weekly PO Visit Count	Peak Correlation	Lead Time of OTC (days)
Richmond	166	61	0.90	0
Eastern Shore	82	137	0.87	2
Western NCA	119	368	0.90	7
Urban NCA	1840	2823	0.93	5
NCA South	104	225	0.91	−2
NCA North	97	499	0.86	5

disease. Furthermore, the OTC sales data gave earlier indications for 12 of 18 out-breaks [10]. In two enteric outbreaks due to *Cryptosporidium*, 5- to 20-fold increases were seen in OTC antidiarrheal sales [5, 7, 8]. Additionally, the OTC sales data gave earlier warning of disease outbreaks by up to 2 weeks before it was noticed by the public health departments. However, because of the confounding factors mentioned previously in this section, it is very important to understand that OTC sales are not consistently the earliest reliable indicator of an outbreak. The confounding factors often vary by region (e.g., snowfall) and by time of year. Thus, the lead times of OTC sales may vary considerably by region and time of year, and may even lag physicians' office visits as an indicator [2, 1], as shown in Table 2.1. It is best to use OTC data along with other data sources, such as hospital and physicians' office visits because having different data sources to corroborate one another can lead to more confidence that a real disease outbreak might be occurring.

Similar to OTC pharmacy sales data, prescription sales data include information on the amount and type of drug, the date it was dispensed, and whether the prescription is new or is a refill. Unlike OTC sales data, where the person may or may not have seen a health care provider, a prescription is written only after the person has seen a physician. Like OTC remedies, a prescribed drug may treat more than one condition. Just as with OTC remedies, prescription drug data are subject to confounding influences. Dispensing of prescriptions is subject to store hours, the day of the week, holidays, and weather conditions. Prescription data may or may not be an early indicator of disease in a community because a visit to a provider occurs prior to prescription purchase. However, if prescription sales data have less of a reporting lag than outpatient visit data, the prescription data may be timelier. For example, the New York State Department of Health receives Medicaid-reimbursed prescription data within 1–2 days of the date in which the prescription was filled [9].

However, timely data collection does not automatically translate into timely de-tection of disease. Detection is also dependent on the statistical algorithms in place. Distinguishing patterns in pharmacy sales due to diseases of concern among the fluc-tuations from non-disease and non-public health factors is a function of how well the data have been characterized and, accordingly, adjusted for these other factors.

2.3 DATA FROM EMS AND 911

Emergency medical services (EMS) are defined as the services needed to provide rapid, appropriate medical care to people in the community who are acutely ill or injured. EMS personnel travel to their patients, provide on-site care, and transport them to a hospital or other health care center for further treatment when needed [11]. In many regions, residents can report emergencies, injuries, or acute illness to authorities via a 911 telephone system. Often, the 911 system is linked directly to local EMS services, so that dispatchers answer the 911 calls and alert and direct EMS personnel as needed. Increasingly, 911 systems are automated. Dispatchers record information from each call directly into a computerized database, producing a single record for each 911 call [12]. These records may be augmented by information recorded directly by the system without dispatcher input, such as the caller's phone number and address. Many 911/EMS systems automatically categorize calls based on the nature of the event or illness/injury being reported. In addition, some systems note when specific hospital EDs begin diverting traffic due to shortages of personnel, beds or supplies [13, 14].

911 and EMS data have been used for syndromic surveillance in a number of regions, including New York City, San Diego County, California, Knox County, Kentucky, Boston, Massachusetts, and Seattle, Washington [12, 15, 18]. In a survey of abstracts submitted to the National Syndromic Surveillance Conference in 2003, 6 of 60 well-described surveillance systems monitored 911/EMS data [19]. Data from automated 911/EMS and ambulance diversions are particularly useful because their data can readily be adapted for use in electronic surveillance systems [20]. The electronic record is completed during or soon after the call [18], so that the latency is nearly zero. Therefore, EMS provides some of the most timely surveillance data available if the data are well integrated into the surveillance system. Depending on needs and resources, the 911/EMS data can be fed into an electronic surveillance system continuously or at discrete intervals. Most systems opt for batch transfer of records at discrete intervals because of limited resources. However, in an emergency situation, a constant feed from the EMS would provide perhaps the timeliest information about serious illness within a community. Calls to a 911 telephone system are often assigned automatically to a symptom or syndrome category, such as difficulty breathing or chest pain. These category labels can be used to select only the records required by syndromic surveillance, minimizing work and time during file creation and transfer. Categories can also be combined to obtain broader illness syndromes [18].

New York City was one of the first localities to develop a syndromic surveillance system with 911/EMS data as one of their sources. Using historical data, city officials adapted a traditional statistical influenza surveillance algorithm for use in a syndromic surveillance system receiving ambulance dispatch data. Their model adjusts for annual periodicity, secular time trends, day-of-week effect, holiday effect, the number of positive influenza A and B isolates reported by the World Health Organization collaborating laboratories in New York City, and outside temperature over the previous 3 days. They calibrated the algorithm by simulating daily forecasts for influenza-like illness (ILI) EMS data to determine alarm thresholds. They found that their algorithm modeled ILI very well in their population, especially when the number of influenza isolates was included as a covariate. Ninety percent of alarms produced by the algorithm occurred shortly before or during a period of peak influenza. Their model generally indicated the start of the flu season in New York City 2 to 3 weeks before traditional influenza surveillance detected widespread influenza activity [12].

The utility of 911/EMS data was also evaluated in San Diego following the major wildfire season in 2003. During the wildfires, personnel at the San Diego County Health and Human Services Agency monitored the 911/EMS data fed into their electronic surveillance system to study the effect of a series of major wildfires on the health of the community. They found increases in fire-related health events, particularly EMS calls for asthma and respiratory illness, which coincided with deterioration in air quality as the wildfires intensified and decreased as the fires were extinguished and air quality improved [17]. Magruder and colleagues [21] also studied the effect of the wildfires in the 2003 San Diego data. They quantitatively compared different data sources used in the San Diego system for signal strength and timeliness and found that EMS asthma data gave the earliest indication of the wildfire event. This study is described in more detail in Section 2.10.

2.4 DATA FROM TELEPHONE TRIAGE HOTLINES

Telephone triage hotlines are facilities that receive telephone calls from persons requiring health care advice or assistance, or who urgently seek to make physician appointments to address an illness or injury. Government agencies [22], health care providers [23], or private contractors may operate these facilities. Triage hotlines gather information about a caller's complaints that enables them to allocate appropriate clinical resources to that patient with appropriate urgency. These hotlines usually produce electronic records that capture syndromic information about calls.

The information available in telephone triage data will vary, but might typically include the time of the call, the caller's identity, age, place of residence, some description of their symptoms, and what advice was given. It may include an assignment of the call to one of a finite list of problems or guideline categories (practice guidelines used by the nurse to manage the call). This categorization is made by a health professional — typically, a registered nurse — based on information provided by the caller.

Triage data that have been placed in standard diagnostic or guideline categories are particularly amenable to syndromic category assignment. The fixed, standard diagnostic categories can be mapped to syndrome groups of interest. In some cases, triage telephone calls can be linked to follow-up physician appointments on a patient-by-patient basis. The call categorizations can then be directly linked to the physician-assigned ICD-9 codes [24]. If the syndrome groups have been defined in terms of ICD-9 codes, syndrome groups for the telephone diagnostic categories can be inferred. Unfortunately, this procedure is complicated by the fact that a given telephone triage category is not always associated with the same office visit ICD-9 code, and a given ICD-9 code is not always associated with a single telephone category. Nevertheless, statistical analysis of these links can provide useful syndrome groupings for triage diagnostic categories [24]. Magruder et al. [24] examined nurse advice calls that could be linked to corresponding physician encounters. Table 2.2 shows the percentage of syndrome groups based on ICD-9 codes that could be linked to specific nurse advice calls and the median lag in hours between the advice call and the linked office visit.

Telephone triage data may contain demographic, geographic and syndromic information that can be used to focus surveillance on relatively small groups of potentially affected individuals. The syndromic information is considered less precise than that obtained from a physician office visit. The Centers for Disease Control and Prevention (CDC) [23] found that the triage data were sensitive for detecting general respiratory and/or gastrointestinal syndromes, but far less sensitive for detecting hemorrhagic

Table 2.2   Percentage of Syndrome Groups Linked to Nurse Advice Calls and Median Lag of Visit Relative to Advice Call, 2002 (*Source*: [24], courtesy of MMWR.)

Syndrome group	% Linked to nurse advice calls	Median lag of visit relative to advice call (hrs)
Botulism-like	58	19
Fever	66	4
Lower GI	75	4
Upper GI	68	5
Hemorrhagic illness	56	14
Localized cutaneous lesion	61	6
Lymphadenitis	51	13.5
Neurologic	57	16.5
Rash	51	7
Respiratory	59	6
Severe illness potentially caused by infectious disease	73	4

conditions. In addition, there was some evidence [23] that telephone triage calls for acute illness were more numerous than office visits, within a population having access to both. Hence, these triage calls may be a more sensitive indicator of disease. In the United States, this advantage tends to be lessened by the fact that telephone triage services are not universally available, even among people who have health insurance. In some other countries, telephone triage services are provided to all citizens by the government health service [22, 25, 26].

Telephone triage data tend to be less specific than physician encounter data because of the relatively imprecise nature of the syndromic information (see section 2.1 for a discussion of data source sensitivity). But the triage data have some advantages with respect to confounding influences. When the triage hotline is operated around the clock, the data are less affected by the day of the week, holidays, or inclement weather than many other sources of syndromic data [24]. Because telephone triage is available immediately to patients with no appointment, the data will typically exhibit a shorter latency than will physicians' office visit information. The CDC [23] reported that for calls indicating respiratory infection, the median time lag between the triage call and the physician encounter was 5 hours. For acute gastrointestinal illness the median lag was 4 hours. These results were based on data from a health maintenance organization (HMO), where the triage nurse could immediately refer patients to schedule acute-care physician appointments. The latency advantage for the telephone data may be greater in other cases.

The usefulness of telephone triage data has been examined for at least three different sources of triage data. The first source was emergency room telephone triage data obtained when patients called their insurance company representatives to obtain permission to go to the emergency room. Some calls could be categorized as respiratory illness, based on the advice guidelines used. A second source of telephone triage data was a nurse advice hotline run by an HMO [23, 24]. In this latter case, physician appointment scheduling and the advice hotline were integrated into a single call center that served as a major entry point into the HMO's health care delivery system. Appointment clerks in the call center scheduled routine appointments, while the nurse advice hotline delivered medical advice and scheduled acute-care office visits when necessary. For this linked data, strong temporal correlations were found between the daily volume of calls meeting respiratory illness guidelines and the daily volume of patients seen with ICD-coded physician office visits falling within the CDC's respiratory illness syndrome group. A similar result held for the gastrointestinal syndrome group and the lower gastrointestinal syndrome group. Other syndrome groups did not correlate as well between the two data sources. An example of the degree of correlation for gastrointestinal (GI) illness is shown in Fig. 2.13 from Magruder.

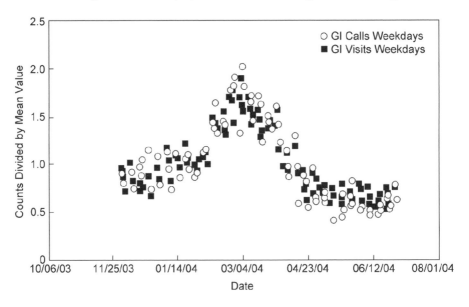

Fig. 2.13   Time series comparing nurse triage calls (GI calls) with physicians' office visits (GI visits) for gastrointestinal syndrome data. (From [21])

In a series of articles, Cooper et al. describe a surveillance system that uses the National Health Service (NHS) Direct telephone service in the UK [22, 26] and noted that spikes in GI and ILI were observed in the NHS Direct data when expected. A second review of the data [28] reported similar results and concluded that the call center data detected substantial levels of illness at both regional and national levels. This report also highlighted one of the problems with using this or any other data source for surveillance. Initially, only a limited proportion of the population was using the NHS Direct service. When data provide only limited coverage of a region, the results seen in the system may present a misleading picture of the health status of the community. For the NHS, the severity of this problem is decreasing as a larger percentage of the population makes use of the system. In their most recent paper Cooper and colleagues injected a historical *Cryptosporidium* outbreak in the UK into their data and analyzed the ability of their surveillance system to detect the outbreak. The probability of finding disease was linked to their assumption of how many people would use the NHS Direct system to seek care for their diarrheal illness; the probability increased as the percentage of the population calling NHS Direct increased [29]. They concluded that the NHS data would probably not have identified the *Cryptosporidium* outbreak as described but maintain that the system is effective in detecting larger, more severe outbreaks. A similar system triage call system, Tele-health, is in use in Ontario, Canada, and is currently undergoing evaluation, although early results suggest that it will be a useful surveillance tool in that setting [30].

2.5 DATA FROM SCHOOL ABSENTEEISM AND SCHOOL NURSES

School systems, especially the public school system, offer an opportunity to monitor the health of a very large fraction of school-aged children in a community. According to the National Center for Education Statistics [31], 90% of elementary and secondary education students in the United States attended public schools in the 2001–2002 school year. Because of the large fraction of school-aged children sampled and the aggregation of the data by individual school district (a natural epidemiological cohort), this data source has the potential to be a very sensitive indicator of illness in the school-agd population, whether the illness is geographically isolated or widespread. This potential is offset, however, by significant differences in absenteeism rates among different school levels (i.e., elementary, middle, and high schools). For a residential county with a population of around 250,000, mean percentages of absenteeism during the first 10 days of November 2000 were 3.5, 4.5, and 5.5% for elementary, middle, and high schools, respectively. Figure 2.14 shows the daily absenteeism for elementary, middle, and high schools divided by these means. The drop in high school absenteeism during school days 47 – 50 is probably associated with required standardized tests occurring on those days. Note in Fig. 2.14 that elementary schools seem to have the highest absentee rate after the holidays, perhaps due to the greater susceptibility of that age group to communicable respiratory illnesses.

School absentee data are less sensitive than school nurse data because there is typically no information about the reason for the absence. Absences could be due to family vacations or other obligations, or simple truancy. If the absence is due to an illness or injury, there is typically no way to separate the different types of illness or injury. Furthermore, there is typically no indication of whether the absence is due to the continuation of a previous illness or injury recovery, or whether it is a new condition. On the other hand, school nurse data include some information about the

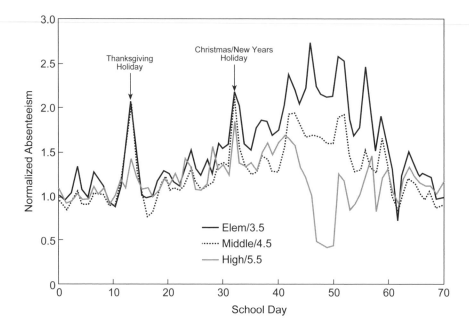

Fig. 2.14 Time series comparing school absenteeism for elementary, middle, and high schools for the first 70 days of the school year. The daily absenteeism percentages are normalized by the mean percent absenteeism during the first 10 school days of November 2000.

nature of the illness. In a school nurse reporting program in one California county, the school nurse reports were separated into 15 categories, including categories such as fever, flu, and diarrhea. If the condition is relatively severe, the student presumably would see the nurse only once or twice before staying home, so that there would be fewer repeat cases to obscure the new cases on each day.

Both school nurse and absentee data exhibit confounding influences related to holidays and to the school schedule. The days before or after holidays, long weekends, or school breaks may have higher absenteeism than other days. News events can also trigger school absenteeism. For example, a high level of school absenteeism was observed in a Maryland county on the day after the September 11 terrorist attack. Such events may be rare, but it is just at such a time that public health surveillance is most critical. Perhaps the most important confounding factor in both school nurse and absentee data is nonreporting. Public health surveillance and absentee reporting are not primary functions of a school system. Data quality and completeness are dependent on the voluntary attention and cooperation of the school system personnel. On some days, some schools simply do not report their data.

The value of school nurse data has been shown in a study of several public health surveillance data sources in San Diego County [32]. School nurse data were compared to school absentee data, military and civilian prescription data, military and civilian physician office encounters, and EMS reports. The school nurse data were normalized by the number of students present by subtracting the absentee numbers from the numbers enrolled.[1] The author compared the data sources both on the basis of signal-to-noise ratio (SNR) and on latency. Reporting delays were not included in the latency measurements (i.e., physician encounters were tagged with the actual day of the encounter, not when the encounter was reported to a public health agency). It was observed that the response of the school nurse data to an influenza outbreak had a higher SNR than any of the other data sources except for the EMS. While the EMS data had a higher SNR, the peak in EMS cases lagged the peak in school nurse cases by approximately 1 week (see Fig. 2.18). Although the EMS cases probably included an older population than the school nurse cases, it is common for many communicable diseases that begin among children to spread to adults.

2.6 DATA FROM HOSPITAL VISITS

Data from hospitals include daily admissions and ED visits. The ED visits typically consist of free text containing chief complaints. A *chief complaint* is a short phrase describing the main concern expressed by a patient as the reason for coming to the ED. If the patient is unable to communicate, the nurse or physician will enter what appears to be the primary presenting sign of the patient. Examples of chief complaints are "abdominal pain," "headache," "blood sugar test," and "gunshot wound," and might include abbreviations or acronyms used by the person recording the chief complaint. These chief complaint texts can be parsed into syndromic categories, taking into account acronyms, abbreviations, and spelling errors. Hospital ED data don't often include discharge diagnoses, but when they do, this additional information can be useful. The discharge diagnosis is usually in the form of an ICD-9 code. One or more ICD-9 codes may be entered for each patient. An ICD-9 code may describe only symptoms and signs (e.g., 786.2, cough) or may indicate a specific disease (e.g., 033.9, whooping cough). However, ICD-9 codes are not always provided in hospital ED data, and when they are, hospital coding of the chief complaints into ICD-9 classification may take several days. In contrast, chief complaints are available at the time the patient is seen. Because they are timelier, chief complaints are the primary ED data used in surveillance systems. Figure 2.6 illustrates how the ED data for ILI tends to lead physicians' office visit data.

As with other data sources, there are different ways of establishing syndromic groupings in ED data, depending on the objectives of the surveillance. A surveillance system that is designed to detect specific diseases may have a syndromic grouping that includes only the leading signs, symptoms, ICD-9 codes, etc., for that one disease. Alternatively, the syndromic grouping could be very general, such as all signs, symptoms, etc., related to the respiratory system representing the respiratory syndrome

---

[1]It should be noted that this normalization method would exclude those students who were ill at home and did not visit the nurse, which potentially could be a large number of excluded cases, thereby reducing the sensitivity of this data source.

group. However, a general syndromic grouping such as GI may include signs and symptoms of diseases that are distinctly not GI. In a hospital emergency department, perhaps the most common chief complaint of patients is abdominal pain. Not only is this complaint not exclusive to the GI system, it is important to realize that it is prevalent in the ED environment. In many surveillance systems, a compromise between the specific and general approaches is used. For example, the same surveillance system could have a syndromic grouping for inhalational anthrax and another for respiratory infections. The former would improve specificity while the latter would be more sensitive.

The correlation between ED chief complaint and ED discharge diagnosis has been studied, but the results differ. One retrospective study [33] comparing ICD-9 diagnosis codes and patient chief complaints found similar patterns in seasonal variation but only fair agreement between the syndromic groupings based on ICD-9 versus those based on ED chief complaints. Another study [34] found good agreement for most syndromic groups but not for all. For the most part, these differing conclusions can probably be explained by the different ways of determining which chief complaint goes into which syndromic grouping.

Because hospital ED data consist mostly of chief complaints, which are in free text and include abbreviations, acronyms, and misspellings, algorithms are used to parse them into syndromic groupings [35]. These algorithms process electronic ED data records by first normalizing the text. One normalization method is to remove punctuation and digits, expand abbreviations and acronyms, and account for misspelled words. Also, the algorithm has to be able to interpret specific in-house or regional abbreviations as well as words and abbreviations that are context-dependent. Next, the resulting chief complaint must be classified into one or more syndromic categories. An individual patient's chief complaint may be placed in several categories, depending on the text that it contains (e.g., fever and runny nose). More details on chief complaint processing are given in Chapter 5.

2.7   DATA FROM PHYSICIANS' OFFICE VISITS

When a patient is examined by a physician, much of the useful information is obtained through a carefully taken history. The history includes answers to questions such as:

- What symptoms bother you the most?

- When did the symptoms first appear?

- Were you well before they appeared?

- How have the symptoms progressed?

- What makes you feel better or worse?

- Have any of your acquaintances or family members had something similar?

- What other medical problems have you had or do you have?

The answers to these questions by the patient are subjective to the patient and are commonly called *symptoms*. The next most useful set of information comes from a careful physical examination. These data are commonly called *signs* because they tend to be more objective than what the patient reports. The history and physical provide important information and useful evidence for developing what is called the *differential diagnosis*. A differential diagnosis is a prioritized list of possible diseases that may explain most, if not all, of the symptoms and signs. The diagnosis at the top of this list is not necessarily the final diagnosis.

Data from physicians' office visits are typically collected by group insurance databases and HMOs. Diagnoses in the form of ICD-9 codes may be obtained from these records. Physicians' office personnel may enter only the ICD-9 code for a patient's primary complaint or sign, or they may enter the ICD-9 code of the primary diagnosis. Even when an ICD-9 code is entered for a specific disease, it may not mean that the patient has this disease. In some instances, the primary diagnosis is not yet known, so either a presumptive diagnosis or a "rule-out" diagnosis may be used. The presumptive diagnosis is based on the physician's experience and best guess that is most likely, given the symptoms and signs. A presumptive diagnosis may be confirmed later by laboratory tests or by the favorable response of the patient to treatment. If the patient fails to respond to therapy, a laboratory test may be ordered and/or the physician may change the diagnosis to the next one on the differential diagnosis list, or revise the differential diagnoses themselves if new information from the patient's history and physical become available. A rule-out diagnosis is one that may fit (though not necessarily be the best fit) the patient's symptoms and signs, but also has the most severe consequences if left untreated. Therefore, a rule-out diagnosis may be used when the physician wants to know as soon as possible if this is the underlying cause of the signs and symptoms. Rule-out diagnoses are typically used to justify ordering laboratory tests or referrals to specialists. A rule-out diagnosis may not be the most likely but is typically a disease with high priority on the physician's index of suspicion. Therefore, an ICD-9 code may not represent the final confirmed diagnosis for a patient and, in that sense, may be considered pre-diagnostic information. Figure 2.6 illustrates how physicians' office visit data can lag other indicators such as ED visits and OTC sales. Nonetheless, physicians' office visit data may corroborate other data sources, leading to higher confidence that a real outbreak is occurring. Furthermore, office visit data may provide more specific clues to the type of outbreak than other data sources.

The ICD-9 codes may be grouped into syndromic categories in a number of ways, depending on the desired specificity and sensitivity. As mentioned above, the ICD-9 code itself may be more general or specific. As an example of the former, a GI syndromic category that includes abdominal pain may include many illnesses not associated with the GI system, thereby making interpretation of an increase in this syndromic category difficult. Therefore, it is important to design syndromic categories balancing sensitivity and specificity with the ultimate goal of the biosurveillance system in mind.

2.8 LABORATORIES ROLE IN PRE-DIAGNOSTIC SURVEILLANCE

Laboratory tests may be ordered by physicians in the community or within hospitals. Some hospitals have their own laboratories for routine tests. Depending on the laboratory test, it may take minutes, hours, days, or even weeks to generate results. These results may be positive, negative, indeterminate, or simply suggestive. Because syndromic surveillance focuses on pre-diagnostic information, requests for laboratory tests are often used as a data source under the assumption that the number of requests for a particular test per unit time indicates the suspected presence of a disease in the community. However, not all test results are positive, so these data have the potential to be misleading. While the *implicit* assumption is that the physician ordered the test because a particular disease was very high on the index of suspicion, a laboratory test may also be ordered to rule-out a disease. In this case, there is a non-trivial possibility that the patient has this disease, and the adverse consequences of a positive diagnosis warrant ruling it out as soon as possible. If the test confirms this diagnosis, the physician can begin treating the patient more expeditiously and, hopefully, with a better outcome for the patient. One must make the *implicit* assumption above because the thinking of the person ordering the test is unknown. Laboratory tests themselves may be nonspecific or specific. A test for anthrax is obviously specific. A complete blood count (CBC) is nonspecific, although it provides useful information to the clinician.

Conventionally, health care providers (physicians, nurses, laboratory personnel, hospital infection control personnel, etc.) report notifiable disease events to state health departments via telephone, e-mail, or facsimile. Large hospital and commercial and national laboratories may also use the Health Level 7 (HL7) standard to transmit data electronically to health departments. The HL7 standard was developed to facilitate communication between health care information systems (http://www.hl7.org). An HL7 message may contain information on one or several laboratory test orders for a patient. There also may be several messages for a single patient in the same transmission. The data may be sent in real time, in batches several times a day, or daily, depending on the receiver and the purpose of the data transmission [36, 37, 38]. The HL7 messages can contain patient identifiers, age, sex, zip code, hospital identification number, physician requesting the order, laboratory identification number, laboratory specimen details, laboratory procedure, results or status of the test request, ICD-9 coded reason for test request, and date and time of the HL7 message and laboratory request. The data contained in the message depends on the variables of interest to the receiver [36, 38]. Many laboratories use the Logical Observation Identifiers, Names, and Codes (LOINC) protocol developed by the Regenstrief Institute for Health Care to encode details about laboratory tests. The LOINC terminology defines standard codes, which are used in interpreting laboratory data for outcomes management, clinical care, research (www.regenstrief.org/loinc/), and syndromic surveillance. These codes also enable lab data to be used across multiple geographic areas, surveillance systems, and jurisdictions [36].

Evaluations comparing electronic versus conventional laboratory reporting systems of notifiable diseases to local and state health agencies indicate that electronic reporting systems are more complete and more timely. An evaluation of the electronic laboratory reporting (ELR) system used by three Hawaiian statewide clinical laboratories indicated that ELR was 3.8 days earlier than the conventional system. In addition, the ELR system resulted in 2.3 times more reports and was 80% more complete for most data fields than conventional reporting [38]. Similar results were reported in an evaluation of a health system in western Pennsylvania [37].

Laboratory tests can be grouped into syndromes like other health indicator data. The CDC convened a panel to group laboratory test orders into syndromes for its national syndromic surveillance system, the BioSense Early Event Detection and Situation Awareness System, which monitors laboratory request data for outbreaks in addition to other pre-diagnostic data [36]. The panel, comprising experts in surveillance, medical informatics, laboratory data, and infectious disease, grouped laboratory requests into eight syndromes: fever, respiratory, GI, neurological, rash, lymphadenitis, localized cutaneous lesion, and specific infection. Laboratory test request data were in HL7 format and were from a large national network of laboratories (Laboratory Corporation of America or LabCorp). To aid in syndromic grouping, the LabCorp codes were classified into five categories: tests for specific and nonspecific infectious diseases, system-specific tests, fluid screening tests, and miscellaneous functional tests. A few of the test requests were in more than one syndrome. For example, tests for *Haemophilus influenzae* were in both respiratory and neurologic syndromes.

Grouping laboratory test requests into syndromes allows these data to be used for surveillance in combination with other health indicator data. For example, syndromic groupings of laboratory test requests from the Department of Defense Composite Health Care System (DoD CHCS) enabled comparison to military prescription pharmacy and clinic visit data in the San Diego area and U.S. National Capital Area (NCA) [39]. The syndrome groups of laboratory test requests developed by the CDC's panel of experts mentioned above were adapted for use in a preliminary grouping of microbiology laboratory tests requested in military treatment facilities in the two metropolitan areas. A preliminary evaluation compared 7-day averages of daily counts of military laboratory test requests, prescriptions, and outpatient clinic visits for 2 months in 2004. Requests for laboratory tests by military physicians were strongly correlated ($\gamma = 0.82$) with GI syndrome in both geographical areas and respiratory syndrome in the U.S. NCA.

A possible limitation of using electronic laboratory test requests for syndromic surveillance is the high rate of false positive reports. In a study that evaluated the reliability of coding of DoD CHCS laboratory test requests, the lab requests were compared with the corresponding ICD-9 code from inpatient and outpatient records [40]. While 61–64% of laboratory test requests were ordered appropriately for the diagnostic code recorded in the patient's inpatient/outpatient electronic record, only 15–19% had confirmatory results. This finding suggests the possibility of a high false positive rate in using test requests alone. Another study, which examined a different surveillance system in the Pittsburgh, Pennsylvania, area [37] found that 8%

of electronic reports were false positives, which is considerably lower than in the DoD CHCS study. The availability of laboratory test requests in electronic format and standardization of laboratory test codes facilitate their use along with other data sources used in syndromic surveillance. However, syndrome groupings of these data to corroborate and confirm disease detection alone or in conjunction with other data sources have yet to be evaluated comprehensively.

2.9   OTHER HEALTH INDICATOR DATA

Other health indicator data include a wide variety of sources, such as environmental and animal health data or more qualitative data such as news articles and reports on moderated list servers (e.g., ProMED). Unfortunately, the earliest news reports about a developing situation frequently include erroneous information that usually, though not always, is removed later. Nevertheless, there may be certain basic information (e.g., time or location of occurrence) that is more likely to be reliable and useful for establishing a timeline or a region of increased scrutiny. While it is important to monitor news sources, it is perhaps as important to prevent erroneous information from entering the data stream. Listservers, especially moderated ones such as ProMED, tend to be more reliable but not as timely as non-moderated sources. As mentioned earlier, OTC ads and circulars may be an important indicator of whether certain OTC product sales are being influenced by promotions or coupons.

2.9.1   Environmental Data

Environmental data may be nonspecific or specific for particular pathogens or toxins. As an example, water utilities routinely measure certain water quality indicators, such as turbidity, total organic carbon (TOC), metals, chlorine, phosphorus, pH and alkalinity. The quantities measured vary from region to region. For example, whereas many regions use chlorine to disinfect their water, some regions use ozone or chloramine. Other measurements made at the water treatment facility may include the percentage of samples that are total coliform positive or the percentage of *E. coli*-positive samples, although these parameters are typically not measured daily. TOC is commonly used as a water quality indicator because organic carbon, in addition to bromide, is a precursor to the formation of harmful disinfection byproducts in municipal water supplies. Therefore, water with high levels of TOC and bromide requires additional and costly treatment steps. From a biosecurity perspective, TOC is important because it includes any source of organic carbon, whether it be rotting vegetation or a deliberately introduced biological organism. Turbidity is another water quality indicator routinely measured. During the 1993 *Cryptosporidia* outbreak in Milwaukee, an increase in turbidity preceded the detected onset of illness by a few days [41]. This outbreak was subsequent to heavy rains that overwhelmed sewage treatment facilities and led to raw sewage entering Lake Michigan in close proximity to the intake of a water treatment plant (*Cryptosporidia* are extremely resistant to commonly used water disinfectants). For these data to be used effectively, a significant quantity of historical data must be collected to understand annual, seasonal, and regional variations and episodic (e.g., heavy rainfall) or longer (e.g., drought) natural events that may affect these measurements. While signals in either syndromic health or water quality data alone may indicate no waterborne health anomalies, contemporaneous anomalies in multiple data streams should lead to a heightened suspicion and perhaps more specific water quality testing at appropriate locations in the distribution system.

The weather is another environmental indicator worth monitoring because there are a variety of ways in which it may affect disease incidence. Certain diseases respond almost directly to environmental parameters (e.g., *Pfiesteria*, vectorborne diseases of humans and animals, crop diseases). Extreme weather events may also affect public health (e.g., flooding overloads sewage treatment facilities and leads to water pollution). A study by the CDC [42] showed significant increases in diarrhea and stomach ailments in the areas flooded by the passage of tropical storm Allison over Texas in 2001. Outside temperature appears to be associated with some variation in disease incidence, although the exact causal mechanisms are not well understood at present. Cold weather could conceivably increase the incidence of disease by several mechanisms, such as inducing people to spend more time indoors, which would increase the indoor population density and thereby promote person-to-person transfer of disease. In addition, cold, dry air may lead to loss of moisture and heat from the bronchial mucosa and thereby increasing disease susceptibility. Studies of exercise-induced asthma have shown that cold dry air may enhance bronchoconstriction, while rapid airway rewarming (e.g., entering a heated building) may cause vascular congestion and transient edema [43]. Falling ambient temperatures may also increase morbidity from chronic obstructive pulmonary disease [44].

Other environmental parameters that are more specific health indicators include aeroallergen (i.e., pollen, mold) concentrations, pollutant (e.g., ozone) concentrations, and biosensor measurements for specific pathogens (e.g., tularemia) or toxins (e.g., ricin). For pathogens and chemical toxins, the fastest response sensors are good for screening but tend to yield higher false positives. Slower response tests, such as polymerase chain reaction (PCR), are very specific but may take a few hours. For example, on February 23, 2006, a suspicious powder was found in a University of Texas dormitory laundromat. The FBI initially confirmed that it was positive for ricin based on state laboratory tests, but on February 26, after slower, more specific tests conducted at a U.S. military laboratory at Fort Detrick, Maryland, the FBI concluded that it was definitely not ricin. Sometimes a test can be inconclusive due to contamination, naturally occurring material, or bad controls. For example, PCR is specific for certain genetic sequences that are presumed to be unique to a particular pathogen. However, PCR cannot distinguish whether such a pathogen is naturally occurring for that region or season, or whether the genetic material identified is associated with a living organism.

Monitoring concentrations of aeroallergens and air pollutants is important for avoiding false alarms from sudden increases in such data as respiratory-related hospital ED visits or OTC sales. In the Washington, DC, region, there are approximately four aeroallergen seasons per calendar year. Tree pollen peaks from March through April, grass pollen peaks around May through June, and weed pollen peaks around August through September. The peaks in pollen concentration tend to be rather narrow, on the order of 2 to 3 weeks. Peaks in mold concentration last longer and are more variable, with annual maxima that may occur in October, August, or as early as May, depending on local rainfall. Each of these aeroallergens may have impacts on hospital ED visits, OTC purchases, and physicians' office visits for respiratory-related illnesses such as asthma.

Air pollution is also associated with increases in hospital and ED admissions [45, 46] and in increased sales of ambulatory respiratory drugs [47]. The primary air pollutants vary among regions and may include ozone, sulfur dioxide, nitrogen oxides, particulates with aerodynamic diameters of 2.5 micrometers or less (called PM2.5), and others. While lightning may produce some ozone, most ground-level ozone results from a photochemical reaction between nitrogen oxides and volatile organic compounds, which come primarily from motor vehicle exhausts. Because sunlight is required for the chemical reaction to produce ozone, ozone levels correlate with the amount of available sunlight. Nitrogen oxides result not only from motor vehicle exhausts, but also from electric utilities and other commercial and industrial sources. PM2.5 includes a variety of particles that come from motor vehicles, factories, construction sites, tilled fields, wood-burning, rock quarries, and roads. Both unpaved and heavily traveled paved roads contribute dust that is included in PM2.5. These small particles may remain suspended in the air for long periods of time.

A sudden increase in respiratory complaints on a given day may be due to increases in air pollutants and/or aeroallergens rather than the onset of an infectious disease outbreak. Poor air quality is associated with stagnant air and temperature inversions that keep polluted air concentrated near the ground. These same environmental effects may enhance an outdoor bioterrorist attack with pathogenic aerosols or toxic gases. Because the effects of a bioterrorist attack may coincide with a day of poor air quality, it is important to understand the environmental data so that the earliest signal of the attack can be detected above the environmental noise.

Knowledge of these environmental factors is important in any effort to detect bioterrorist-induced or other anomalous disease outbreaks in at least two ways. First, because they don't always occur exactly within the same time period every year, these factors may explain increases over the expected disease incidence background that would otherwise trigger false alarms. Second, they can present as confounding factors that may hide a natural or human-made disease outbreak. Therefore, knowledge of environmental effects may help reduce false alarms and increase the sensitivity of a biosurveillance system to true positive alarms.

2.9.2   Animal Health Data

Because most diseases are specifically adapted to their hosts, in general, humans don't contract animal diseases and vice versa. There are however, important *zoonotic diseases*, so called because of their ability to infect both humans and animals. These diseases include rabies, West Nile virus, monkeypox, and most of the diseases considered to be bioterrorist threats, such as plague and anthrax. Therefore, domestic animals and wildlife may serve as early warning indicators or sentinels of naturally occurring or bioterrorism-caused zoonotic disease outbreaks. For example, in 1999, an unexpectedly high number of crows and zoo birds were found dead in New York City. A subsequent outbreak of encephalitis in humans was noted in the same communities. These bird cases signaled the introduction of West Nile virus into the United States. Animals can serve as sentinels for zoonotic disease outbreaks if they are exposed to the agent simultaneously with humans, if they are at least as susceptible to the disease as humans, and if the disease has a shorter incubation period in animals than in humans and leads to identifiable disease signs in the animals. Figure 2.15 shows how these properties influence the usefulness of animal data in biosurveillance. The figure illustrates the most useful surveillance data on animals is collected automatically on animals that are in close proximity to humans. In order to be use for early detection of disease in humans, the signs of disease in animals must occur before signs of disease in humans.

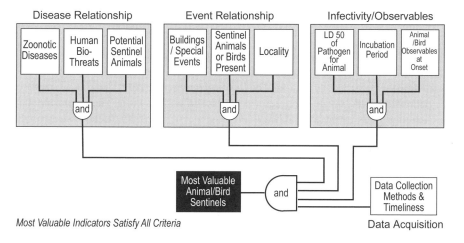

Fig. 2.15   The relationships of animal health to human disease determines how valuable it may be for early detection of that disease.

Among the indications in animals that a zoonotic agent might be present is an increase in numbers of certain signs of disease above a pre-established level. The normal or expected rate and frequency of specific disease signs or syndromes in the community's animal population must be determined quantitatively over a long period of time to account for natural phenomena such as seasonal changes. Knowing this normal spatial and temporal "background" in the region will permit statistical recognition of an "abnormal" or unexpected number of these occurrences, i.e., a possible outbreak. Other clues that something unusual is happening in animals include the occurrence of disease in a species in which it is not normally observed, the occurrence of a disease that is not responsive to normal treatment modes, the occurrence of a disease in a location where it is normally not seen, or a disease appearing at the "wrong" time of year. To use animals as sentinels, we should be able to recognize a zoonotic disease outbreak in the animal population before it affects humans. For example, sheep, cattle, goats, and horses are more susceptible than humans to anthrax [48, 49]. Cats, rats, prairie dogs, chipmunks, and ground squirrels may be useful as sentinel animals for plague [50, 51]. The 1994 pneumonic plague outbreak in India was preceded by a large urban rat die-off a few weeks earlier than the first reported human case [52, 53]. Rohrbach [54] suggested that local die-offs of rabbits or rodents should be investigated for possible tularemia.

Several animal data sources may be available, including private veterinary practices, veterinary clinic chains, wildlife rehabilitators, and livestock sales barns. Unlike human health data, most of these animal health data are not maintained in electronic databases suitable for surveillance. Even when they are available, electronic veterinary databases can yield a variety of unflagged and unexplained artifacts (e.g., 50% drops in data perhaps due to changes in personnel) that may compromise its use for biosurveillance. Local departments of agriculture inspect animals at sales barns, but many of these records are not computerized. Furthermore, because of these inspections, animals showing any obvious signs of being unwell are typically not presented for sale.

The minimum data characteristics for all types of animal sources include number of animals, species, date of examination, location, and syndrome. The specific data characteristics will vary by source. The location may be the zip code; county; name of the pet owner, farm, ranch, care facility; or place of examination. The syndrome may be entered directly by the animal health professional or derived indirectly based on the primary presenting signs of the animal. Because many veterinary health professionals still maintain primarily paper health records and any animal health databases are small, specialized, or nonexistent, the establishment of health databases similar to those used for humans is a challenge. Furthermore, such data must be collected consistently over a long period of time to track normal seasonal and periodic patterns.

Therefore, despite its potential, using animals for early detection of bioterrorism poses unique challenges. The pathogen may be introduced directly into a part of an urban area where many potential animal sentinels are likely to be absent (e.g., a commercial district with office buildings and restaurants). The large historical databases of health data that exist for humans because of insurance requirements are not typically kept for animals. For all these reasons, using animal surveillance to provide early warning of zoonotic diseases that are intentionally introduced into the human population is limited at the present time, but may become more prevalent as animal health data become more computerized.

2.10   DATA SOURCE EVALUATION

Three public health events in San Diego are used [21] to illustrate an approach to evaluating some of the data sources discussed above. These events are varied enough to capture a range of outbreak signals and conditions. The public health events type and month/year of the event were:

- Wildfires (October 2003)

- Influenza Outbreak (December 2003)

- Gastrointestinal Outbreak (January–February 2004)

Various types of data were compared for each of the three public health events. These data sources varied in the timeliness of availability to public health professionals, the population represented, and the level of fidelity for capturing health behavior. The data sources compared were:

- EMS reports

- Civilian physician encounters (ICD-9) ("Civ Dx")

- Military treatment facility encounters (ICD-9) ("Mil Dx")

- OTC pharmaceutical sales

- Civilian prescriptions ("Civ Rx")

- Military prescriptions ("Mil Rx")

- School absenteeism

- School nurse reports

Note that all the data sources were included in the analysis, although not all were compared for all public health events. The ambulatory encounter data are labeled by the day of the encounter, and the prescription drug data are labeled by the day the prescription was filled. This analysis did not address possible reporting latencies for any of the data sources.

2.10.1 Approach and Methodology

The approach to each public health event comprised two primary phases: data processing and data comparison. The objective of the data processing phase was to prepare the data to improve the likelihood of detecting the outbreak in a given data source. Data processing entailed development of data filters for each data source and data smoothing via application of a 7-day smoothing window. The objective of the data comparison phase was to identify data source(s) for each outbreak that were the best indicator of the event. Both visual and analytical comparisons of data source signal strength and timeliness were performed.

Data sources were first filtered to extract the types of symptoms associated with each outbreak. In some cases, such as EMS data, the categories were broad and readily mapped to the outbreak event. As an example, the Fever/Flu/Rash EMS category was mapped to the influenza outbreak. In other cases, such as physicians' office ICD-9 codes, data were analyzed prior to developing the filter to select ICD-9 codes that were likely to respond to that event and exhibit a response during the time of the event.

Data were then processed to eliminate effects, such as day-of-week cycles. Discovering the best possible processing method and then demonstrating that it is in fact the best method is difficult as well as potentially time and cost prohibitive. However, by applying a simple and uniform process to each data channel, one can learn to remove some of the strongest correctable effects. In this case, the strongest confounding effect was the day-of-week cycle. In addition, some of the data sources suffered from relatively low daily counts. Both of these problems were addressed by smoothing the data using a 7-day moving average, where each day's count is replaced by the average count over a week centered on that day.

Following the processing step, the data sources were compared based on timing and SNR for their ability to signal these public health events. The data were first inspected visually to identify peaks and other characteristics of the time series. This step provided essential information that might not stand out in the statistics — which are represented by a single response value — along with a calculation of the outbreak time span.

Three measures were utilized for data source comparison: SNR, minimum date, and maximum date. These measures require the use of mean and standard deviation calculations over a baseline period, where the baseline time periods are outside the primary outbreak events and vary by event. Note that given the length of the baseline periods selected for each event, an SNR greater than 2 is associated with a p-value of approximately 0.03. The SNR provides a measure of the strength of the data source response to the event. SNR is defined as:

$$SNR = \frac{peak_{count} - \mu_{count}}{\sigma_{count}} \tag{2.1}$$

where $peak_{count}$ is the daily count at the peak of the event, μ_{count} is the mean for the baseline period, and σ_{count} is the standard deviation for the baseline period. The minimum and maximum dates (Min Date and Max Date), which provide a sense of relative timeliness of the data sources, were reported for the first and last days, respectively, when the 7-day average count reached within 1 standard deviation of the peak level for each data source type.

2.10.2   Example: Wildfires (October 2003)

EMS, civilian physician encounters, military treatment facility encounters, and military prescription data sources were analyzed for the wildfire event. OTC, civilian prescription, and school data were not included. The EMS categories examined for the wildfire event were asthma and respiratory distress. For civilian and military treatment facility encounters, data were analyzed prior to development of the filter. The method for selecting ICD-9 codes was to examine all the codes that showed particularly high counts during the week of the wildfires compared with the previous and following weeks. After review of this initial list of ICD-9 codes, only those that seemed to be related to poor air quality were retained. Table 2.3 lists the office visit ICD-9 codes (and their descriptions) used to filter data for the wildfire event.

Table 2.3   Wildfire Event ICD-9 Codes Used

ICD-9 Code	Description
464.00	Acute laryngitis, without mention of obstruction
493.0	Extrinsic asthma
493.12	Intrinsic asthma with acute exacerbation
508.8	Respiratory conditions due to other specified external agents
518.82	Other pulmonary insufficiency, not classified elsewhere
785.50	Unspecified shock
786.05	Shortness of breath
786.52	Painful respiration

Similarly, military prescription data were analyzed prior to development of the filter. As a result of the preliminary analysis, two military prescription drug classes that displayed a signal corresponding to the fire event were identified: beta-adrenergic agent and glucocorticoid. Note that results were reported for individual EMS and military prescription categories, whereas office visit data were reported collectively.

Figure 2.16 displays the normalized October 2003 wildfire daily counts for EMS, civilian physician encounters, military treatment facility encounters, and military prescription data sources. The raw counts were scaled by the mean daily count over a common time interval so that the time-series data could be plotted on a comparable y-axis. The daily counts for the wildfire event, shown in Fig. 2.16, reached a local maximum during the same time period. Note that the times-series data indicate that the EMS-asthma data source had the strongest absolute response as well as the timeliest response to the wildfire event.

Figure 2.17 displays the normalized October 2003 7-day average counts for EMS, civilian physician encounters, military treatment facility encounters, and military prescription data sources. In this view, each day's count was replaced by the average count over a week centered on that day. After smoothing using a 7-day average, the behavior of each data source over time was more apparent, enabling a straightforward visual comparison. The EMS-asthma data source had the strongest absolute response as well as the timeliest response to the wildfire event.

Table 2.4 summarizes the SNR and timeliness performance for EMS, civilian physician encounters, military treatment facility encounters, and military prescription

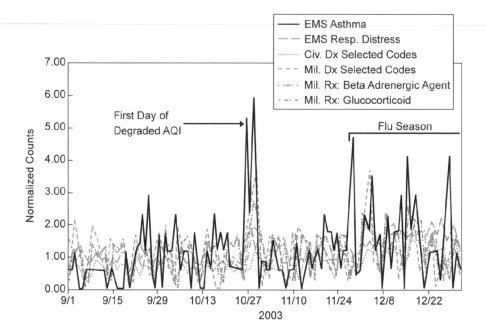

Fig. 2.16 Wildfire event: normalized daily counts by data source type.

data source types. The baseline period for the mean and standard deviation calculations was July 1, 2003, through October 21, 2003.

Table 2.4   Wildfire Event: Data Source Performance Summary

	SNR	Min Date (within 1 σ of peak)	Max Date (within 1 σ of peak)
EMS asthma	3.9	Oct 25	Oct 29
EMS Resp. distress	9.5	Oct 27	Oct 29
Civ Dx	1.9	Oct 27	Nov 1
Mil Dx	6.6	Oct 28	Oct 30
Mil Rx: BAA	5.6	Oct 27	Oct 31
Mil Rx: glucocortic	4.4	Oct 29	Oct 31

The EMS respiratory distress data had the highest SNR and the military treatment facility encounters data the second highest. Using the minimum date as the basis for comparison, the EMS data, especially the asthma calls, showed the earliest response

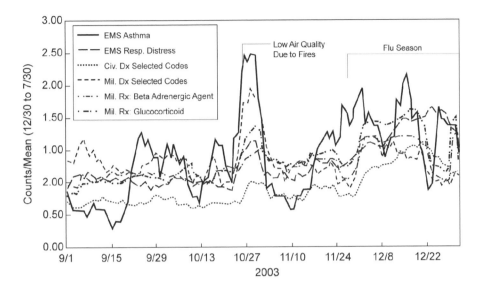

Fig. 2.17 Wildfire event: normalized 7-day average counts by data source type.

to the event. Note that the shapes of the peaks may differ as a function of data source, and a data source may show an earlier indication of an event even though it has a later peak.

2.10.3   Example: Influenza Outbreak (December 2003)

EMS, civilian and military treatment facility encounters for the ILI and fever syndrome groupings, military prescription, school absenteeism, and school nurse data source types were included in the influenza evaluation. OTC data were not available for this time period. The EMS category for the influenza event was fever/flu/rash. Civilian and military treatment facility encounters data were filtered for two syndrome groups: influenza-like-illness (ILI) and fever. Tables 2.5 and 2.6 provide a list of ICD-9 codes for each group. Note that some ICD-9 codes appear in more than one syndrome group.

Military prescription data used for treating cough and cold symptoms were examined first. Subgroups were then identified that had the strongest peak during the time of the influenza outbreak. The groups were: bronchial mucolytics, cough preparations only with codeine, cough preparations only without codeine, cough/cold with expectorant, cough/cold without expectorant, oral cold preparations with analgesics, and oral cold preparations without analgesics.

School absenteeism data were the percent of students absent based on enrollment. School health nurse data describe the number of students that reported flu and respiratory symptoms.

Figure 2.18 displays the normalized December 2003 influenza 7-day average counts for EMS, civilian and military treatment facility encounters for the ILI and fever

Table 2.5   Influenza Event: Influenza-Like Illness (ILI) Syndrome ICD-9

ICD-9	ICD-9 Description
079.89	Viral infection NEC
079.99	Viral infection NOS
460	Nasopharyngitis, acute
462	Pharyngitis, acute
464.00	Laryngitis, acute w/o obstruction
464.10	Tracheitis, acute w/o obstruction
464.20	Laryngotracheitis, acute w/o obstruction
465.0	Laryngopharyngitis, acute
465.8	Infct up rsprt mlt sites, acute NEC
465.9	Infct up rsprt mlt sites, acute NOS
466.0	Bronchitis, acute
466.11	Bronchiolitis d/t RSV
466.19	Bronchio acute d/t oth infct orgnsm
478.9	Disease, upper respiratory NEC/NOS
480.0	Pneumonia d/t adenovirus
480.1	Pneumonia d/t RSV
480.2	Pneumonia d/t parainfluenza
480.8	Pneumonia d/t virus NEC
480.9	Viral pneumonia unspecified
484.8	Pneumonia in oth infct disease CE
485	Bronchopneumonia, organism, NOS
486	Pneumonia, organism NOS
487.0	Influenza w/pneumonia
487.1	Influenza w/rsprt mnfst NEC
487.8	Influenza w/manifestation NEC
490	Bronchitis NOS
780.6	Fever
784.1	Pain, throat
786.2	Cough

Table 2.6   Influenza Event: Fever Syndrome ICD-9

ICD-9	ICD-9 Description
038.8	Septicemia NEC
038.9	Septicemia NOS
066.1	Fever, tick-borne
066.3	Fever, mosquito-borne NEC
066.8	Disease, arthpd-borne viral NEC
066.9	Disease, arthpd-borne viral NOS
078.2	Sweating fever
079.89	Infection, viral NEC
079.99	Infection, viral NOS
780.31	Convulsions, febrile
780.6	Fever
790.7	Bacteremia
790.8	Viremia NOS
795.39	Nonsp positive cult NEC

syndrome groupings, military prescription, school absenteeism, and school nurse data sources. This view represents the 7-day average, where each day's count is replaced by the average count over a week centered on that day. School nurse flu and respiratory reports and the EMS fever/flu/rash reports stand out as influenza indicators here because the reporting rate during flu season was a very high multiple of the background rate outside the flu season.

Table 2.7 summarizes the SNR and timeliness performance for EMS, civilian and military treatment facility encounters for the ILI and fever syndrome groupings, military prescription, school absenteeism, and school nurse data source types. The baseline period for mean and standard deviation calculations was February 1, 2004, through June 15, 2004.

The most sensitive indicator for the flu, as measured by the SNR, was the EMS data source. However, the outbreak peaked 6 days earlier, on December 6, 2004, in the School nurse flu and respiratory data. Military treatment facility encounters also provided strong evidence of an outbreak, showing a high SNR and an early indication of outbreak. Although the military prescription data exhibited the earliest indication of an outbreak as measured by the minimum data statistic, the relative weakness of the

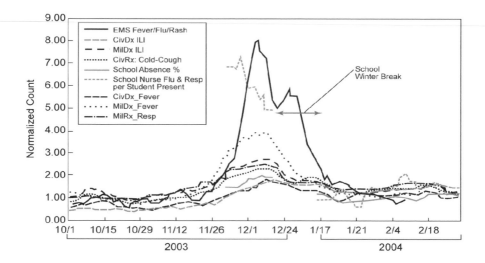

Fig. 2.18   Influenza event: normalized 7-day average counts by data source type.

Table 2.7   Influenza Event: Data Source Performance Summary

	SNR	Min Date (within 1σ of peak)	Max Date (within 1σ of peak)
Civ Dx–ILI	2.2	Dec 12	Jan 9
Civ Dx–fever	5.9	Dec 15	Dec 20
Mil Dx–ILI	6.7	Dec 9	Dec 20
Mil Dx–fever	16.9	Dec 11	Dec 17
EMS Fever/Flu/Rash	36.3	Dec 12	Dec 13
Civ Rx–/cough	5.0	08 Dec	20 Dec
School absence %	11.1	13 Dec	19 Dec
School health nurse–flu and resp	18.2	Dec 6	Dec 6
Mil Rx resp	4.3	Dec 2	Dec 20

signal suggests an increased risk of contamination of the leading edge by unrelated illnesses.

2.10.4   Example: Gastrointestinal Illness (January–February 2004)

EMS, civilian, and military treatment facility encounters, OTC, school absenteeism, and school nurse data source types were analyzed for the GI illness event. Civilian and military prescription data were not included. For EMS, school nurse, and OTC data source types, the mapping of diagnostic code or category to the gastrointestinal illness event was straightforward:

- *EMS*: GI/GU

- *School health nurse*: diarrhea

- *OTC*: electrolytes

However, for civilian and military treatment facility encounters, data were analyzed prior to development of the filter. For the GI analysis, the GI syndrome grouping was utilized initially. After data analysis revealed that the early stages were dominated by a peak in the military treatment facility encounters, the peak was analyzed to identify which codes contributed most. Subsequent analysis included this subset in addition to the GI group. Table 2.8 lists the codes that comprised the majority of this early peak, labeled "Dx Selected Codes."

Table 2.8   Gastrointestinal Event: DX Selected Codes ICD-9

ICD-9 Code	Description
008.00	Intestinal infection due to unspecified E. coli
008.69	Intestinal infection, enteritis due to other viral enteritis
009.2	Infectious diarrhea
535.50	Unspecified gastritis and gastroduodenitis, without obstruction
558.9	Other and unspecified noninfectious gastroenteritis and colitis
787.02	Nausea alone

Figure 2.19 displays the normalized January–February 2004 GI 7-day average counts for EMS, civilian and military treatment facility encounters for the GI and selected codes, OTC, school absenteeism, and school nurse data sources. This view represents the 7-day average, where each day's count is replaced by the average count over a week centered on that day.

When both the GI and Select Codes filters were applied, the military treatment facility encounters data suggested two outbreaks: one in mid-to-late January and the other in late February. The first peak was identified as a *Norovirus* outbreak in the military population. The corresponding civilian data mostly indicated the second peak in late February, although there also appeared to be a general rise in GI illness

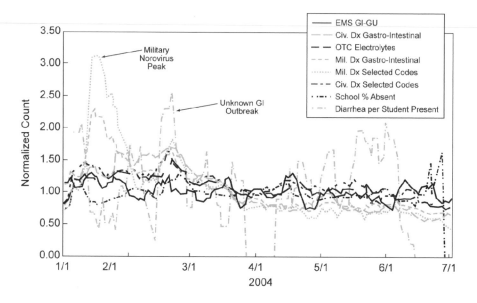

Fig. 2.19   Gastrointestinal event: normalized 7-day average counts by data source type.

throughout the January–February time period. This GI illness appeared weakly or perhaps not at all in the EMS, school nurse and OTC data.

Table 2.9 summarizes the SNR and timeliness performance for EMS, civilian and military treatment facility encounters for the GI and selected codes, OTC, school absenteeism, and school nurse data source types for the second peak of the GI event. The baseline period for mean and standard deviation calculations was April 1, 2004, through July 15, 2004.

The military treatment facility encounters data showed the strongest indication of the second GI event for both GI and selected codes groups. The civilian physician encounters data also produced a signal, although it might be difficult to discern the event given the typical variance in the background data. Also, when SNR was used as a measure, the school health nurse, school absenteeism, and EMS data gave only a weak signal.

Although a visual inspection of the time series might indicate that the OTC data source did not respond to the GI event, the SNR indicated a strong response. For these data, the baseline period for the mean and standard deviation that was input to the SNR calculation was an approximately 3.5-month period following the GI event, where the average daily OTC count was substantially lower than prior to the event. When viewing the data in real time, the epidemiologist would probably not notice any response to the event because of the higher background level.

Table 2.9   Gastrointestinal Event: Data Source Performance Summary

	SNR	Min Date (within 1σ of peak)	Max Date (within 1σ of peak)
Civ DX–GI	3.9	Feb 20	Feb 23
Civ Dx–selected codes	4.8	Feb 20	Feb 23
Mil Dx–GI	12.2	Feb 20	Feb 21
Mil Dx–selected codes	10.8	Feb 20	Feb 22
EMS Gi-GU	2.3	Feb 14	Feb 19
OTC electrolytes	10.0	Feb 16	Feb 23
School % absent	3.0	Feb 20	Feb 27
School health nurse–diarrhea	2.3	Feb 16	Feb 21

2.10.5   Conclusions

The three major disease outbreaks were each observable in multiple data sources, while the most useful data source varied with the event. EMS, military ambulatory encounters, OTC, and school nurse reports each proved especially useful for different illness events. For example, the EMS data showed the strongest SNR for disease caused by wildfires, the school nurse data gave an early indication of influenza, and the military treatment facility encounters data showed the strongest indication of an outbreak of GI illness. These results illustrate that a system that integrates multiple syndromic data streams into a single prospective surveillance tool will enhance the ability of military and civilian authorities in a locality to detect bioterrorist or other disease outbreaks in a timely fashion.

2.11   STUDY QUESTIONS

Health Indicator Properties:

2.1 As discussed in this chapter, when evaluating a health indicator, many factors are considered. From a quantitative perspective, some of the most important measures are sensitivity, specificity, and timeliness. These measures can all be calculated for an indicator with respect to individual cases or outbreaks. *Q: Consider how sensitivity and specificity of an indicator for individual cases is related to the sensitivity and specificity of the indicator for outbreaks. Does accuracy for individual cases have a direct and consistent effect on accuracy for outbreaks? Explain why or why not.*

2.2   The indicators discussed in this chapter are mainly relevant to automated surveillance in systems that operate continuously. Another venue for automated surveillance is following disasters or around large gatherings. In these "drop-in" settings, systems are implemented rapidly and data are often collected by health care staff using standardized forms. *Q: What types of indicators might be useful in a drop-in setting? Would any of the indicators described in this chapter be useful?*

Modeling Individual Events:

2.3   Most of the indicator evaluations in this chapter examined the relationship between two time series of different indicators. Each of these time series is the aggregated count of individual events. Research in epidemiology and other fields has shown that relationships between aggregate data do not always hold for individual events. In other words, if a rise in OTC sales tends to precede a rise in ED visits, this does not necessarily imply that a person will visit a pharmacy before an ED. *Q: Describe one possible scenario where a relationship between aggregate indicators does not hold for individual events.*

2.4   One method for attempting to understand the timing and relationship of indicators is to develop a graphical model of events for individuals. In such a model, events are denoted by circles and the influence of one event on another is indicated by an arrow from the first event to the second. *Q: Develop a model of the events that might occur for a person following the onset of symptoms. Consider how the events you have identified might influence aggregate indicators.*

Coding of Events in Health Indicator Data:

2.5   Events followed in surveillance systems, such as visits to an ED, may be recorded using standardized codes or free text. Coded data are generally considered easier to handle because the analyst knows in advance the possible codes that may be used and the codes are easily grouped into syndromes. An important consideration, however, is the validity of the code for a particular event. In other words, does the code truly represent the event? *Q: Suggest reasons why a code for an ED visit might not accurately represent the event. For which of the reasons, if any, might free-text data represent an event with greater accuracy?*

2.6   For some indicators, the coding system used was not developed for the purpose of surveillance. Codes for OTC data, for example, were developed for product tracking and logistics. *Q: What problems might be encountered when reusing a code set developed for another purpose for surveillance? In the particular case of OTC data, can you think of any solutions to the problems that you identified?*

REFERENCES

1. Magruder SF, Lewis SH, et al. Progress in understanding and using over-the-counter pharmaceuticals for syndromic surveillance. MMWR. 2004; 53(suppl): 117-122.

2. Magruder SF. Evaluation of over-the-counter pharmaceutical sales as a possible early warning indicator of human disease. Johns Hopkins APL Tech. Dig. 2003;24(4):349-354.

3. Zhang X, Fiedler R, et al. A biointelligence system for identifying potential disease outbreaks. IEEE Eng Med Biol. 2004;23(1):58-64.

4. Wagner MM, Tsui FC, et al. National retail data monitor for public health surveillance. MMWR. 2004;53(suppl):40-42.

5. Stirling R, Aramini J, et al. Waterborne *Cryptosporidiosis* outbreak, North Battleford, Saskatchewan, Spring 2001. Can Commun Dis Rep. 2001;27(22):185-192.

6. Welliver RC, Cherry JD, et al. Sales of nonprescription cold remedies: a unique method of influenza surveillance. Pediatr Res. 1979; 13(9): 1015-1017.

7. Proctor ME, Blair KA, et al. Surveillance data for waterborne illness detection: an assessment following a massive waterborne outbreak of *Cryptosporidium* infection. Epidemiol Infect. 1998; 120(1): 43-54.

8. Rodman J, Frost F. Pharmaceutical sales: a method of disease surveillance? J Environ Health. 1997; 60(4): 8-14.

9. Chen JH, Schmit K, et al. Use of Medicaid prescription data for syndromic surveillance, New York. MMWR. 2005; 54(suppl): 31-34.

10. Hogan WR, Tsui FC, et al. Detection of pediatric respiratory and diarrheal outbreaks from sales of over-the-counter electrolyte products. J Am Med Inform Assoc. 2003; 10(6): 555-562.

11. Suburban Emergency Management Project (SEMP). Glossary of disaster management, emergency medical service. July 27, 2002. Accessed March 28, 2006. Available at http://www.semp.us/htmlpages/glossarye1.html.

12. Mostashari F, Fine A, Das D, Adams J, Layton M. Use of ambulance dispatch data as an early warning system for community wide influenzalike illness, New York City. J Urban Health. 2003; 80(2 suppl 1): 43-49.

13. Foldy SL. Linking better surveillance to better outcomes. MMWR. 2004; 53(suppl): 12-17.

14. Foldy SL, Barthell E, Silva J, et al. SARS surveillance project: Internet-enabled multiregion surveillance for rapidly emerging disease. MMWR. 2004; 53(suppl): 215-219.

15. Johnson J, Gresham L, Browner D, McClean C, Ginsberg M, Wood S. From data sources to event detection: summary of the Southern California Regional Surveillance Summit. MMWR. 2004; 53(S1): 244.

16. Coberly JS, Holtry R, Feighner B, Tokars J, Lombardo J. Standard methods for early event detection and situational awareness in electronic biosurveillance. 2005 National Syndromic Surveillance Conference, Seattle, WA, September 14-15, 2005.

17. Johnson J, Hicks L, McClean C, Ginsberg M. Leveraging syndromic surveillance during the San Diego wildfires, 2003. MMWR. 2005; 54(S1): 190.

18. Lawson B, Fitzhugh EC, Hall SP, et al. Multifaceted syndromic surveillance in a public health department using the early aberration reporting system. J Public Health Manage Pract. 2004; 11(4): 274-281.

19. Sosin D, DeThomasis J. Evaluation challenges for syndromic surveillance: making incremental progress. MMWR. 2004; 54(suppl): 125-129.

20. Heffernan R, Mostashari F, Das D, et al. New York City syndromic surveillance systems. MMWR. 2004; 53(Suppl): 25-27.

21. Magruder S, Marsden-Haug N, Hakre S, et al. Comparisons of timeliness and signal strength for multiple syndromic surveillance data types, San Diego County, July 2003 – July 2004. MMWR. 2005; 54(S1): 193.

22. Baker M, Smith GE, Cooper D, et al. Early warning and NHS Direct: a role in community surveillance? J Public Health Med. 2003; 25(4): 362-368.

23. Centers for Disease Control and Prevention. Comparison of office visit and nurse advice hotline data for syndromic surveillance: Baltimore – Washington, DC, metropolitan area, 2002. MMWR. 2004; 53(SU1): 112.

24. Magruder SF, Henry JV, Snyder M. Linked analysis for definition of nurse advice line syndrome groups, and comparison to encounters. MMWR. 2005; 54(SU1): 93.

25. Cooper DL, Smith GE, et al. Use of NHS direct calls for surveillance of influenza: a second year's experience. Commun Dis Public Health. 2002; 5(2): 127-131.

26. Cooper D, Smith GE, O'Brien SJ, Hollyoak VA, Baker M. What can analysis of calls to NHS Direct tell us about the epidemiology of gastrointestinal infections in the community? J Infect. 2003; 46(2): 101-105.

27. Magruder SF. Linked analysis for definition of nurse advice line syndrome groups, and comparison to encounters. Presented at the 2004 National Syndromic Surveillance Conference, Boston, MA, November 3-4, 2004.

28. Cooper D, Smith G, Baker M, et al. National symptom surveillance using calls to a telephone health advice service, United Kingdom, December 2001 – February 2003. MMWR. 2004; 53(S1): 179-183.

29. Cooper D, Verlander NQ, Smith GE, et al. Can syndromic surveillance data detect local outbreaks of communicable disease? A model using a historical *Cryptosporidiosis* outbreak. Epidemiol Infect. 2005; 134(1): 1-8.

30. Moore K. Real-time syndrome surveillance in Ontario, Canada: the potential use of emergency departments and Telehealth. Eur J Emerg Med. 2004; 11: 3-11.

31. Bielick, S, Chapman C. Trends in the use of school choice 1993 to 1999. Publication NCES 2003031. Washington, DC: US Department of Education National Center for Education Statistics. Available at http://nces.ed.gov/pubs2003/schoolchoice/. Accessed March 24, 2006.

32. Magruder S, Marsden-Haug N, Coberly J, et al. Comparisons of timeliness and signal strength for multiple data types in San Diego County. Presented at 2004 Syndromic Surveillance Conference, Boston, MA, November 3-4, 2004.

33. Mocny M, Cochrane DG, Allegra JR, et al A comparison of two methods for bio-surveillance of respiratory disease in the emergency department: chief complaint vs. ICD-9 diagnosis code. Acad Emerg Med. 2003; 10(5): 513.

34. Begier EM, Sockwell D, Branch LM, et al. The National Capital Region's emergency department syndromic surveillance system: Do chief complaint and discharge diagnosis yield different results? Emerg Infect Dis. 2003; 9(3): 393-396.

35. Sniegoski CA. Automated syndromic classification of chief complaint records. Johns Hopkins APL Tech Dig. 2004; 25(1): 68-75.

36. Ma H, Rolka H, et al. Implementation of laboratory order data in BioSense Early Event Detection and Situation Awareness System. MMWR. 2005; 54(suppl): 27-30.

37. Panackal AA, M'ikanatha NM, et al. Automatic electronic laboratory-based reporting of notifiable infectious diseases at a large health system. Emerg Infect Dis. 2002; 8(7): 685-691.

38. Effler P, Ching-Lee M, et al. Statewide system of electronic notifiable disease reporting from clinical laboratories: comparing automated reporting with conventional methods. JAMA. 1999; 282(19): 1845-1850.

39. Olsen C, Hakre S, Pavlin J. A preliminary evaluation of laboratory test order data for medical surveillance. Presented at 2004 Syndromic Surveillance Conference, Boston, MA, November 3-4, 2004.

40. Riegodedios AJ, Ajene A, et al. Comparing diagnostic coding and laboratory results. Emerg Infect Dis. 2005; 11(7): 1151-1153.

41. MacKenzie WR, Hoxie NJ, Proctor ME, et al. A massive outbreak in Milwaukee of *Cryptosporidium* infection transmitted through the public water supply. NEJM. 1994; 331: 161-167.

42. Centers for Disease Control and Prevention. Tropical storm Allison rapid needs assessment, Houston, TX, June 2001. MMWR. 2002; 51: 365-369.

43. Tan RA, Spector SL. Exercise-induced asthma. Sports Med. 1998; 25: 1-6.

44. Donaldson GC, Seemungal T, Jeffries DJ, Wedzicha JA. Effect of temperature on lung function and symptoms in chronic obstructive pulmonary disease. Eur Respir J. 1999; 13: 844-849.

45. Frischer TM, Kuehr J, Pullwitt A, et al. Ambient ozone causes upper airways inflammation in children. Am Rev Respir Dis. 1993; 148: 961-964.

46. Simpson RW, Williams G, Petroeschevsky A, Morgan G, Rutherford S. Associations between outdoor air pollution and daily mortality in Brisbane, Australia. Arch Environ Health. 1997; 52: 442-454. A

47. Zeghnoun A, Beaudeau P, Carrat F, et al. Air pollution and respiratory drug sales in the city of Le Havre, France, 1993–1996. Enviro Res. 1999; 81: 224-230.

48. Pipkin AB. Anthrax. In: Smith BP, editor. Large nimal Internal Medicine. 2nd ed. St. Louis, MO: Mosby – Year Book; 1996: 1246-1250.

49. Aiello SE, ed. The Merck Veterinary Manual. 8th ed. Whitehouse Station, NJ: Merck and Co.; 1998.

50. Leib MS, Monroe WE, Eds. Practical Small Animal Internal Medicine. Philadelphia, PA: WB Saunders; 1997.

51. Acha PN, Szyfres B. Zoonoses and Communicable Diseases Common to Man and Animals. 2nd ed. Pan American Health Organization Scientific Publication 503. Washington, DC: World Health Organization; 1987.

52. Centers for Disease Control and Prevention. Human plague: India, 1994. MMWR. 1994; 43(38): 889.

53. John TJ. Learning from the plague in India. Lancet. 1994; 344:972.

54. Rohrbach BW, Tularemia. J Am Vet Med Assoc. 1988; 193(4): 428-432.

3 Obtaining the Data

Richard Wojcik, Logan Hauenstein, Carol Sniegoski, Rekha Holtry

Chapter 2 examined various types of data that can contain early indicators of a community's changing health status. The utility of these data types can be measured using metrics such as timeliness, specificity, and completeness. Data that come from clinical settings such as hospital emergency departments and laboratories, tend to have higher utility than non-clinical data. These data can be obtained in real-time and reflect the initial comments and insights of knowledgeable health care workers who enter the data. Other data streams often lack the timeliness and specificity of clinical data and may not be as useful as a primary source of surveillance data. Non-clinical sources can, however, provide value by corroborating initial trends found in more specific data sources.

Once the desired data sources are identified for a surveillance system, the system developer must find an efficient way to obtain the data. This chapter presents the basic knowledge needed to acquire the data for an automated disease surveillance system using the data sources described in Chapter 2. This knowledge includes basic information technology concepts required for the transfer and storage of the acquired health data. Current and emerging standards used to communicate health care information, as well as the basics of the privacy constraints imposed by the Health Insurance Portability and Accountability Act of 1996, are reviewed. Finally, examples are given of a system implementation used to acquire data from a hospital that is supporting its local health department in performing surveillance within its community.

3.1 INTRODUCTION TO DATA COLLECTION AND ARCHIVING

Our modern information technology (IT) infrastructure serves an integral role in today's society. Computers driven by fast and inexpensive processors sift through untold amounts of data every second in an effort to enhance our lives. In the realm of medical informatics, a wide array of technologies must work together hand-in-hand to fully leverage the power provided by modern computers: databases store and process large volumes of medical data; the Internet enables users to find data from nearly any location; web applications provide users with interfaces to the medical data; mapping applications provide a geographical context for the data. The careful application of these modern technologies can greatly enhance the collection, preparation, and analysis of important medical data.

The Internet connects our computers together, enabling worldwide connectivity of computer networks. This level of connectivity enables us to exchange information quickly and easily through the use of e-mail, websites, instant messaging, and a variety of other technologies.

Databases make it very easy to store large amounts of data electronically. Since databases can store and organize data so efficiently, engineers, scientists, economists, and nearly everyone can easily collect all sorts of measurable data. Once stored, the data can be pulled back out quickly for analysis.

These two major technologies comprise the core building blocks that enable powerful informatics-based disease surveillance. The following sections introduce some of the fundamental technical concepts relating to the Internet and databases. Chapter 5 expands on these IT-related concepts and provides more information on how these technologies can be used to enhance disease surveillance.

3.1.1   The Internet: Universal Connectivity

Most early computer systems were isolated, with data movement limited by portable media (disks, tapes, etc.). Early computer networks rarely communicated beyond the confines of the organization. Sharing data often meant that someone physically transported data on a portable disk from one computer to another. The Defense Advanced Research Projects Agency (DARPA), originally known as ARPA, developed technology that allowed computers to communicate with each other through existing telecommunication lines. Their system, called ARPANET, was the predecessor to the modern Internet [1]. Soon, fast and inexpensive technologies such as Ethernet and the Asymmetric Digital Subscriber Line (ADSL) spurred the rapid growth of the Internet. Now personal computers routinely connect to the Internet, where they can access a worldwide network of information.

Universal connectivity provides computers with a simple mechanism for information exchange. The ever-growing popularity of the Internet is responsible for increased worldwide economic development. At the same time, security issues such as recent high-profile computer virus scares have highlighted the importance of software security.

3.1.1.1   The Internet: How It Works   Modern networked computers use the Internet Protocol (IP) language to communicate with other computers on the network. Many organizations allow their computers to communicate freely over an organizational *intranet*, the local organization's network. Data exchanged between intranet computers never leave the organization's network. Computers in an intranet that wish to communicate with computers on the Internet may need to send their data through the organization's firewall (Fig. 3.1). A *firewall* is a special piece of computer hardware designed to protect the organization's intranet from the potentially hostile traffic that flows through the Internet. Most corporations follow this general network design style. Many modern home networks even follow this design by using a Distributed Subscriber Line (DSL) or cable modem as a simplified firewall. Once connected to the Internet, a computer has access to many different information services, including e-mail services, the World Wide Web, instant messaging, and many others.

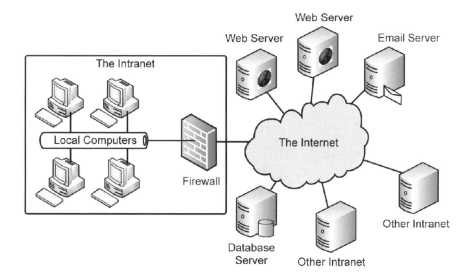

Fig. 3.1   Internet connectivity.

Internet connection speeds have improved dramatically in the recent past. *Internet service providers* (ISPs) provide high-speed Internet connections to nearly all modern organizations. Internet connections are most often measured in terms of their band-width, which is their capacity for data throughput. Some organizations only require the relatively low bandwidth supplied by simple DSL modems. Others, however, may need the higher bandwidth supplied by a T1 connection to support communications-intensive IT applications.

Computers that connect to the Internet have a unique number assigned to them — called an IP address — that allows them to be identified to the rest of the Internet. To communicate with another computer, your computer must know the IP address of the other computer. Computers are very good in working with IP addresses, but people generally have a hard time dealing with these complicated-looking numbers. To solve this problem, a group called the Internet Corporation for Assigned Names and Numbers (ICANN) took responsibility for maintaining a list of *domain names* and the corresponding IP addresses to which the domain names are mapped. Figure 3.2 depicts the general process through which computers communicate with each other over the Internet. First, the computer asks the domain name server (DNS), provided by its Internet provider, to find the IP address associated with an Internet site (e.g., www.google.com). The computer receives the IP address and then sends a request to the address to transfer the contents of the webpage. The computer hosting the site identified by this IP address, receives this request and returns the content of the webpage back to the requesting computer. Although it seems complicated, the entire exchange happens quite quickly. Advances in technology have streamlined the entire process to the point of near transparency.

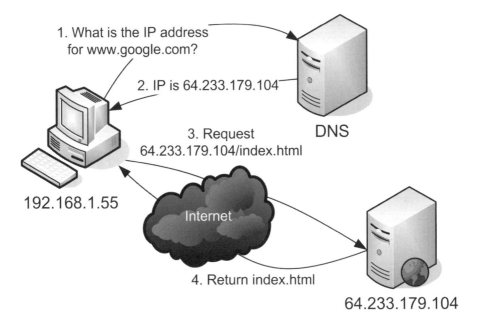

Fig. 3.2   A computer requests www.google.com using a domain name server lookup.

Computers that listen and respond to requests sent through a computer network are called *servers*. Servers are usually high-powered machines that are finely tuned to respond quickly to requests from clients. Servers are not, however, required to be particularly high-powered. In fact, software such as Microsoft's Personal Web Server, included with newer versions of Windows, allows users to turn their personal computers into small-scale web servers. A collection of electronic data hosted on the Internet often relies on one or more different types of servers. For example, file transfer protocol (FTP) servers allow clients to store and retrieve files on the server, and database servers (explained in greater detail in Section 3.1.2) provide flexible mechanisms for storing, querying, and modifying data.

FTP servers are used to store and share files on the Internet. Users can log-in and upload files from their local computer onto the server, where they are made available to other users of the FTP server. The FTP server software is responsible for authenticating the users who connect to the server and for determining the permissions assigned to the user — such as what files they may access and what file operations they may perform. Secure FTP (SFTP) servers build upon the FTP server functionality by adding an additional layer of security around the system via encryption of data transmissions and stronger password authentication mechanisms. Organizations will often use FTP or SFTP to share files across the Internet because the overall system is quite simple to operate and maintain [2].

Even though FTP servers make it easy to exchange individual files or data, most IT applications require a more flexible way to access and modify sets of structured data. Database servers provide a popular and useful solution to this problem. The next section gives a basic overview of databases.

3.1.2   Databases: Flexible Data Storage

Before the development of the first electronic databases, data were generally stored on paper in files. These files were manually stored and retrieved by staff members who were trained in filing. When companies increased the volume and variety of data stored, they had to hire more filing staff and find more space in which to store the data. Human error complicated the manual storage process — even the most meticulous file clerk occasionally misplaced a file. The cost associated with increased data storage soon became unmanageable.

In the 1970s, a company called IBM understood that computers could be used to store and organize large amounts of data efficiently. Their research team developed a method based on relational calculus for quickly storing and retrieving data in electronic form. The original vision of their database project was to allow users to interact directly with a database using English-like commands.

Today, the word *database* generally refers to a system of structured, organized, and persistent data. Manual paper filing systems are technically databases, but the term almost always implies a computer-managed system. The program responsible for the organization and management of a database is called a *database management system* (DBMS). A DBMS provides mechanisms that enable users to find and store data, in addition to controlling the low-level details concerning the physical storage of data.

Databases have become a critical part of an IT infrastructure. There are great volumes of data in the world — far too much to collect by hand. Often, though, there is value in collecting all of these data. For example, companies can analyze their customers' purchasing trends to spot patterns and provide an intelligent direction for their marketing campaign. Databases make information available in a flexible manner so that the data can be used to make well-informed decisions.

3.1.2.1   Databases: How They Work   The DBMS organizes sets of data using a description of the overall structure, called a *schema*. A schema describes the structure of sets of data, in addition to describing the relationships between individual sets of data. There are a number of different styles of databases — network, hierarchical, and relational, for example — which have different ways of handling data relationships and data navigation. The relational database style is by far the most popular.

The functionality of the relational database style is based on relational calculus. The fundamental idea behind relational databases is that data are organized in sets of tables that consist of a number of rows and columns. The items in a single row of data are assumed to be related to each other. Relationships between tables are expressed through common values.

For example, say a company wanted to create a simple database to keep track of employees (Table 3.1). An employee table contains data about the company's employees. Each row of the employee table holds information about a single employee — in this example, the employee ID, first name, last name, and a sectionID column that represents the section to which an employee belongs. The section table represents the different sections of the company: human resources, accounting, engineering, etc. Each row contains the name of a section along with a section ID number that uniquely identifies a section. A relationship between the employee table and the section table is expressed through their common SectionID column. For example, employee 2296 belongs to the section with SectionID 4. This value links into the section table, where SectionID 4 corresponds to the Engineering section of the company.

Table 3.1   Example of Table Relationship in Simple Database

Employee Table

EmployeeID	FirstName	LastName	SectionID
2295	Robert	Brown	4
2296	Amanda	Smith	4
2297	Nicholas	Williams	7
...	...	...	...

Section Table

SectionID	SectionName
1	Accounting
4	Engineering
7	Human Resources
8	Sales
...	...

This method may seem like a roundabout way of expressing a simple relationship, but it greatly simplifies the process of maintaining very large sets of data. If the company wanted to change the name of the Engineering section to Scientific Application Development, only a single value in the section table would need to be updated. Conversely, if the actual name of the section were stored in the employee table instead of a reference to a record in the section table, potentially thousands of records would need to be updated for a large company (one for every employee in the Engineering section).

Some database vendors develop software that provides a visual front end for accessing the database. At the most basic level, though, users interact with databases using a query language. Nearly all modern databases understand a variant of a declarative language called the *Structured Query Language* (SQL), a standard of the American National Standards Institute (ANSI) and the International Organization for Standardization (ISO). SQL contains a number of language subsets [3]. The most commonly used subset, the *Data Manipulation Language* (DML), defines a general grammar used to retrieve, insert, delete, and update data in the database. An example DML statement that retrieves a list of employees from the database would be:

```
Select emp.EmployeeID, emp.LastName, sect.SectionName

From Employee emp

INNER JOIN Section sect

ON (emp.SectionID = sect.SectionID)
```

This query pulls data from the employee table and matches up each employee row with its related section row in the section table. Because SQL is such a fundamental part of database systems everywhere, many technical resources are available for learning more about the language.

The *Data Definition Language* (DDL) subset of the SQL language enables database schema information to be created, altered, and removed. Essentially, the DDL is used to define the database structure and organization from the creation, augmentation, and removal of tables and relationships all the way down to the physical ordering of data. The following simple DDL statement would create the section table:

```
CREATE TABLE Section

    (SectionID INT NOT NULL, SectionName VARCHAR(50) NOT NULL)
```

Most database vendors also support another subset of SQL called the *Data Control Language* (DCL). The DCL provides functionality for defining users, user roles, and access privileges so that the database administrator has control over who can access and control different parts of the database.

The various components of a DBMS combine to form a flexible tool that makes it easy to store, modify, and access data in an organized fashion. Nearly all modern IT applications are driven by databases in one way or another.

3.1.3   Summary

The universal connectivity provided by the Internet and the organized storage capabilities provided by database servers form two critical building blocks for data collection systems. These technologies leverage the power afforded by the modern computing infrastructure to improve communications and increase data availability. Disease surveillance applications must keep these technologies in mind in order to provide optimal utility for the medical community.

3.2   OBTAINING ACCESS TO SURVEILLANCE DATA

The health indicator data used in syndromic surveillance can take many forms: hospital emergency department chief complaint records, nurse call center data, pharmacy sales data, outpatient insurance claims records, and others. Determining which types of health indicator data provide the greatest value is only one step in establishing an operational disease surveillance system. Actually obtaining the necessary access to real-world data streams can pose a significant challenge. For each data type, access and ongoing collection processes must be negotiated, established, and maintained. The nature of the negotiations and their accompanying concerns may differ according to the type of data, the type of institution providing the data, and the provider's location.

Because data access is such a fundamental aspect of surveillance, it is important to understand and respect the factors that motivate data owners to share their data for surveillance. It is important as well to understand the increasingly complex legal and proprietary issues pertaining to data disclosure and use. Although some of the concerns are familiar from traditional disease surveillance, others are less so. Unlike traditional surveillance, syndromic surveillance requires the collection of much larger quantities of data, data transmission on a real-time or near-real-time basis, data types from outside the traditional healthcare system, and data collection before any specific disease outbreak or health threat has been identified. In agreeing to participate, the institutions providing data are making a nontrivial commitment to setting up and maintaining steady data feeds for the foreseeable future, potentially in the absence of any serious community outbreaks to provide motivation. The importance of maintaining positive relationships with data providers cannot be overemphasized. Whether a legal mandate for data collection exists or not, the success of the system depends on their ongoing cooperation. As one factor in preserving cohesive relationships, it is important that all parties involved become familiar with their responsibilities related to issues of data privacy and data proprietorship. The overview in this section should not be considered a substitute for knowledgeable legal counsel. Parties who are considering disclosing, receiving, or using data for surveillance purposes are advised to obtain current legal advice before proceeding.

3.2.1   Sharing Health Indicator Data

Due to the wide variety of data types used in surveillance, the institutional owners of data streams of interest cover the spectrum. They may be local or national; commercial, nonprofit, or governmental; or inside or outside the traditional health care industry. Not every institution is guided by the same legal requirements, motivations, and concerns. To obtain desired data streams successfully, it is important to understand the legal requirements pertaining to data access as well as the informal concerns and motivations of the data providers. Some of the factors that commonly motivate data owners to participate in public health surveillance are discussed here.

3.2.1.1 Supporting the Community

The terrorist attacks of September 11, 2001, and the subsequent anthrax mail incidents that followed left communities anxious about the possibility of bioterrorism and motivated some in the private sector to do their part to protect the public. Recognizing that enhancing public health surveillance makes a critical contribution to preparedness, some private health care agencies and nontraditional data providers began to share their data for use in surveillance. Examples of such providers include hospitals and pharmacy chains.

3.2.1.2 Obeying Legal Mandates

In the United States, there are no federal laws currently obliging data owners to supply data for syndromic surveillance. Although some mandatory federal disease reporting requirements exist, they are generally limited to morbidity and mortality reports for passengers on cruise ships and other types of transport [4]. The Centers for Disease Control and Prevention (CDC), in conjunction with the Council of State and Territorial Epidemiologists (CSTE), produces a yearly list of federal notifiable diseases for which it requests reporting by each state and territory. Diseases are put on the list when it believes that their prevention and control will benefit from timely and regular information collection. Federal notifiable disease reporting, however, is voluntary rather than mandatory, and is acknowledged to be incomplete [5].

The bulk of the mandatory disease reporting requirements in the United States lie at the state level. Each of the 50 states has mandatory reporting laws that require health care providers and private laboratories to report diseases of public health significance to state, local, or county agencies. Some statues are couched as specific notifiable disease listings and some as broader reporting requirements. The nature of the reporting requirements and the specific diseases that must be reported differ by state. Although state-level notifiable disease reporting is an accepted practice, data collection for syndromic surveillance is less well established. Many states are reviewing the language in their existing broad disease reporting laws to determine whether it may apply to syndromic surveillance as well [4]. The following (Adapted from Broome et al. [4]) lists the language in each of the 50 states' broad disease reporting laws that may provide statutory authorization for syndromic surveillance, as of 2002:

Alabama: "cases of diseases of potential public health significance"

Alaska: "epidemic outbreaks"; "an unusual incidence of infectious disease"

Arizona: "Outbreaks of foodborne/waterborne illness."

Arkansas: "Occurrences which threaten the welfare, safety, or health of the public such as epidemic outbreaks."

California: "OCCURRENCE of ANY UNUSUAL DISEASE"; "OUTBREAKS of ANY DISEASE."

Colorado: "any unusual illness, or outbreak or epidemic of illnesses which may be of public concern."

Connecticut: "other condition of public health significance."

Delaware: "Any disease outbreak in a community, a hospital, or other institution or a foodborne, or waterborne outbreak."

Georgia: "Outbreaks or unusual clusters of disease (infectious and noninfectious)."

Hawaii: "Any communicable disease . . . occurring beyond usual frequency or of unusual or uncertain etiology, including diseases which might be caused by a genetically engineered organism."

Idaho: "Rare diseases and unusual outbreaks of illness which may be a risk to the public."

Illinois: "Any unusual case or cluster of cases"; "any suspected bioterrorist threat of events."

Indiana: "Unusual occurrence of disease"; "any disease . . . considered a bioterrorism threat."

Iowa: "Outbreaks of any kind unusual syndromes, or uncommon diseases."

Kansas: "Any exotic or newly recognized disease, and any disease unusual in incidence or behavior, known or suspected to be infectious or contagious and constituting risk to the public health"; "The occurrence of a single case of any unusual disease or manifestation of illness that the health care provider determines or suspects may be caused by or related to a bioterrorist agent or incident."

Kentucky: "an extraordinary number of cases or occurrences of disease or condition."

Louisiana: "all cases of rare or exotic communicable disease, unexplained death, unusual cluster of disease and all outbreaks."

Maine: "Any pattern of cases or increased incidence of illness beyond the expected number of cases in a given period, or cases which may indicate a newly recognized infectious agent, or an outbreak or related public health hazard."

Maryland: "Outbreaks and Single Cases of Diseases of Public Health Importance."

Massachusett: "Illness Believed to be Part of an Outbreak or Cluster."

Michigan: "the unusual occurrence of any disease, infection or condition that threatens the health of the public."

Minnesota: "Any pattern of cases, suspected cases, or increased incidence of any illness beyond the expected number of cases in a given period."

Mississippi: "Any Suspected Outbreak."

Missouri: "The occurrence of an outbreak or epidemic of any illness, disease or condition which may be of public health concern . . . [and] public health threats that could result from terrorist activities such as clusters of unusual diseases or manifestations of illness and clusters of unexplained deaths."

Montana: "Any unusual incident of unexplained illness or death in a human or animal."

Nebraska: "Clusters, outbreaks or epidemics of any health problem, infectious or other, including food poisoning, influenza or possible bioterrorist attack; increased disease incidence beyond expectations; unexplained deaths possibly due to unidentified infectious causes; any unusual disease or manifestations of illness."

Nevada: "Extraordinary occurrence of illness."

New Hampshire: "Unusual occurrence or cluster of illness which may pose a threat to the public's health,"

New Jersey: "Any outbreak or suspected outbreak, including but not limited to food-borne, waterborne, or nosocomial disease or a suspected act of bioterrorism."

New Mexico: "Illnesses suspected to be caused by the intentional or accidental release of biologic or chemical agents"; "Acute illnesses of any type involving large numbers of persons in the same geographic area"; "Other conditions of public health significance."

New York: "Any disease outbreak or unusual disease."

North Carolina: "all outbreaks or suspected outbreaks of foodborne illness"; "a cluster of cases of a disease or condition . . . which represents a significant threat to the public health."

North Dakota: "Unusual cluster of severe or unexplained illness or deaths."

Ohio: "Any unexpected pattern of cases, suspected cases, deaths or increased incidence of any other disease of major pubic health concern because of the severity of disease or potential for epidemic spread, which may indicate a newly recognized infectious agent, an outbreak, epidemic, related public health hazard or act of bioterrorism."

Oklahoma: "Outbreaks of apparent infectious disease."

Oregon: "Any known or suspected common-source outbreaks; Any Uncommon Illness of Potential Public Health Significance."

Pennsylvania: "Unusual occurrence of a disease, infection or condition."

Rhode Island: "an outbreak of infectious disease or infestation, or a cluster of unexplained illness, infectious or noninfectious . . . Exotic diseases and unusual group expressions of illnesses which may be of public health concern."

South Carolina: "all cases of known or suspected contagious or infectious diseases . . . all cases of persons who harbor any illness or health condition that may be caused by chemical terrorism, bioterrorism, radiological terrorism, epidemic or pandemic disease, or novel and highly fatal infectious agents and might pose a substantial risk of a significant number of human fatalities or incidents of permanent or long-term disability."

South Dakota: "Epidemics or outbreaks . . . and Unexplained illnesses or deaths of humans or animals."

Tennessee: "disease outbreaks foodborne, waterborne, and all other."

Texas: "any outbreak, exotic disease and unusual group expressions of disease which may be of public health concern."

Utah: "Any sudden or extraordinary occurrence of infectious or communicable disease" and "Any disease occurrence, pattern of cases suspect cases, or increased coincidence of any illness which may indicate an outbreak, epidemic or related public health hazard, including but not limited to suspected or confirmed outbreaks of foodborne or waterborne disease, newly recognized or re-emergent diseases or disease producing agents."

Vermont: "Any unexpected pattern of cases, suspected cases, deaths or increased incidence of any other illness of major public health concern, because of the severity of illness or potential for epidemic spread, which may indicate a newly recognized infectious agent an outbreak, epidemic, related public hazard or act of bioterrorism."

Virginia: "Outbreaks, all (including foodborne, nosocomial, occupational, toxic substance-related, waterborne, and other outbreaks)."

Washington: "Disease of suspected bioterrorist origin", "Other rare disease of public health significance."

West Virginia: "An outbreak or cluster of any illness or condition — suspect or confirmed.", "Unexplained or ill-defined illness, condition, or health occurrence of potential public health significance."

Wisconsin: "Suspected outbreaks of . . . acute or occupationally related diseases."

Wyoming: "A cluster of unusual or unexplained illnesses or deaths and suspected biological incidents."

Only a few states have laws that explicitly require hospitals to support syndromic surveillance. A revised Nevada statute, which became effective in July 2003, lists regulations for the "use of syndromic reporting and active surveillance to monitor public health," including policy for "(a) the manner in which and situations during which the system actively gathers information; (b) the persons who are required to report information to the system; and (c) the procedures for reporting required information to the system" [5]. Maryland's Catastrophic Health Emergency Disease Surveillance and Response Program allows a directive to be issued in certain circumstances mandating that health care providers report to public health authorities "(i) the presence of an individual or group of individuals with specified illnesses or symptoms; (ii) diagnostic and laboratory findings relating to diseases caused by deadly agents; [and] (iii) statistical or utilization trends relating to potential disease outbreaks" [6]. Revised Arizona statutes allow health information to be gathered in the event of a suspected bioterrorism attack [7].

3.2.1.3 *Boosting the Bottom Line*   Syndromic surveillance systems frequently use nontraditional health indicator data. The technology creates a new demand for data types not traditionally used in conventional surveillance. Proprietors of these previously untapped data sources may recognize the growing value of their data archives. Within the limits of federal regulations, they may be willing to supply selected data elements from their proprietary data warehouses to public health agencies in return for a fee. Types of data that may be purchased in this way include health maintenance organization (HMO) data, laboratory requisition records from privately owned laboratories, and physician office visit data from health insurance claims clearinghouses.

A data provider may charge fees based on the duration of the feed, such as a monthly or yearly rate, or on the gross number of data records provided. In the latter case, the costs may rise with seasonal disease fluctuations or in the case of an actual outbreak. To cut down on costs, data purchaser can often arrange to receive only those data records that contain values of particular interest to surveillance. Examples include purchasing only pharmacy sales records that contained designated National Drug Code (NDC) codes or only insurance claims records that contain certain International Classification of Disease, Ninth Revision, Clinical Modification (ICD-9-CM) codes. The cost of purchasing data streams can be significant over time and should not be overlooked when calculating the total cost of establishing and maintaining a surveillance system.

3.2.2   Data-Sharing Issues

Although some providers may agree to provide data for surveillance, others are understandably apprehensive. Some of the factors that tend to deter data owners from participating in syndromic surveillance are discussed below.

3.2.2.1 *Cost and Inconvenience*   Even otherwise willing data providers can be justifiably wary of the time, effort, and resources needed to establish and maintain surveillance data feeds. To establish a feed, the scope of the effort must be negotiated,

data use agreements drawn up and approved, and technical staff time devoted to planning and implementation. To maintain the feed, resources must be set aside more or less in perpetuity to provide upkeep and to fix any problems that might arise. Designing a data feed that places the least burden on the data provider, for both setup and maintenance, can substantially contribute toward allaying such fears.

3.2.2.2   Protecting Proprietary Information   Much of the data used in syndromic surveillance are proprietary. Both traditional and nontraditional health indicator data may contain information that the owning entity may be unwilling to make available in the public domain. Schools, for example, may not want their absenteeism levels publicly known to avoid political repercussions. Commercial pharmacies are unlikely to want their sales data available to investors or competitors. Because of the proprietary nature of many types of surveillance data, potential data recipients must be prepared to address issues of nondisclosure. These issues are commonly approached using formal, legally binding data use agreements. The agreement should clearly delineate which data or data elements are considered proprietary, and it should state who is allowed to see the data and under which circumstances. Generally, such an agreement includes language to the effect that while the data provided may be used internally by public health agencies for matters of public health, no proprietary data should be released into the public view unless written authorization is received from the data provider. Most owners of proprietary data are unlikely to consent to releasing it for public health purposes without such an agreement firmly in place.

3.2.2.3   Privacy Concerns   The Health Insurance Portability and Accountability Act of 1996 (HIPAA) has increased health care providers' concerns about privacy issues [8]. The act contains privacy rules that govern the manner and circumstances in which health care providers are allowed to release patients' health care information. The rules carry civil and criminal penalties for violation, including fines of up to $250,000 and up to 10 years of imprisonment [9]. If a health care institution that is covered by HIPAA is approached about supplying surveillance data, it is likely to raise concerns about HIPAA compliance. To gain the cooperation of potential data providers, it is important to understand the legal restrictions that the HIPAA privacy rules place on health data disclosure.

3.2.3   HIPAA and Disease Surveillance

HIPAA consists of two major parts. Title I addresses health insurance portability, protecting coverage for workers and their families when they change or lose their jobs. Title II has three parts: transaction standards, security rules, and privacy rules. The transaction standards, sometimes referred to as the *administrative simplification provisions*, require health organizations to adopt a common set of codes and protocols to transmit health data in electronic form. The security rules require the adoption of appropriate policies, procedures, and technical security measures for protecting electronic health data. The privacy rules mandate federal privacy protections for certain types of individually identifiable health information.

The privacy rules, approved in 2001 and effective two years later, are most pertinent with respect to obtaining access to data for public health purposes. They describe in detail which types of health information must be protected, which institutions must protect them, and from whom and under what circumstances they must be protected. All parties that disclose, receive, or use surveillance data should understand the implications of these rules for public health surveillance.

3.2.3.1   *Who Must Protect Private Health Information?*   HIPAA requires all covered entities to protect health information. The definition of covered entities includes all health plans, healthcare clearinghouses, and health care providers that transmit health information in electronic form for certain specified transactions (45 CFR §160.103) [10]. Clearinghouses are defined to include "public or private entities, including billing services, re-pricing companies, community health management information systems or community health information systems, and 'value added' networks and switches" (45 CFR §160.103) [10]. Many major sources of data for public health surveillance are covered entities under HIPAA, including hospitals, HMOs, health care clearinghouses, and laboratories. HIPAA legally binds each of these institutions to protect the privacy and security of its health care information.

A public health agency generally does not qualify as a covered entity under HIPAA, except in special circumstances, such as when the agency engages in covered functions, the fundamental activities of a health care provider, health plan, or health care clearinghouse. Examples of covered functions related to public health include Medicaid administration and immunization programs. The flowcharts provided in Figs. 3.3 and 3.4, developed by the CDC, can be used by a public health agency to determine whether it qualifies as a health plan or a health care provider under HIPAA.

A public health agency that does not engage in covered functions is not bound by the HIPAA privacy rule. This means that once a health data set is transferred from a covered entity to a noncovered public health agency, HIPAA no longer applies to it directly. The public health agency must still adhere to any privacy policies and procedures for its jurisdiction, however, and must obey any data use agreements into which it has entered with the data provider [4].

3.2.3.2   *What Kinds of Health Information Are Protected?*   HIPAA defines *health information* as any data related to a patient's health status, treatment, or payments [12]. The act aims to protect patient privacy by restricting access to those aspects of health information that could be used to identify an individual patient.

Individually identifiable health information is defined as information "(i) which identifies the individual, or (ii) with respect to which there is a reasonable basis to believe that the information can be used to identify the individual" [45 CFR §164.514 (a)] [10]. *Protected health information* (PHI) is defined as "individually identifiable health information that is or has been electronically maintained or electronically transmitted by a covered entity" (45 CFR §164.501) [10]. Although the HIPAA

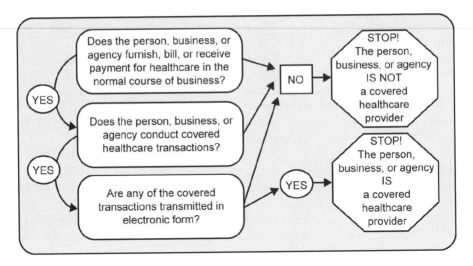

Fig. 3.3 Flowchart for determining whether a business, agency, or person is a covered health care provider under the HIPAA privacy rules. (From the Centers for Medicare and Medicaid Services of the U.S. Department of Health and Human Services [11])

privacy rules were originally developed to protect health information used in electronic transactions, they cover health data transmitted or maintained in any form, electronic or otherwise [12]. The HIPAA privacy standards apply to all individually identifiable health information [45 CFR §164.506 (d)] [10].

Under HIPAA regulations, the protected status of health information can be nullified if the information is de-identified. The act provides two ways to de-identify health data [45 CFR §164.514(b)] [10]. The first approach, the *safe harbor method*, consists of stripping out 18 specific types of information, listed in Fig. 3.5. If these elements are removed, and if the covered entity has no other reason to believe the remaining data elements can be used to identify individual patients, the HIPAA privacy requirements are considered to be met. The second approach, *statistical de-identification*, is more complex. In this approach, statistical analysis determines which data elements, either alone or in combination with other information, pose a nontrivial risk of allowing individual patients to be identified. These elements are then aggregated or removed [12]. The statistical de-identification process must be documented and certified by an expert. Regardless of how de-identification is achieved, the resulting data set no longer qualifies as PHI and is not subject to the HIPAA privacy rules.

Because situations might arise in which establishing identity is important, HIPAA allows a de-identified data set to contain a special identifier that can be used later to re-identify the data [45 CFR §164.514 (c)] [10] . The identifier must not be derived from any information related to the person and may not be used or disclosed for any other purpose. The process for assigning the identifier may not be revealed.

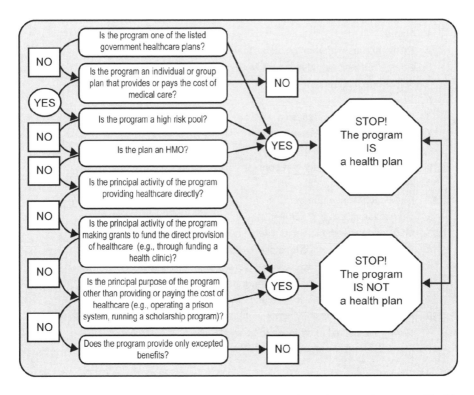

Fig. 3.4   Flowchart for determining whether a government-funded program is a covered health plan under HIPAA privacy rules. (From the Centers for Medicare and Medicaid Services of the U.S. Department of Health and Human Services [11])

3.2.3.3   *When Can Protected Health Information Be Disclosed?*   When one interprets the HIPAA privacy rules, it is important to distinguish between required and permissible data disclosures. *Required disclosures* are those that are mandated by law. *Permissible disclosures* are those that are allowed by law but are left up to the data owner's professional judgment, ethics, and discretion. From the public health perspective, HIPAA describes only which disclosures are permissible. Nothing in the act requires data disclosure for public health purposes [12]. Required disclosures are generally mandated by individual state laws, as discussed in Section 3.2.1.

- *Required disclosures.*   There are only two circumstances under which HIPAA requires disclosure of PHI: first, to patients themselves upon request; and second, to the U.S. Department of Health and Human Services to determine HIPAA compliance (45 CFR §164.502) [10] . If other laws require disclosure, HIPAA does not bar such disclosures [45 CFR §164.512(a)] [10].

- *Permissible disclosures.*   HIPAA discusses at great length which PHI disclosures are permissible. Under HIPAA, covered entities may use or disclose PHI for purposes of health care treatment, payment, or operations. Most other uses or

1. Names.
2. Postal address information, other than town or city, state, and zip code.
3. Ages > 89, including dates from which age can be determined.
4. Telephone numbers.
5. Fax numbers.
6. Electronic mail addresses.
7. Social Security numbers.
8. Medical record numbers.
9. Health plan beneficiary numbers.
10. Account numbers.
11. Certificate/license numbers.
12. Vehicle identifiers and serial numbers, including license plate numbers.
13. Medical device identifiers and serial numbers.
14. Web universal resource locators (URLs).
15. Internet Protocol (IP) address numbers.
16. Biometric identifiers, including finger and voice prints.
17. Full face photographic images and any comparable images.
18. Any other unique identifying attributes, with the exception of codes assigned to allow de-identified information to be re-identified.

Fig. 3.5   The 18 types of health care information that must be removed in the safe harbor method of de-identifying protected health information under HIPAA.

disclosures of PHI that are not otherwise required by law are forbidden unless written authorization is obtained from the patient [12].

HIPAA does, however, acknowledge the need to balance personal privacy with the public good. Certain types of data collection are considered too important to public welfare to be contingent on the express authorization of each patient. Twelve specific activities of public interest or benefit are granted exceptions to the written authorization requirement, including law enforcement, reporting of domestic violence, judicial proceedings, and public health (45 CFR §164.512) [10].

The public health exceptions written into HIPAA permit, for certain purposes, the disclosure of PHI without patient authorization to a *public health authority*, defined as an "agency or authority of the United States, a state, a territory, [or] a public subdivision of a state or territory... that is responsible for public health matters as part of its official mandate" (45 CFR §164.501) [10]. The public health authority that receives the information must be "authorized by law to collect or receive such information for the purpose of preventing or controlling disease... including, but not limited to... the reporting of disease... and the conduct of public health surveillance, public health investigations, and public health interventions" [45 CFR §164.512(b)(1)(i)] [10]. Examples of legitimate public health authorities include state and local public health authorities, the CDC, the National Institutes of Health (NIH), the Federal

Drug Administration (FDA), and the Occupational Safety and Health Administration (OSHA) [12].

The public health exceptions in HIPAA also permit data to be disclosed to a person or entity, which, although not itself a public health authority, has received a grant of authority from one (45 CFR §164.501) [10]. In the context of surveillance, this permission allows a public health authority to authorize a third party to perform designated aspects of data collection, data archiving, or data monitoring on its behalf. Because the HIPAA rules on data disclosure are not always well understood, the CDC provides sample letter templates (Figs. 3.6 and 3.7) that a public health authority can use to clarify data disclosure rules to a covered entity or to extend a grant of authority to an external agency.

To Whom it May Concern:

[*Public health authority*] is an agency of [*parent authority*] and is conducting the activity described here in its capacity as a public health authority as defined by the Health Insurance Portability and Accountability Act (HIPAA), Standards for Privacy of Individually Identifiable Health Information; Final Rule (Privacy Rule) [45 CFR § 164.501]. Pursuant to 45 CFR § 164.512(b) of the Privacy Rule, covered entities such as your organization may disclose, without individual authorization, protected health information to public health authorities "... authorized by law to collect or receive such information for the purpose of preventing or controlling disease, injury, or disability, including, but not limited to, the reporting of disease, injury, vital events such as birth or death, and the conduct of public health surveillance, public health investigations, and public health interventions ..."

[*Public health authority*] is conducting [*project*], a public health activity as described by 45 CRF § 164.512(b), and is authorized by [*law or regulation*]. The information being requested represents the minimum necessary to carry out the public health purposes of this project pursuant to 45 CFR § 164.514(d) of the Privacy Rule.

If you have questions or concerns please contact [*project leader*].

Fig. 3.6 Example of a letter from a public health authority to a covered entity, clarifying rules regarding disclosure.

3.2.3.4 How Much Health Information Can Be Disclosed? Even when it makes a permissible disclosure of information, a covered entity is usually required to disclose only the minimum necessary amount of information, described as the "amount reasonably necessary to achieve the purpose of the disclosure" [amended 2002 version,

---

Dear [*Authorized Agency*]:

This letter serves as verification of a grant of authority from [*public health authority*] for you to conduct the public health activities described here, acting as a public health authority pursuant to the Standards for Privacy of Individually Identifiable Health Information promulgated under the Health Insurance Portability and Accountability Act (HIPAA) [45 CFR Parts 160 and 164]. Under this rule, covered entities may disclose, without individual authorization, protected health information to public health authorities "... authorized by law to collect or receive such information for the purpose of preventing or controlling disease, injury, or disability, including, but not limited to, the reporting of disease, injury, vital events such as birth or death, and the conduct of public health surveillance, public health investigations, and public health interventions ..." The definition of a public health authority includes "... and individual or entity acting under a grant of authority from or contract with such public agency ..."

[*Authorized agency*] is acting under [*contract, grant, or cooperative agreement*] with [*public health authority*] to conduct [*project*], which is authorized by [*law or regulation*]. [*Public health authority*] grants this authority to [*authorized agency*] for purposes of this project. Further, [*public health authority*] considers this to be [*activity type*], for which disclosure of protected health information by covered entities is authorized by 45 CRF § 164.512(b) of the Privacy Rule.

Fig. 3.7   Example of a letter from a public health authority to an authorized agency, providing a grant of authority.

45 CFR §164.514 (d)] [10]. When making a permitted disclosure to public officials, such as public health authorities, a covered entity is allowed to assume that the amount of the information requested is the minimum amount necessary for the stated purpose [13].

Also in the context of permissible disclosure, HIPAA introduces the concept of a *limited data set* [amended 2002 version, 45 CFR §164.514 (e)(1)] [10]. This type of dataset may be used or disclosed without patient authorization for purposes of research, public health, or health care operations. It excludes specific identifying information pertaining to the person or to any of the person's relatives, employers, or household members. The identifiable elements that must be removed to create a limited data set are listed in Fig. 3.8. These are identical to the elements removed to de-identify data, with the exception of the age restriction and the medical device identifiers or serial numbers (items 3 and 13 in Fig. 3.5).

Because a limited data set may still contain identifiable information, it continues to qualify as PHI. Before releasing it, a covered entity is required to put into place a data use agreement ensuring that the new owner will maintain certain privacy and

1. Names.
2. Postal address information, other than town or city, state, and zip code.
3. Telephone numbers.
4. Fax numbers.
5. Electronic mail addresses.
6. Social security numbers.
7. Medical record numbers.
8. Health plan beneficiary numbers.
9. Account numbers.
10. Certificate/license numbers.
11. Vehicle identifiers and serial numbers, including license plate numbers.
12. Device identifiers and serial numbers.
13. Web universal resource locators (URLs).
14. Internet protocol (IP) address numbers.
15. Biometric identifiers, including fingerprints and voiceprints.
16. Full-face photographic images and any comparable images.

Fig. 3.8   The 16 types of health care information that must be removed from protected health care information to create a limited data set under HIPAA.

security protections. The required terms of the agreement are outlined in Fig. 3.9. Any covered entity that receives a limited data set and violates the data use agreement is considered to be in violation of HIPAA. Any covered entity that releases a limited data set to a recipient that it knows is not obeying the data use agreement is also in violation of HIPAA [13].

3.2.3.5   *What Types of Health Information Does Syndromic Surveillance Need?*
Although traditional disease outbreak investigations have an inherent need to gather detailed patient health data, syndromic surveillance may have limited need for many of the details. Detecting a suspicious increase in disease counts does not require directly identifiable information such as name, street address, or medical record number. Most syndromic surveillance systems focus on core information about syndrome, date, zip code or larger region, age group, and sex. The data elements that are needed to support these analyses are permitted to appear in both de-identified and limited data sets. Anomaly detection methods in syndromic surveillance systems can function effectively without further personal details. Some systems are developing the capability to use only aggregate-level or summary data, moving a step farther from HIPAA's protected health information.

Effective public health disease surveillance requires having the tools and capabilities to monitor community health indicators and detect abnormal health events quickly. Beyond having the proper tools, it is as important for public health entities to have

The data use agreement must:

A. Establish the permitted uses and disclosures of the health information.

B. Establish who is permitted to use or receive the limited dataset.

C. Provide that the limited dataset recipient will do the following:

    i. Not use or further release the information other than as allowed by the data use agreement or as may be required by law;

    ii. Use proper safety measures to prevent use or disclosure of the information other than as allowed by the data use agreement;

    iii. Inform the covered entity if the recipient becomes aware that data is being used or disclosed in any way not described in the data use agreement;

    iv. Make sure that any agents including subcontractors to whom the limited dataset is provided agrees to the same restrictions and conditions that apply to the recipient;

    v. Does not identify the information or contact the individuals.

Fig. 3.9 Provisions of the data use agreement required by HIPAA when a covered entity discloses a limited data set. (From the 2002 amended version, 45 CFR §164.514(e)(2) [10])

the authority to conduct detailed investigations when needed. If an unusual disease cluster is detected by a surveillance system, public health personnel will generally need identifiable health information in order to follow up on the potential outbreak. In a known or suspected emergency, it may be crucial to have HIPAA-permitted re-identification codes available that allow investigators to re-identify health records of interest quickly and reliably. A thorough understanding of the rules governing the privacy and confidentiality of health care information can help to design surveillance systems that are able provide maximum public health benefit while respecting legal and ethical limitations.

3.2.4 Summary of Data Sharing

Reliable data streams of health indicator data are a foundation of operational syndromic surveillance. Obtaining access to the necessary types of data often poses one of the major early challenges of establishing an operational surveillance system. It is important to understand the factors that motivate data owners to share their information and the legal and proprietary issues pertaining to data disclosure and use.

Many of the nontraditional health indicator data types used in surveillance have not historically been needed for public health purposes. Access to these types of data must generally be obtained either through purchase or through voluntary disclosure by their owners. In either case, due to the proprietary nature of the data, data providers commonly require a data use agreement that limits the ways in which the recipient can use or further disclose the data received.

Traditional health care data, on the other hand, are subject to numerous rules and regulations. All states have laws that grant state and local public health authorities the power to gather health information for local public health activities. In some cases, these laws might be interpreted as providing legal authority for syndromic surveillance as well.

The privacy rules of HIPAA primarily restrict the use and disclosure of traditional health care information. HIPAA does provide exceptions for data disclosure for public health purposes, however, and it does not block data disclosures that are otherwise required by law. Permissible data disclosures designed to support surveillance will most likely be one of the following types: disclosure of a de-identified data set that is no longer protected by HIPAA; disclosure of a protected data set that consists of the minimum data needed for public health purposes; or disclosure of a limited data set that is still considered protected and must be accompanied by a data use agreement that limits how the data recipient can use or further disclose the data.

Regardless of the data type, the data source, or the existence or absence of legal mandates, maintaining the goodwill and cooperation of data providers is an enormous asset for practitioners of syndromic surveillance. Accommodating concerns about privacy and proprietorship, respecting data use agreements, and working to minimize cost and inconvenience all contribute to developing the positive long-term relations needed to establish and maintain the level of data access required to support operational syndromic surveillance systems for the benefit of the community.

3.3   THE ROLE OF STANDARDS IN DATA EXCHANGE

Much of the health indicator data used for surveillance already exist within health care institutions in electronic form. In normal daily business operations, these institutions enter, retrieve, view, and exchange electronic data. It also has become increasingly important for these institutions to be able to exchange their data with external organizations responsible for protecting the health of the nation. To exchange data electronically, each aspect of the exchange needs to be defined in some way using either ad hoc approaches or existing standards. Using existing standards can help improve efficiency and lower implementation cost when sharing data with national health information systems. Because surveillance applications collect electronic data from other systems, builders of electronic surveillance systems need to understand electronic data standards used by data provider institutions and industries. Efforts are under way, through organizations such as the American National Standards Institute (ANSI) [14] and the Healthcare Information Technology Standards Panel (HITSP) [15], to standardize for the collection and exchange of public health data. Data standards are the principal informatics component necessary for information flow through the national health information infrastructure. With common standards, clinical and patient safety systems can share an integrated information infrastructure whereby data are collected and reused for multiple purposes to meet more efficiently the broad scope of data collection and reporting requirements [16]. This section focuses primarily on health care industry data standards that are related to public health surveillance.

3.3.1 Types of Standards

In information technology, data standards are the common language that allows information to be shared across systems. They can be formally defined as "documented agreements containing technical specifications or other precise criteria to be used consistently as rules, guidelines, or definitions of characteristics, to ensure that materials, products, processes and services are fit for their purpose" [17]. In the context of health care, data standards encompass the broad range of methods, protocols, terminologies, and specifications for the collection, exchange, storage, and retrieval of information associated with health care applications, including medical records, medications, billing, and administrative processes [17].

Consider the standards used when communicating laboratory test results using paper-based forms.

- Words and numbers are written on a standardized report form. They come from the standard set of English words and Arabic numerals.

- The layout of the form dictates the placement of words and numbers in a way that allows their meanings to be interpreted (e.g., the number in the box labeled "Zipcode" should be interpreted differently from the number in the box labeled "Blood Cholesterol").

- An understanding of the relationships between the various words and numbers on the form allows the viewer to recognize, for instance, that the person whose name appears on the form is the person to whom the results on the form pertain.

- The form is transmitted via the postal system mail, a complex system that involves standardized packaging in envelopes, standardized payment via stamp, standardized routing using a written address, and standardized drop-off and pickup locations.

- The laboratory transmits the form to a clinician's office in response to the clinician's previous request for laboratory testing, and the staff member that receives the form understands why it has arrived and files it appropriately.

The numerous kinds of informal standards used in the above scenario parallel the formal standards needed for exchanging electronic data. Standards exist to codify each aspect of data exchange. Unfortunately, competing or overlapping standards commonly exist for each type. When one is trying to make sense of the large number of existing standards, it helps to understand the aspects of data exchange that each covers. Some address only one aspect, such as vocabulary or record format, while others bundle several into a single package, such as data format and transmission.

This section focuses on standards for surveillance data. Other standards for electronic data exchange more pertinent to basic computer science issues, such as network protocols and security, are not covered here. The major types of standards covered are terminologies, message formats, message protocols, and knowledge models. Of these, terminologies and message formats are most pertinent to surveillance.

Several terms with similar meanings are commonly employed to designate a finite set of defined terms used to describe, classify, and encode the concepts in a domain.

- *Vocabulary, terminology*: the terms and their definitions only.

- *Codeset*: a terminology whose terms are numeric or alphanumeric strings rather than words.

- *Classification*: a terminology organized for easy retrieval, such as by major and minor categories.

- *Nomenclature, taxonomy*: the terms, their definitions, and an associated hierarchical scheme specifying "is-a" relations among terms.

- *Ontology*: the terms, their definitions, and an associated scheme describing more complex semantic relations among terms. Although sometimes used as simple vocabularies, ontologies properly belong to the category of knowledge models.

- *Message format*: the structure of a data message. The message format typically specifies the data elements that appear in the message, their data types, their order of appearance, and any headers, trailers, and delimiters.

- *Message protocol*: an agreed-upon format for transmitting data between two devices. Although the term is often used loosely for any type of electronic communication, a protocol typically specifies the following:

  - The message format
  - Error checking methods
  - When messages are sent
  - How a device indicates that it has finished sending a message
  - How a device acknowledges having received a message.

- *Knowledge model*: a formal representation of the knowledge proper to a domain. A knowledge model typically includes terms, their definitions, and a logic that describes semantic relations among terms and supports reasoning.

3.3.2   Standards Development

Standards are developed and gain acceptance de facto, de jure, or by consensus. *De facto standards* are typically not developed or endorsed by an official standards body but have gained acceptance because of their wide use. *De jure standards* are those whose use is required by law. *Consensus standards* are developed and approved by official standards bodies through collaborative processes among working groups of stakeholders. An enormous number of government and industry standards organizations are involved in developing standards related to health data. The two major organizations in consensus standards development are the International Standards Organization (ISO) [18] and the American National Standards Organization (ANSI) [14].

The ISO, an international agency headquartered in Geneva, is broadly tasked with advancing worldwide standardization for trade and cooperation in intellectual, scientific, technological, and economic activity. Its members are the national standards institutes of some 150 countries, and it presently comprises over 2000 technical committees, subcommittees, and working groups. The ISO itself does not develop standards or dictate who uses them. It coordinates the development processes for international standards and publishes the finished standards. ISO standards related to health care data include the electronic business mode using eXtensible Markup Language (ebXML) protocol [19], Health Level Seven (HL7) [20], and the Electronic Health Record (EHR) [21].

ANSI, a private, nonprofit organization dating back to 1918, is the U.S. national standards body belonging to the ISO. Like the ISO, ANSI does not develop standards itself or mandate their use. It acts primarily as a coordinator to designate official ANSI-accredited standards development bodies, such as the HITSP mentioned earlier, to ensure that the processes they use meet ANSI criteria for openness and accountability, and to accredit the results as American National Standards.

As broadly outlined by the Public Health Data Standards Consortium [22], the process for creating consensus-based standards consists of the following steps:

1. First, an appropriate ANSI-accredited or other organization must be convinced of the need for the new standard.

2. An appropriate standards development organization (SDO) is then designated to develop the standard.

3. The SDO drafts the standard, ensuring that appropriate participation opportunities are provided, feedback is obtained and incorporated, and consensus has been reached among stakeholders.

4. After completing the initial development process, the standard is approved and published.

5. Post publication, the SDO may collect further comments about the implementation of the standard and revise it accordingly.

3.3.3   Standards for Health Indicator Data in Biosurveillence

Many standards exist for the health care data. This section covers a representative handful of standards related to the leading types of health indicator data used in biosurveillance. The list is organized by data type.

- **Pharmacy Data (Over-the-Counter and Prescription)**

  - **UPC (Universal Product Code)** The UPC is an 8- or 12-digit identifier that is unique for every commercial product, including OTC pharmacy products. In the United States, UPC codes are managed by the Uniform Code Council [23] and are assigned upon application from the manufacturer.

  - **NDC (National Drug Code)** The NDC is a three-segment, 10-digit unique identifier for every human prescription drug product manufactured for commercial sale in the United States. NDC codes are assigned by the FDA and maintained in its NDC directory, as mandated by the Drug Listing Act of 1972 [24].

- **Laboratory Data**

  - **LOINC (R) (Logical Observation Identifiers, Names, and Codes)** The LOINC code is a five- to six-digit alphanumeric identifier for laboratory and clinical observations. The approximately 30,000 laboratory codes cover chemistry, hematology, serology, microbiology (including parasitology and virology), toxicology, drugs, cell counts, and antibiotic susceptibilities. The approximately 10,000 clinical codes cover vital signs, hemodynamics, intake/output, EKG, obstetric ultrasound, cardiac echo, urologic imaging, gastroendoscopic procedures, pulmonary ventilator management, selected survey instruments, and other clinical observations. Originating in 1994, LOINC is a proprietary, copyrighted standard owned by the nonprofit Regenstrief Institute for Health Care, associated with Indiana University. It is available free due to financial support from the National Library of Medicine (NLM). The standard's continued development is overseen jointly by Regenstrief and the ANSI-accredited LOINC standards development committee. LOINC enjoys significant market penetration. In 1999, it was identified by the HL7 Standards Development Organization as a preferred code set for laboratory test names in health care transactions. Under HIPAA, LOINC has been designated for use in the HL7 messages included in claims attachments [25].

- **Hospital Emergency Department and Physicians' Office Visit Data**

  - **ICD-9-CM (International Classification of Diseases, Ninth Revision, Clinical Modification)** The ICD-9-CM code is an alphanumeric code, at most five digits long, used to uniquely represent clinical diagnoses and procedures. A semihierarchical classification system, ICD-9-CM represents similar diagnoses and procedures with similar codes and represents subclasses with additional digits beyond the decimal point. Based on the World Health Organization (WHO) standard of the same name, the ICD-9-CM system is maintained within the United States by the government's National Center for Health Statistics (NCHS) and Centers for Medicare and Medicaid Services (CMS) and is freely available. Historically developed as a classification system for statistical compilation of data in inpatient settings, ICD-9-CM is now the cornerstone of health care reimbursement. In 2000, the U.S. Department of Health and Human Services (DHHS) designated it as one of the five code sets that must be used to encode diagnoses and procedures in health care transactions under HIPAA. ICD-9-CM volumes 1 and 2 are designated for diagnosis codes, and ICD-9-CM volume 3 is designated for inpatient hospital services. In 1994, the WHO replaced the aging Version 9, first implemented in 1979, with an expanded and more detailed Version 10. Several countries, including Australia and Canada, have converted to ICD-10, but conversion is still under evaluation in the United States. [26, 27].

– **CPT-4 (Current Procedural Terminology, Version 4)** The CPT code is a five-digit code used to uniquely represent medical, surgical, and diagnostic services and procedures. Originally developed in 1966 with a focus on surgical procedures, it has greatly expanded over the years — a 2006 version contains 8568 codes and descriptors. The CPT standard is copyrighted and maintained by the American Medical Association (AMA), which charges a modest licensing fee for its use. In the 1980s, CMS, then known as the Health Care Finance Administration (HCFA), mandated use of CPT codes for Medicaid and Medicare reporting. CPT-4 is another of the five code sets mandated by the DHHS in 2000 for encoding diagnoses and procedures in health care transactions under HIPAA [28].

– **HL7** The common format and protocol for exchanging health care information is through Health Level Seven (HL7). HL7 is a set of implementation specifications at the highest level (application or level 7) of the ISO communications model for open systems interconnection (OSI) [29]. It defines the record structure and transfer protocols for exchanging information between health care information systems. HL7 was initially introduced in 1987 and is copyrighted and maintained by Health Level Seven, a not-for-profit volunteer organization comprising commercial and government groups. Its mission is to create standards for the exchange, management, and integration of electronic health care information. Several versions of HL7 exist. HL7 v2.5 is the latest approved ANSI standard (June 2003); however, a newer version, v3.0, is still evolving and will significantly depart from the current version's structure and implementation.

3.3.4   National Health Information Systems — Implementing Standards

In addition to creating standards, tools must be provided to implement the standards. The CDC has developed many public health-related tools that have adhered to many standards for IT, security, and public health. Systems such as the National Electronic Disease Surveillance System (NEDSS) [30], the Laboratory Response Network (LRN) [31], and BioSense [32] are part of the CDC's Public Health Information Network (PHIN) [33]. PHIN provides an overarching framework for not only helping forge new standards, but also implementing them in the field. In addition to complete systems, other aspects of standards are being implemented by tools such as the Public Health Information Network Messaging System (PHIN-MS) [34] and the Public Health Information Network Vocabulary Access and Distribution System (PHIN-VADS) [35] to allow these surveillance systems and others to adhere to set standards.

The tools themselves adhere to IT, security, and public health standards. The PHIN-MS implements ebXML message service specification [36], XML encryption requirements [37], XML signature syntax processing [38], and the simple object access protocol (SOAP) [39], among others. The PHIN-VADS is an application that provides PHIN, application-based, message-based, and standards-based vocabularies to users. These vocabularies include the standards put forth by HL7, LOINC, and ICD-9 among others.

So while the creation of standards is extremely important for public health and electronic disease surveillance systems, it is equally important for key institutions to recognize these standards and implement them in their applications and systems.

3.4   ESTABLISHING THE DATA FEEDS

Data are an important fundamental building blocks of a medical surveillance system. The success of the system is highly dependent on the data that it collects. Chapter 2 provided detail about many different types of health indicator data and their relative merits. This section discusses the technical considerations involved with obtaining and working with these data sources. In particular, special attention is given to four widely available and highly useful data sources: emergency department patient visits, school absenteeism reports, OTC pharmacy sales, and physicians' office visits.

The data may come from many disparate sources, may be formatted in peculiar ways, and may be transmitted by an assortment of different protocols. Some of the popular emerging data format and communication protocol standards currently used in the medical industry are highlighted. In many instances, however, a surveillance system will need to interact with source systems that implement all, some, or none of these standards; therefore, it is in the best interest of the developers to be flexible.

3.4.1 Information Systems of the Data Provider or Source

Hospitals, schools, pharmacies, and physician's offices use information systems to gather and process data in their day-to-day operations. Fortunately, most of these information systems have existing report generation or data export capabilities that can be leveraged to provide data to the surveillance system. The information system of the provider of the data will be referred to here as the *source information system*.

Data collected directly from their source have the advantage of being very timely. Establishing and maintaining a multitude of individual data sources can be overwhelming, but one solution is to leverage hierarchical sources of data that act as a central collection or accumulation node. This approach has two primary advantages. First, it is easier for the surveillance system to collect data from one central node than from each source separately. Second, the individual sources that send their data to a central node often do so as part of their existing daily routine — so no extra effort is required from the individual sources.

For example, hospitals may belong to hospital groups where the individual hospitals feed their data to a central system of the hospital group. Schools may provide their daily absentee reports to the school district's central office. Individual pharmacies may provide their daily sales to a regional central office. Finally, individual physicians' offices may send their data to an insurance claims processor for payment reimbursement. Figure 3.10 provides an approach for collecting data for use in a health department's electronic surveillance system. This data acquisition strategy consists of collecting as much data as possible from central collection offices. Because not all data sources belong to a larger group, individual providers — in this case private hospitals — send their data to the surveillance system directly.

The primary disadvantage with this approach is that the data may be delayed for a period of time while they are being accumulated by the central node. Depending on how and when the data are collected, the delay may be minutes, hours, or, for some sources, even days.

Once it has been determined that the data are useful, that the source agrees to provide the data, and that the data can be easily obtained from a collection node, the next issue to consider is the cost to the provider for transmitting the data. To succeed, the burden on the data provider for establishing a data feed must be minimal. In many cases, data providers will not willingly provide their data if doing so is labor and resource intensive or otherwise costly. For this reason, imposing requirements outside the providers' immediate capabilities will result in failure, unless the data providers are compensated or mandated by law to supply their data. Success is more likely if the requesting organization can be flexible and leverage the provider's assets and resources as much as possible. Often, once the data providers see the merits of their participation, they will be willing to supply their data. Similarly, providing routine feedback to data providers after a system is established can aid in maintaining the relationship.

Information needed to help understand current trends in health indicator data may be available and relatively simple to collect. The National Weather Service data can be

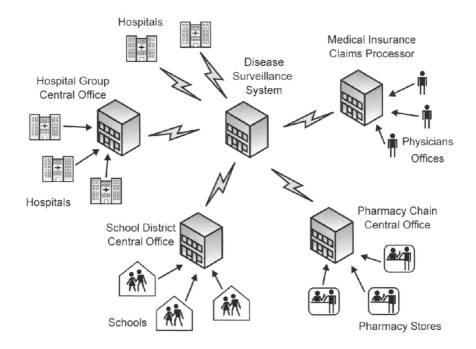

Fig. 3.10   Data acquisition strategy leveraging central collection sites.

accessed via the Web to provide environmental information for surveillance analysis. Reference information sources, such as the U.S. Census Bureau or the U.S. Postal Service, can also be accessed periodically to provide current reference information for the surveillance system.

3.4.2   Setting Up the Data Feed

A critical step in the process of setting up a data feed is finding a person who knows the technical details of the data repository of the provider. Unfortunately, in many cases, this person is not included in discussions until it is time to implement the data feed; IT staff should be included in early discussions to identify any immediate technical obstacles in setting up a data feed.

Information systems vary from organization to organization. For example, some hospitals may have a hospital information system that integrates the emergency department registration application tightly with other hospital applications; others may have a stand-alone emergency department registration application that operates separately from the other hospital applications. The information required for the data feed may need to come from more than one application or information system within the hospital. Additionally, the hospital's source information system may not provide data in an established standard, such as HL7, but instead may provide data through a report generator. Electronic surveillance systems must be flexible enough to adapt to the idiosyncrasies presented by many different data sources.

Data feeds can be transmitted using a "push" or "pull" method. In a *push Transmission*, the data source pushes data onto the surveillance system by initiating the data transfer and copying the data over. Alternatively, the surveillance system initiates the data transfer in a *pull Transmission* by pulling the data from the data provider, often querying the provider directly for the data. In almost all cases, the source information system will push the data to the surveillance system. Data providers rarely allow an external system to query or pull data directly from the provider's information system.

3.4.2.1 *Batched and Real-Time Feeds*   Once the format of the data feed has been determined, the next step is to establish the frequency of the data collection. There are essentially two types of data feeds: batched or real time. From a network implementation perspective, the fundamental tradeoff between batched and real-time data feeds is network infrastructure implementation costs versus data immediacy.

A *batched feed* usually implies that the data will be sent at a scheduled time interval, which could vary from once every 5 minutes to once a day. These data feeds do not require continuous network bandwidth. The advantage of a batch feed is that most, if not all, of the network infrastructure required to establish a data feed may already be in place. There are few disadvantages from an analytic perspective if the batched data are sent frequently, such as several times an hour.

A *real-time feed* usually implies that the data will be sent at roughly the same time that they are processed by the provider. However, establishing a real-time data feed requires a network infrastructure with enough network bandwidth to support these continuous data streams. Although any source information system can potentially provide a real-time data stream, hospital HL7 messages are primarily the format considered for real-time data feeds. Conceptually, the advantage of a real-time feed is the immediate availability of the data. However, in most instances, real time data transfer is limited to the real-time transfer of the data from the source provider to the surveillance system and not the actual availability of the data to the end user. The data may sit in the surveillance system's archive waiting for processing for several minutes or hours before they are processed by surveillance algorithms.

A batched feed that processes the data upon receipt and makes them available to the user may provide more timely information than a system that receives a real-time data feeds that are directed to the archive for processing at a predetermined interval. The necessary network infrastructure to maintain the continuous data stream required by a real-time data feed can also be expensive to establish and maintain. Batched feeds that are sent every 15 minutes require very little extra network bandwidth and provide a real-time-like level of data immediacy without the expense of a real-time connection.

Not every source system will be able to provide the data the same way. A surveillance system will very likely use a mixture of batched and real-time feeds. Ultimately, the budget for implementing a surveillance system will dictate which type of data feeds can be supported. The cost to implement the data feeds depends upon the type of data feed, the level of IT staff resources needed to extract the data from the source information system, and the state of the existing hardware and network infrastructure of both the data provider and the surveillance system. The cost associated with extracting data from the source information system depends on the IT programming and network capabilities of the provider. In most instances, hospitals use their own IT staff to set up the data feed. In some cases, however, hospitals use turnkey information systems and will need the system's vendor to create the data feed. Other hospitals outsource their IT and network staff and will need to contract with them for the creation of the data feed.

The amount of time needed to develop the extract software for the data feed may range from one to two days to several weeks or months depending on the complexity of the data source's information system. This setup is usually a one-time cost in IT resources. Additional IT resources are occasionally needed afterward for maintenance or troubleshooting problems.

For a batched data feed, the hardware costs incurred by the source provider are minimal. If the health department already has a server infrastructure that can receive these batched files, the hardware and network costs for the health department will be minimal. If the health department does not have a server infrastructure, startup hardware costs are usually limited to the cost of acquiring a low- to mid-range server ($2000–$5000) and server software ($100–$1000) to accept files from providers.

The hardware costs are minimal for real-time data feeds if both the source provider and health department already have the hardware and network infrastructure in place. If not, startup hardware and network costs are usually higher than those for batched feeds. The source provider may need to install a security network device (e.g., virtual private network router) to communicate with the health department. The health department will need to acquire a mid- to high-range server to receive the real-time data, one or more secure network devices (e.g., virtual private network concentrator at $4000 – $5000) each, and possibly an Internet connection with sufficient bandwidth to handle the increased network traffic ($200–$2000 per month).

3.4.3 Data Characteristics

From a surveillance perspective, the data collected by the system should provide representative coverage of the population. Although ideal, complete coverage is unlikely due to restricted budgets, unwillingness of the data providers to participate, and limitations of the automated collection capabilities of the data sources.

A typical question encountered when a system is being developed is how much disk space does the surveillance system require? The answer depends on the geographic area and number of data sources. Metropolitan, suburban, and rural areas will vary in the number of hospitals, schools, pharmacy chains, and physician offices. A large metropolitan hospital may see 200–500 patients in the emergency department a day, whereas a small suburban hospital may see 50–100 patients a day in its emergency department.

For purposes of discussion on disk capacity, assume that the surveillance system has established data feeds from 10 hospitals, three pharmacy chains, five school districts, and a central medical insurance claims processor who provides data for 100 local physicians.

Table 3.2 presents rough estimations of the number of individual data sources, number of records, record sizes, and file storage requirements per day and per year for each of the different types of data feeds. The following calculations were used to populate the table:

- Records per site $\times$ bytes per record => bytes per day

- Bytes per day $\times$ number of aggregated sites => bytes per day per site

- Bytes per day per site $\times$ days per year => bytes per year per site

- Bytes per year per site/1,048,576 => Mbytes per year per site

- Mbytes per year per site $\times$ number of data providers => total Mbytes per year

The daily total file sizes are in bytes and the yearly totals are in megabytes (Mbyte $= 2^{20} = 1,048,576$ bytes) and do not reflect any additional overhead bytes needed by the disk storage system.

Assumptions:

- Each of the 10 hospitals sees, on average, 150 patients each day.

- Each of the five school districts has 100 schools per district that report student attendance during a 170-day school year to each of their respective central district offices.

- Each of the three pharmacy chains averages 10 individual stores, each of which sells 100 products of interest per day and reports the sales to each of their respective central regional offices.

- Eeach of the 100 individual physician offices sends an average of eight insurance claims per day during the work week (Monday – Friday) to one central claims processor.

Summing the individual sources together gives the total for one day as 400,000 bytes, or approximately 0.38 Mbytes daily and 390 Mbytes annually. With current off-the-shelf technology, an entry-level server may have anywhere from 300 to 600 gigabytes of disk space capacity and could comfortably store 390 Mbytes a year. Commercial and noncommercial (i.e., freeware) utilities are available to compress the data files after they have been processed to reduce the amount of disk space consumed.

Table 3.2 **Example of Disk Storage Estimates for a Small Surveillance System**

Data	Records per Site	Bytes per Record	Bytes per Day	Aggregated Sites	Bytes per Day per Site
Hospital	150	100	15,000	1	15,000
School district	1	50	50	100	5,000
Pharmacy chain	100	300	30,000	10	300,000
Physician office	8	100	800	100	80,000
Totals					400,000

Data	Days per Year	Bytes per Year per Site	Mbytes per Year	Number of Data Providers	Total Mbytes per Year
Hospital	365	5,475,000	5.22	10	52.21
School district	170	850,000	0.81	5	4.05
Pharmacy chain	365	109,500,000	104.43	3	313.28
Physician office	260	20,800,000	19.84	1	19.84
Totals			130.30		389.39

3.4.4 Data Fields or Elements

The primary goal of collecting surveillance data is to gather enough information to help answer the basic questions of when, where, who, and what relating to a potential public health event. The amount of data that the system can collect may be governed by local and federal privacy regulations and laws such as HIPAA. Also, commercial competitive market concerns may limit the data collected from both health and nonhealth data providers.

HIPAA restricts not only specific protected health information (PHI), such as a person's name and residence address, but also potentially identifying information, such as dates when a service was performed. However, HIPAA does allow for a limited data set that includes service dates, such demographics as birth dates, and such geographic information as five-digit zip codes, counties, or cities. However, address and account information is still excluded from the limited data set [10, 40].

The following list contains the bare minimum PHI data fields needed to ascertain when an event is occurring, where it is occurring, who is involved, and what is involved:

- Date

- Time

- Location (e.g., a hospital name, a store name, a school name)

- Residence (e.g., census tract, residential zip code)

- Item (e.g., an emergency department initial complaint, product UPC code)

Other data fields (such as age and sex) provide more granular stratification of the data to help determine if an event involves a particular demographic group. PHI data elements (e.g., medical record number, transaction number) provide information for further follow-up with the data provider. These fields are also extremely useful in reducing duplicate records ingested by the surveillance system. In real-time data feeds, providers will include "updates" to records that have already been transmitted to the surveillance system. If the provider includes a unique account identifier, the surveillance system will be able to identify and update these records. Otherwise, it is very difficult to distinguish "new" records from duplicate "update" records.

A provider may be reluctant to provide a unique account identifier field because of HIPAA, but at least one data element needs to be included that uniquely identifies the data event or record. Demographics may be enough to uniquely distinguish individual hospital patients in most instances. However, if two people with the same demographic profile are seen at the same time, then distinguishing them uniquely is much more difficult.

With the sample data fields listed above as a foundation, Table 3.3 presents fields that might be part of a surveillance system data feeds. The data fields are divided into basic, account, and supplementary information categories. By no means is this is an exhaustive list of all possible data elements. It does, however, represent a list of data fields that a provider may reasonably be able to provide.

Table 3.3   Basic Surveillance System Data Elements

Hospital Emergency Department	Pharmacy Chain	School Absenteeism	Physician Office Visits
Basic Information:			
Date of encounter;	Date of sale;	Date of attendance;	Date of encounter;
Time of encounter;	Store identification;	School identification;	Provider identification;
Name of hospital;	Store location;	School location;	Provider zip code;
Primary complaint of patient;	Product UPC;	Number of students enrolled;	Patient residence zip code;
Residence zip code	Product Name	Number of students absent	ICD-9 diagnosis codes
Age	Number of units sold		Age
Sex	Product category		Sex
Account Information:			
Medical record number			Transaction number
Visit number			
Supplementary Information:			
Mode of arrival	Promotion indicator	Planned event	
Work zip code	Product regular price	Weather event	
Discharge diagnosis	Product promotion price		
Discharge disposition			

For hospital emergency department encounters, the basic data fields may include the date, time, and location of the patient's encounter; such patient demographic information, as age, sex, and residence zip code; and the primary reason (chief complaint) for going to the emergency department. Account information can be used to update existing records with newer information. The account information includes the patient's medical record number, which is usually a unique account number that is associated with the patient across visits to the hospital, and a visit number, which is usually a unique account number associated with the specific hospital visit. The visit number is useful to determine if a patient was seen in the emergency department more than once during a particular day.

Other hospital visit data fields that provide supplementary information are also useful. It is useful to know how patients arrived at the emergency department (e.g., ambulance, walk-in), work zip codes, their diagnoses, and disposition after being seen in the emergency department (e.g., admitted as inpatient, released, left before being seen). Hospital registration protocols vary greatly, so these additional data items may not be collected or transmitted to other hospital applications.

For OTC self-medication information, a pharmacy chain's basic data fields could include the date of purchase, the purchase location, the product purchased, and the number of units sold. An extremely useful piece of information is the chain's internal categorization of the product (e.g., beauty, cough and cold). However, this piece of information may be retained in a separate system from an inventory system and be very difficult to obtain as part of the extract.

Pharmacy chains may also be able to include information about their current store promotions. Additionally, some pharmacy chains can include the difference in price between the regular and promotional prices for the items sold. Although these two promotional indicators are not definitive, they help to determine if an increase in the number of units sold can be attributed to a promotion instead of an illness. For example, a healthy person may be induced to stockpile a product available at 50% off the regular price, whereas a product at 10% off the regular price may not explain as much of a spike in sales. These additional informative data items may be difficult to obtain, however, because of competitive market concerns. Other pharmacy data, such as prescription drugs, may be available and may include the date the prescription was written, the prescription drug, the dosage, the number of refills, and the date filled.

A school's attendance extract from the school district may include the basic data fields of the attendance date, the school location, the number of students enrolled, and the number of students absent. Other information that is useful to know is sanctioned school or weather events, such as field trips or snow delays that can account for absent students. Although not definitive, this information helps to determine if an increase in the number of absent students can be attributable to a sanctioned school event, such as a field trip, or a weather event, such as a snowstorm delay. Other school data, such as health office visits, may be available. However, in many cases, these data are not stored electronically or collected centrally.

For physicians' office visits, an insurance claim broker's extract may contain the patient's encounter date, the location where the patient was seen, the patient's demographics, and the ICD-9 diagnosis codes submitted for payment. As with hospital emergency department data, a unique account number is useful for follow-up and for reducing duplicate records.

3.4.5   Data Transfer Format

Source information systems generally use a variety of different operating systems and applications to store their data. This variety can make it difficult for source providers to package the data in a common format that is understandable by both the source and destination systems.

Two of the most common data file formats are structured *fixed width* and *delimited* ASCII text files (i.e., files with suffixes of .csv, .txt, or .tab). These types of files are commonly referred to as *flat files* because all the data elements for a single record are specified on single line or row. The data content of this type of file can be viewed easily with any text editor. Data elements in a fixed-width ASCII text file are placed at specific column positions for every line in the file. The first line of a file may contain an optional header record that describes the data in each column. For field content clarity, a header record should be included whenever possible.

Excerpt of data elements in a fixed-width file (MRN = Medical Record Number)

Date	Time	Age	Sex	Complaint	MRN
03/11/2006	12:00:00	25	F	Has an "upset stomach"	M2400
03/11/2006	12:00:01	30	M	Fever, sore throat	M2401
:	:	:	:	:	:

Data elements in delimited ASCII text files are separated by a delimiter character. Common character delimiters are a tab or comma. Commas, tabs, or quotes may be embedded in the actual data element and may cause problems while importing the data.

Excerpt of data elements in a comma(,)-delimited file:

Date,Time,Age,Sex,Complaint,MRN

03/11/2006,12:00:00,25,F,Has an "upset stomach",M2400

03/11/2006,12:00:01,30,M,Fever, sore throat,M2401

:

Note that the second record in the excerpt contains an embedded comma in the chief complaint, a condition that would likely cause a data ingestion routine to fail. To avoid problems with embedded commas, the data elements may also be surrounded by double quotes.

"Date","Time","Age","Sex","Complaint","MRN"

"03/11/2006","12:00:00","25","F","Has an "upset stomach"","M2400"

"03/11/2006","12:00:01","30","M","Fever, sore throat","M2401"

:

Note, however, that the first record now has double quotes embedded within its chief complaint field. Some import routines have problems distinguishing the embedded quotes from the quotes surrounding the field. The delimiter character chosen should be one that will not be found in the data elements, such as a pipe character (|).

Excerpt of data elements in of a pipe(|)-delimited file:

Date|Time|Age|Sex|Complaint|MRN

03/11/2006|12:00:00|25|F|Has an "upset stomach"|M2400

03/11/2006|12:00:01|30|M|Fever, sore throat|M2401

Other common data exchange file formats are Microsoft Excel (.xls) and dBASE or xBASE (.dbf) files. These types of files are similar to an ASCII text flat file in that all the data elements for a single record are nominally on a single line or row. However, they are different in that the individual data elements are stored in the file in a format that is unique or proprietary to the application that created it. The data content cannot be viewed easily with a text editor and must be imported into an application that can translate the proprietary format.

More recently, source information systems are able to package their data as an eXtensible Markup Language (XML) document (.xml). For this discussion, XML, is conceptually similar to a flat file in that it contains records of data. Individual data elements are surrounded by "tags" (e.g., <Age>25</Age>) and are components of a parent structure such as a record.

Excerpt of data elements of a XML payload document:

<Hospital Chief Complaint>
<Date>03/11/2006</Date>
<Time >12:00:00</Time>
<Age>25</Age>
<Sex>F</Sex>
<Complaint>Has an "upset stomach"</Complaint>
<MRN>M2400</MRN>
< /Hospital Chief Complaint>
<Hospital Chief Complaint>
<Date>03/11/2006</Date>
<Time >12:00:01</Time>
<Age>30</Age>
<Sex>M</Sex>
<Complaint>Fever, sore throat</Complaint>
<MRN>M2401</MRN>
< /Hospital Chief Complaint>
⋮

This excerpt provides a very simplistic example of an XML document. An XML document is more than just a set of data elements. XML documents can also describe what the data elements represent and how they relate to other data elements and structures [41, 42].

In all of the examples given, the data package, field names, order, and form of the data elements are mutually agreed upon by both the sending and receiving organizations and do not adhere to a universal standard. Alternatively, the data can be packaged to adhere to a specified standard. The CDC, for example, has established PHIN implementation and specification guides for various data types [43]. As of this writing (September 2006), the PHIN specification guide uses HL7 version 2.3.1 ADT (admit, discharge, transfer) A04 register patient messages for healt care-related encounter information. This specification defines the structure, layout, and arrangement of the data needed to process an ADT message. Any system that adheres to this specification should be able to read and process these types of messages.

The following is an excerpt of an HL7 ADT A04 (version 2.3.1) message stream for emergency department encounters with the chief complaint in the PV2 segment. For readability, the MSH and PV1 segments in this excerpt are not complete and have been altered to fit the page. This excerpt is only meant to provide a general understanding of the format.

```
MSH|^~\&|ADT|Hospital||||200611031200||ADT^A04|142248||2.3.1|142248||
EVN|A04|200603111200||
PID|1||M2401|||||19810311|F||||||||||||||
PV1|1|E|||||||||||||||||ER|||||||||||||||||||||Hospital...
PV2|1||Has an "upset stomach"
MSH|^~\&|ADT|Hospital||||200611031201||ADT^A04|142249||2.3.1|142249||
EVN|A04|200603111201
PID|1||M2402|||||19760311|M|||^^^^||||||||||
PV1|1|E|||||||||||||||||ER||||||||||||||||||||||||Hospital . . .
PV2|1||Fever, sore throat
```

There are other types of messages and segments of the HL7 specification that can provide additional information, such as messages that provide updated patient information (A08) or additional segments that provide diagnosis information (DG1). Starting with HL7 version 2.3.1, messages may also be expressed as an XML document.

As with all standards, the HL7 specification is evolving to incorporate newer methodologies and technologies. HL7 version 3 will use the reference information model (RIM) and will be very different in structure than earlier versions [19].

Established standards should be used whenever possible. However, if not available, a format can be selected to maintain structure across the same type of data. For example, use the same flat file format, data element order, and data format for every hospital that will supply a flat file. The majority of hospitals will be able to accommodate the format specified, but there will always be hospitals that cannot provide the data in the format requested.

3.4.6 Data Transfer Protocol

As mentioned in Section 3.4.5, data are commonly packaged in files. Data packaged as files can be transferred from the source information system in various ways. Figure 3.11 illustrates various data transfer options available to health departments establishing a surveillance system.

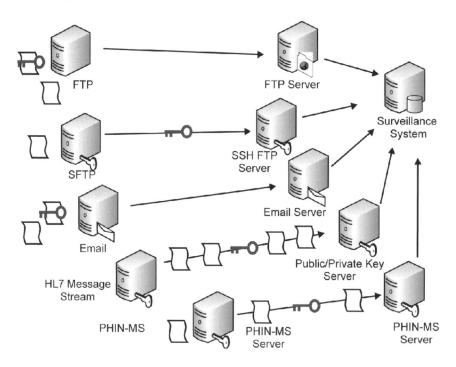

Fig. 3.11 Data transfer options available to health departments for acquiring surveillance data.

One of the most common data transfer protocols is the file transfer protocol (FTP). This protocol operates on the open network and does not encrypt usernames, passwords, or file payloads during transmission. This protocol does not include sender integrity, encryption, or file transfer validation. If encryption of the payload is required, the file must be encrypted separately prior to its transmission.

This protocol is used mostly for FTP "deposit only" sites, which restrict the sender to write-only privileges. With this type of server, files can be written by the sending organization to the FTP site but cannot be read. The sending organization is responsible for validating the success of the transfer. The receiving organization must have an FTP server, and the sender must have an FTP client. Both commercial and noncommercial (i.e., shareware and freeware) versions of FTP client software are available to perform file transfer verification.

Although the FTP payload may be encrypted, the FTP protocol is inherently insecure because it does not encrypt the FTP account's user name or password during transmission. It is possible for malicious users on the Internet to steal user names and passwords by looking for these unencrypted FTP transmissions and then using the account information to gain unauthorized access to the FTP server. To help reduce the risk of compromise, many FTP servers will accept files only from specific network addresses. Malicious users, however, can still gain access to the server by "spoofing" the data source provider's network address, so this approach to FTP server security is not perfect. More information about FTP vulnerabilities can be found at the CERT Coordination Center [44].

A more secure data transfer protocol similar to FTP is the SSH (secure shell) secure file transfer protocol (sFTP). This protocol provides for public key infrastructure (PKI) certificates for sender integrity, encrypted user names and passwords for account access, and encryption of the data file payloads prior to transit. This protocol does not include file verification. The receiving organization must have an SSH server, and the sender must have an sFTP client. Commercial and noncommercial (i.e., shareware and freeware) versions of SSH client software are available to perform file transfer verification [45].

Alternatively, data can be transfered via e-mail. The data payload may be sent as part of the e-mail body or as a file attachment. The receiving system must be able to process the content of the e-mail body or attachment. As with FTP, if the payload or file must be encrypted, the file must be encrypted separately prior to its transmission. Commercial and noncommercial versions of e-mail text body extraction, attachment extraction, and encryption utilities are available.

Although the e-mail payload may be encrypted, privacy concerns have been raised about sending sensitive information in e-mail messages. The message may pass through and be saved on several intermediate e-mail servers along its transmission route. The message may reside on the intermediate servers long enough to be compromised. Transferring data through e-mail has become increasingly difficult as organizations grapple with security policies to restrict data transmissions (e.g., compressed .zip files) in an effort to stave off spam and malicious payloads.

Real-time HL7 data may also be sent as network packet payloads using the minimal lower layer protocol (MLLP, which connects the sending system application directly to the receiving system application through the network. The HL7 specification not only specifies the structure and format of the data (as mentioned in Section 3.4.6, but also defines how the sending and receiving systems communicate with each other. The receiving organization must have an application or "listener" waiting for HL7 messages to arrive on the network.

HL7 messages are sent to the receiver one at a time. The receiver listens for a message, and after a message is received, the listener sends an acknowledgment back to the sender to confirm receipt of the message. If a connection to the listener cannot be made, or the last message was not acknowledged, newer messages will be buffered and queued by the sender until the receiver is ready to receive the messages. The sender will continue to attempt to send unacknowledged messages.

HL7 messages almost always travel securely over virtual private networks (VPNs) that connect the sending and receiving organizations securely. The VPN infrastructure is used to validate the account and encrypt network messages prior to transit. The sending and receiving organization must have a network infrastructure capable of establishing a continuous VPN connection between them.

HL7 messages may also be transmitted through the electronic business mode using the eXtensible Markup Language (ebXML) protocol. This protocol, used in the PHIN-MS architecture, provides for sender integrity through certificates, data encryption in transit, and message acknowledgment or file verification. It is similar in concept to the "acknowledgment and retry" scheme of HL7, where negative receipt of messages or files will cause the ebXML message service to attempt to resend the message or file. However, it is also different in that the protocol does not specify the structure or format of the message being delivered. The data payload is decoupled from the delivery, which allows any type of payload (text files, binary data or XML documents) to be transferred. This protocol requires both the sending and receiving organizations to have an ebXML Message Server. The CDC provides a no-cost ebXML server for organizations that will be transferring files to or from CDC through PHIN-MS [18, 33].

Some nontraditional information sources may have a really simple syndication (RSS) service available, such as syndicated news agencies. An RSS service provides brief or summary data in XML documents to subscribers. An RSS reader or aggregator periodically polls the RSS service site for data content. The National Weather Service has an experimental RSS service available that lists various weather-related items, such as temperature, relative humidity, and heat index [46, 47]. A less desirable means of obtaining nontraditional information is through a technique called *screen scraping*. Basically, screen scraping parses the HyperText Markup Language (HTML) of a website's web page for information. This method is prone to frequent problems and is not a very desirable means of obtaining consistent data because of the high rate of change in the source's web page content. Without approval from the information source, the ethics and legality of obtaining information in this manner are also questionable.

3.4.7   Security Considerations

After the data arrive at the health department, they must be stored in an appropriate manner. HIPAA applies to covered entities that collect public health information (PHI). The security standard offers sound guidance for the administrative, physical, and technical aspects of storing and accessing the data [48]. Access to the PHI data must be traceable and limited physically and electronically to only those persons and programs that process or analyze the data.

The standard's physical safeguards include guidelines for access control to the facility and equipment, data tampering, data restoration, personnel validation, maintenance records, appropriate workstation access controls and locations, removable media storage, data disposal, accountability, and data backups. The standard's technical safeguards include guidelines for access control to programs and data, unique user names per user, emergency access procedures, automatic log-off, encryption/decryption, audit controls, data tampering, data validation, personnel validation, network security, and data integrity.

3.4.8   Data Import Methods

In previous sections, several types of data formats and transport protocols were mentioned. For data packaged as data files using FTP or sFTP, the files may either be sent or "pushed" from the sending system to the receiving system server or retrieved or "pulled" by the receiving system from the sending system's server.

In almost all cases, the source information system will push the data to the surveillance system. Rarely will the data provider allow an external system to pull data directly from the provider's information system. Even if the file is "pulled" from the source, the data are first exported to a file within the source system for pickup. Most surveillance systems will probably use a mixture of pushed and pulled data files. The file transfers may occur once or multiple times throughout the day. For files that are pulled from a remote site, the system must know the exact time when a file is ready or must occasionally look or "poll" for the file on the remote site. Most operating systems have schedulers that can schedule tasks or "jobs" to automate the process. Data files transferred through PHIN-MS are always pushed from a sending system to a receiving server.

Once the data files reside on the local system, the contents of the files must be stored where an analyst or application can access them. In most cases, the files will be read into a database management system (DBMS) or other analysis application. Where appropriate, a consistant filename convention should be used, such as `provider_yyyymmdd_hhmmss.csv`, where "provider" in the filename is replaced with the name of the data provider, and `yyyymmdd_hhmmss` is replaced with the current date and time specified as a four-digit year, two-digit month, two-digit day, two-digit 24 hours, two-digit minutes, and two-digit seconds. Using the date and time in the file name will allow the data files to be organized by provider and file date and time.

Just as the system polls for remote files, the operating system or DBMS can be programmed to poll a local directory folder periodically for files to process. Routines to import or ingest the data files will read the contents of the data files and place the contents into the local data repository or database archive. This process is referred to as extract, transform, and load (ETL). The DBMS may have a native ETL product for importing the data. Commercial and open-source ETL products are available as well.

3.4.9   Data Cleaning

The same data element from different sources may have its value represented in different ways. To use the data effectively in the surveillance system, the source's data elements need to conform to the surveillance system's data format, representation, and vocabulary. The PHIN and NEDSS vocabulary standards and specifications provide a foundation for a health care-related vocabulary across systems [35].

Systems that collect data across date and or time zones may need to convert date and time data to a common time zone. Hospitals may represent their patients' ages by a date of birth or as an age listed in years. For younger children, the age might be listed in months or even weeks and days. The surveillance system may need the date of birth or age converted to years or placed into an age groups. The source system may list patient sex as male, female, or unknown (M, F, U). Occasionally, the sex field may be empty. Zip codes may be listed as 5 digits or 5 + 4 digits. The 5 + 4-digit zip code may be formatted with a dash (e.g., 12345-6789) or without a dash (e.g., 123456789).

Data cleaning also includes detecting duplicate records. Duplicate records may occur if the sending system inadvertently or unexpectedly sends a duplicate extract or data record. Duplicate or updated records may also occur when the sending system, such as a hospital, sends multiple records for the same patient throughout the patient encounter. For example, a hospital may send a record when the patient first registers, another when a diagnosis is determined, another after the patient is discharged, and, a final record, after ICD-9 diagnosis codes are assigned several days later. Removing duplicate data or updating existing data is more difficult if a specific identifier, such as the medical record number or visit identifier, is not provided. If an identifier is not included, duplicates can enter the archive and impact the overall results provided by the surveillance system.

3.4.10   Data Quality

Even though the data format and file structure may arrive as expected, the quality of the data may be poor. OTC pharmacy records are typically very predictable because they are produced from scanned items at the point of sale. The data fields supplied by other sources that enter data into the source system manually are not always so predictable, however.

Obvious data quality problems arise when erroneous or mistyped information is entered into the source system. All data entries that are not generated automatically are potential sources of error. For example, items selected from pulldown lists or data entered in free-text fields are prone to error. If a hospital's data entry system requires the user to enter the date manually, the resulting data will occasionally include dates in the future or dates a century in the past. Even with automatically generated values, it is possible (although to a lesser extent) that the source system may be incorrectly programmed.

Other data quality problems arise when data are not received when expected. Failure to receive automated data feeds may be caused by internal or external server crashes, network outages, or power outages. Without expensive and extensive redundancy throughout the data flow, these events are bound to happen, and unfortunately, they happen more than one would like. Manual data feeds are subject to the same problems as automated feeds but are extremely dependent on personnel availability and are prone to schedule fluctuations.

Problems also arise when a single source, such as a pharmacy chain, accumulates the data for its individual stores. Although this is the best way to collect the data, it can lead to fluctuations in the number of individual stores providing data on a daily basis. Just like any other data source, a connection problem may prevent an individual store from reporting to the central node.

Less obvious data quality problems can occur. Although the data supplied may not be erroneous, per se, they may not provide enough detail. For example, a hospital's registration protocol may list a patient's chief complaint as "Sick" for every patient who does not feel well, instead of being more descriptive. This type of problem can be mitigated if the hospital is willing to change its registration protocol.

Content problems can also occur due to changes in the data provider's environment. Over time, new schools, pharmacy stores, pharmacy products, ICD-9 codes, or registration protocols may be added or existing ones removed. All of these changes may affect the surveillance system.

3.4.11   Summary

Obtaining data for an automated surveillance system requires numerous considerations on the part of both the data providers and the system developers. To ensure strong provider participation and sustainability, the system must be flexible enough to receive data of differing frequency and format, using the method that best suits the provider. Furthermore, due to security concerns, standards for the transmission, use, and protection of health information must be taken into consideration at every step of the data transmission process.

3.5   STUDY QUESTIONS

3.1 Consider the laws and regulations in your locality or jurisdiction. *Q: What specific legislative regulation, code, or authority governs your ability to collect health care data for surveillance? How much detail about the patient can be obtained? Under what circumstances or situations are you able to collect more detailed patient information?*

3.2 *Q: Which people and resources in your organization would you need to engage to initiate an automated disease surveillance program?*

3.3 *Q: Which data sources and data elements in your jurisdiction would you consider to be crucial to a surveillance program? Where would you obtain the data? How would you go about requesting the data? What nonlegislative issues or barriers will you need to consider?*

3.4 For a surveillance program, the ability to exchange data is extremely important. Several representative standards organization and standards are available. *Q: Given the types of data that you would like to collect, which of the standards bodies, committees, organizations, and consortiums mentioned should you consider for the implementation of your system? What other organizations not mentioned are you aware of? How do their decisions affect your surveillance efforts?*

3.5 Various methods for formatting and transmitting data were mentioned in this chapter. *Q: What are the tradeoffs in IT resources and infrastructure between receiving transmissions once a day, several times a day, and in realtime? What day-to-day operational issues will you need to consider?*

3.6 *Q: Given your organization's existing IT resources and infrastructure, which data formats and transmission methods would best fit within your organization? What day-to-day operational issues will you need to consider?*

REFERENCES

1. Roberts L. Multiple computer networks and intercomputer communication. In: ACM Symposium on Operating Systems Principles, Proceedings of the First ACM Symposium on Operating System Principles, Gaitlinburg, TN, October 1–4;1967: 3.1-3.6.

2. Postel J, Reynolds J. RFC 0959: File Transfer Protocol (FTP). October 1985. Available at `http:\\www.ietf.org/rfc/rfc0959.txt`. Accessed July 23, 2006.

3. Chamberlin DD, Boyce RF. SEQUEL: a structured English query language. In: International Conference on Management of Data, Proceedings of the 1974 ACM SIGFIDET (now SIGMOD) Workshop on Data Description, Access and Control, Ann Arbor, MI, May 1–3; 1974: 249-264.

4. Broome CV, Horton HH, Tress D, Lucido SJ, Koo D. Statutory basis for public health reporting beyond specific diseases. J Urban Health. June 2003; 80(suppl 1): i14-i22.

5. Nevada Revised Statutes, NRS-441A.125, Title 40, Chapter 441A.125, Communicable Diseases, General Provisions. Use of syndromic reporting and active surveillance to monitor public health; regulations. Available at `http://www.leg.state.nv.us/NRS/NRS-441A.html#NRS441ASec125`. Accessed July 2006.

6. Title 10 Department Of Health And Mental Hygiene, Subtitle 5, Catastrophic Health Emergencies, Chapter 1, Care of Individuals Isolated or Quarantined Due to a Deadly Agent Authority. Health General Article, §18-904–18-907, Annotated Code of Maryland; Chap 1, Sect 4, Acts of 2002. Available at `http://www.dsd.state.md.us/comar/subtitle_chapters/10_Chapters.htm#Subtitle59`. Accessed July 14, 2006.

7. Arizona Revised Statutes, Article 9, Enhanced Surveillance Advisories and Public Health Emergencies, Subtitle 59, Title 36-782, Enhanced surveillance advisory. Available at `http://www.azleg.state.az.us/FormatDocument.asp?inDoc=/ars/36/00782.htm&Title=36&DocType=ARS`. Accessed July 14, 2006.

8. Public Law 104-191. Health Insurance Portability and Accountability Act of 1996. 104th Congress. August 21, 1996. Available at `http://aspe.hhs.gov/admnsimp/pl104191.htm`. Accessed July 23, 2006.

9. US Department of Health and Human Services, Office of Civil Rights. OCR privacy brief: Summary of the HIPAA privacy rule. Last revised May 2003. Available at `http://www.dhhs.gov/ocr/privacysummary.pdf`. Accessed July 23, 2006.

10. US Department of Health and Human Services, Office for Civil Rights. Standards for privacy of individually identifiable health information; security standards for the protection of electronic protected health information; general administrative requirements including civil money penalties: procedures for investigation, imposition of penalties, and hearings. Regulation text (Unofficial Version) (45 CFR §160 and 164). December 28, 2000, as amended: May 31, 2002, August 14, 2002, February 20, 2003, and April 17, 2003. Available at `http://www.dhhs.gov/ocr/combinedregtext.pdf`. Accessed July 23, 2006.

11. U.S. Department of Health and Human Services, Centers for Medicaid and Medicare Services. Covered entity charts: guidance on how to determine whether an entity is a covered entity under the administrative simplification provisions of HIPAA. Last modified July 2003. Available at `http:www.cms.hhs.gov/apps/hipaa2decisionsupport/CoveredEntityFlowcharts.pdf`. Accessed July 23, 2006.

12. Thacker SB. HIPAA privacy rule and public health: guidance from CDC and the US Department of Health and Human Services. MMWR. May 2, 2003; 52(suppl 1): 1-12. Available at `http://www.cdc.gov/mmwr/preview/mmwrhtml/su5201a1.htm`. Accessed July 23, 2006.

13. US Department of Health and Human Services, National Institutes of Health. Protecting personal health information in research: understanding the HIPAA privacy rule. April 14, 2003. Available at `http://privacyruleandresearch.nih.gov/pdf/HIPAA_Booklet_4-14-2003.pdf`. Accessed July 23, 2006.

14. American National Standards Institute. Available at `http://www.ansi.org`. Accessed September 14, 2006.

15. American National Standards Institute Healthcare Information Technology Standards Panel, Technical Committee. Selected standards, Version 1.1. June 9, 2006.

Available at `http://public.ansi.org/ansionline/Documents/`
`Standards%20Activities/`
`Healthcare%20Informatics%20Technology%20Standards%20Panel/`
`Standards%20Selection%20June%206,%202006/`
`_BIO%20Selected%20Standards%20June%206.doc`. Accessed September 14, 2006.

16. Board on Health Care Services, Institute of Medicine, National Academies. Patient Safety: Achieving a New Standard for Care. Washington, DC: National Academies Press; 2004. Available at `http://www.nap.edu/books/` `0309090776/html/`. Accessed September 14, 2006.

17. Overview of Healthcare EDI Transactions: A Business Primer. Rockville, MD: Washington Publishing Company, 1998. Available at `http://www.wpc-edi.com/` `Default_40.asp`. Accessed February 2002.

18. International Organization for Standardization. Available at `http://www.osi.org`. Accessed September 14, 2006.

19. OASIS Open. ebXML (Electronic Business using eXtensible Markup Language). Available at `http://www.ebxml.org/`. Accessed July 25, 2006.

20. Health Level Seven, Inc. Health Level 7 (HL7). Available at `http://www.hl7.org`. Accessed July 23, 2006.

21. International Organization for Standardization. Health informatics electronic health record. ISO/TS 18308:2004, ISO/TR 20514:2005. Available at `http://www.iso.org/iso/en/CombinedQueryResult.` `CombinedQueryResult?queryString=Electronic+Health+Record`. Accessed September 14, 2006.

22. Public Health Data Standards Consortium. Available at `http://www.phdatastandards.info`. Accessed 2006 Sep 14.

23. Uniform Code Council. Available at `http://www.uc-council.org/`. Accessed September 14, 2006.

24. Federal Drug Administration. The National Drug Code Directory. Available at `http://www.fda.gov/cder/ndc/`. Accessed September 14, 2006.

25. Logical Observation Identifiers, Names, and Codes (LOINC). Available at `http://www.regenstrief.org/loinc/`. Accessed September 14, 2006.

26. Hazlewood, A. ICD-9-CM to ICD-10-CM: implementation issues and challenges. Available at `http://library.ahima.org/xpedio/groups/public/` `documents/ahima/bok3_005426.hcsp?dDocName=bok3_005426`. Accessed September 2006.

27. US Department of Health and Human Services, Centers for Medicare and Medicaid Services. ICD-9 Provider and Diagnostic Codes. Available at

http://www.cms.hhs.gov/ICD9ProviderDiagnosticCodes. Accessed September 14, 2006.

28. American Medical Association. CPT (Current Procedural Terminology). Available at http://www.ama-assn.org/ama/pub/category/3113.html. Accessed September 14, 2006.

29. International Organization for Standardization. Open systems Interconnection, ISO/IEC 7498-1:1994. Available at http://isotc.iso.org/livelink/livelink/fetch/2000/2489/Ittf_Home/PubliclyAvailableStandards.htm. Accessed September 14, 2006.

30. Department of Health and Human Services, Centers for Disease Control and Prevention. National Electronic Disease Surveillance System, The Surveillance and Monitoring Component for the Public Health Information Network. Available at http://www.cdc.gov/nedss/. Accessed September 14, 2006.

31. Laboratory Response Network Partners in Preparedness. Available at http://www.bt.cdc.gov/lrn/. Accessed September 14, 2006.

32. US Department of Health and Human Services, Centers for Disease Control and Prevention. BioSense. Available at http://www.cdc.gov/biosense/. Accessed September 14, 2006.

33. US Department of Health and Human Services, Centers for Disease Control and Prevention. Public Health Information Network (PHIN). Available at http://www.cdc.gov/PHIN/. Accessed September 14, 2006.

34. US Department of Health and Human Services, Centers for Disease Control and Prevention. Public Health Information Network Messaging System (PHIN-MS). Available at http://www.cdc.gov/phin/software-solutions/phinms/index.html. Accessed September 14, 2006.

35. US Department of Health and Human Services, Centers for Disease Control and Prevention. Public Health Information Network Vocabulary Access and Distribution System (PHIN-VADS). Available at http://www.cdc.gov/PhinVSBrowser/StrutsController.do. Accessed September 14, 2006.

36. OASIS ebXML Messaging Services Technical Committee. Message Service Specification, Version 2.0. Available at http://www.ebxml.org/specs/ebMS2.pdf. Accessed September 14, 2006.

37. XML encryption requirements. Available at http://www.w3.org/TR/xml-encryption-req. Accessed September 14, 2006.

38. XML. Signature syntax processing. Available at http://www.w3.org/TR/xmldsig-core/. Accessed September 14, 2006.

39. SOAP Version 1.2 Part 0: Primer. Available at http://www.w3.org/TR/soap12-part0/. Accessed September 14, 2006.

40. Code of Federal Regulations, Title 45: Public Welfare and Human Services, Part 164–Security and Privacy, Subpart E–Privacy of Individually Identifiable Health Information, Sect. 164.514, other requirements relating to uses and disclosures of protected health information (45 CFR §164.514). Revised as of October 1, 2003: 741-745. Available at http://frwebgate4.access.gpo.gov/cgi-bin/waisgate.cgi?WAISdocID=71281716916+30+0+0&WAISaction=retrieve. Accessed July 23, 2006.

41. W3C Architecture Domain Working Group. Extensible Markup Language (XML). Last modified: April 22, 2006. Available at http://www.w3.org/XML/. Accessed July 23, 2006.

42. W3Schools. Online Web tutorials, 1999–2006. Available at http://www.w3schools.com/default.asp. Accessed July 23, 2006.

43. US Department of Health and Human Services, Centers for Disease Control and Prevention. PHIN: implementation guides. Available at http://www.cdc.gov/PHIN/architecture/implementation_guides/index.html. Accessed July 23, 2006.

44. Carnegie Mellon University, Software Engineering Institute, CERT Coordination Center. Anonymous FTP abuses. Available at http://www.cert.org/tech_tips/anonymous_ftp_abuses.html. Accessed July 25, 2006.

45. SSH Communications Security. What is your FTP and telnet lock-down plan? Available at http://www.ssh.org/. Accessed July 25, 2006.

46. Winer D. RSS 2.0 Specification. Cambridge, MA: Berkman Center for Internet and Society at Harvard Law School. Available at http://blogs.law.harvard.edu/tech/rss. Accessed July 25, 2006.

47. National Oceanic and Atmospheric Administration, National Weather Service. Experimental XML feeds of current weather conditions. Available at http://www.weather.gov/data/current_obs/. Accessed July 25, 2006.

48. Department of Health and Human Services, Office of the Secretary. Health insurance reform: security standards; final rule (45 CFR §160, 162, and 164). Fed Reg. February 20, 2003; 68(34): 8334-8381. Available at http://www.cms.hhs.gov/SecurityStandard/Downloads/securityfinalrule.pdf. Accessed July 25, 2006.

4 Alerting Algorithms for Biosurveillance

Howard Burkom

Chapter 3 addressed several issues that developers and operators of disease surveillance systems must consider to acquire data automatically for the purpose of conducting disease surveillance. Included were basics of the Internet for beginners in the field as well as more in-depth examples of data transfer between data providers and surveillance systems.

This chapter discusses the analytic processes that can be applied to the data once they are acquired and archived into a database. The analytic processes described here are intended to provide an earlier notification of a change in the normal levels of observed counts of the desired health indicator. These indicators include a variety of data types, such as patients seen for a syndrome of interest, the number of OTC products sold that relieve certain disease symptoms, and the number of students absent from classes. The emphasis here is on the importance of matching the analytic process to the data type so as to achieve the performance needed for early identification of the event with minimum false alarms. The chapter ends with examples of how to evaluate the performance of these analytic processes using accepted metrics.

4.1 NEED FOR STATISTICAL ALERTING ALGORITHMS

A primary goal of an automated health surveillance system is to enable early recognition of disease outbreaks. The only information accessible to these systems is the data streams described in Chapters 2 and 3. In other words, the only evidence of the desired epidemiological truth available to the system is contained in these data streams, as illustrated in Fig. 4.1.

The background disease levels (i.e., actual levels in the absence of an outbreak) determine the customary scale and distribution of data observed in the system. The surveillance system is based on the premise that when an outbreak occurs, the care-seeking behavior of an infected population will add a signal to the background data that will be recognizable if the data are processed appropriately. The value of the

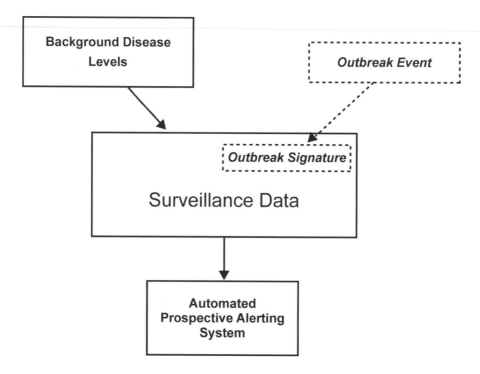

Fig. 4.1   In the automated health surveillance, understanding the data is crucial because they are the only link between the system users and epidemiological reality.

system for outbreak detection depends on its capability for prompt signal alerting without excessive false alarms (i.e., without alerts in the absence of an outbreak). The analyst might naively hope to visually inspect a data time series or group of series each day and start an investigation when observed data levels were high according to some heuristic condition, such as:

more than 10 respiratory diagnoses in a day

a 50% increase in diagnoses over counts from the previous day

However, with the variety of data types to monitor for multiple syndromic signals on a daily or more frequent basis, visual inspection could be too labor intensive and subjective. A simple alerting algorithm might be envisioned that would trigger an investigation whenever the specified condition is observed. Although the simplicity of that approach is appealing, there are several reasons why such an algorithm would be inadequate:

1. *Evolving data streams.* Data streams evolve because of changes in the under-lying population, including care-seeking behavior, and the changes in the data-processing steps producing the surveillance data streams. Examples of such

changes are modifications in hospital information systems, insurance plans, care providers, coding practices, and product groupings.

2. *Required detection performance.* The dilemma in infectious disease surveillance is that the system must be sensitive to early signs of an outbreak, especially threats related to bioterrorism or pandemic influenza, but if false alarm rates are excessive, alerts will eventually be ignored. The example in Fig. 4.2 shows regional counts of a GI syndrome group comprising only relatively rare diagnoses. No diagnoses are recorded on many days, and the maximum on any day is 3. The plot shows the effects of a single outbreak beginning in mid-April of 1999 and continuing for about 6 weeks. A simple data threshold criterion would yield poor detection performance. For example, if the rule were to alert when the number of daily cases exceeded a threshold of 2, the event would be missed completely. If the threshold were dropped to 1 case, there would be 44 alerts outside the outbreak interval.

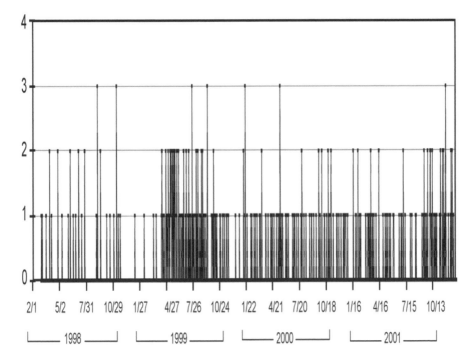

Fig. 4.2 Daily time series of regional counts of a GI syndrome group limited to relatively rare diagnoses. When a denominator variable (such as total of all diagnoses) is available, the proportion of syndromic counts can be more effective than the actual counts for distinguishing an outbreak signal.

Several simple strategies could overcome this problem — for example, a moving- average filter could be used to detect the outbreak signal with fewer false alarms. The point is that an algorithm must be chosen that is appropriate for both the data background (here, a small-count series with many zeros) and the signal of interest (here, a distributed cluster of rare diagnoses). It might be argued that a more inclusive syndrome grouping could yield higher daily counts that might permit more accurate data forecasts. However, if the outbreak were confined to the rare cases included in Fig. 4.2, the daily variability of the more general diagnoses would probably mask the 6-week outbreak. Furthermore, if an epidemiological investigation yielded a restrictive case definition, the sparse time series should dictate the algorithmic detection approach. Thus, the algorithms discussed in this chapter should not be chosen in a vacuum but as part of an overall surveillance plan.

3. *Systematic data features.* Simplistic alerting methods cannot account for predictable data features that generate nuisance alarms irrelevant to monitoring objectives. For example, suppose that visit counts are being monitored at a clinic that is known to be closed on Sundays and holidays, and visits rise sharply at the start of each school year. Ignoring the resulting frequent statistical alerts on Mondays, after holidays, and at certain times of year would result in a loss of sensitivity to true health events, undermining the utility and credibility of the system. Modeling or other means of accounting for seasonal trends, day-of-week effects, and other known features in alerting algorithms can provide sustained sensitivity through repeated cycles of data behavior.

4. *Multiplicity of data types, substreams, and classifications.* These issues are exacerbated by the general nature of syndromic surveillance, where there is no single public health threat or case definition of concern. When systems monitor multiple syndrome groups in multiple subregions, a multiple testing problem results. For example, from the discussion of Fig. 4.2, an alarm on any day with more than a single syndromic visit count would have caused 44 false alarms in about 1360 nonoutbreak days. One might argue that this rate is less than one false alarm per month and might be acceptable, depending on the cost of an investigation. However, if n independent syndrome/subregion data streams are monitored with this false alarm rate, the probability of at least one false alarm is $1 - [1 - (44/1360)]^n$, so that the rate doubles for two streams, exceeds one alarm per week for five streams, and produces more nuisance alarms as more data sources are monitored. As the number of data sources and ways of monitoring them increase, statistical methods must be applied to retain sensitivity while both minimizing false alarm rates and controlling for the multiple testing problem.

Statistical algorithms may thus be seen as more sophisticated alerting criteria or as data filters to achieve the required sensitivity while reducing the number of false alerts to manageable levels. The algorithm yielding optimal detection performance depends on the data background and other factors. Most surveillance algorithms are based on statistical hypothesis tests or process control charts, as discussed in section 4.4. Such methods cannot eliminate alerts when no outbreak is in progress—alerts that may be correct mathematically but are still false alarms in the surveillance context. As illustrated in Fig. 4.1, the data can contain only the footprint of a health event of concern. In view of this gap between statistical and epidemiological significance, alerting algorithms form one link in the surveillance chain; their role is to focus the attention of health monitors on data features or combinations of features that merit further investigation. The accuracy of this filtering is important for directing subsequent investigations and conserving resources.

4.2 FEATURES OF ALERTING ALGORITHMS

4.2.1 Expected Data Behavior and the Denominator Problem

The algorithms described in this chapter are intended to detect statistical behavior that is in some sense anomalous or unusual enough to indicate a possible public health threat among the cases contributing to this behavior. The detected behavior may take the form of a time-series spike, or the changes may be more subtle. Whatever the trigger, recognition of unusual data requires an estimate of baseline or expected behavior for comparison with the data being tested.

Epidemiology employs rates to compare data across geographic regions, time periods, and other strata. For example, the prevalence of a disease in a population at a given time is the number of cases of that disease in that population at that time divided by the population size at that time [1]. Uniform comparisons are enabled by good estimates for the denominator, which in the prevalence example is the count of the population of interest at the time of interest. Whereas obtaining direct estimates of the population may be difficult and expensive in classical epidemiology, in syndromic data, it is often impossible. Examples of such estimates include:

- The current population of the catchment area of a hospital emergency department

- The current number of consumers using physician practices that subscribe to a data warehouse; even more difficult, the number using practices whose data have been reported in time for current monitoring

- The current number of consumers eligible for a medical insurance plan whose data are used for health monitoring

Without these estimates, recognition of anomalous counts in the numerator (i.e., the observed case count) may be biased by changes in the denominator. For example, a sudden jump in influenza-like illness (ILI) diagnoses in a military treatment facility may be the natural result of a large influx of recruits and standard examinations and may be independent of any increase in disease incidence. Conversely, a drop in the monitored population could mask an actual outbreak.

Several solutions to this denominator problem have been attempted; a practical, effective solution in a given situation depends on the data and processing resources available. Basic approaches include:

- *Monitoring syndromic counts relative to other information internal to the data source.* Such approaches use information contained within the data records to derive an inherent denominator instead of using classical rates. For example, suppose that the total number of facility encounters is recorded in addition to the number of ILI diagnoses. One can then monitor the proportion

(number of ILI diagnoses on day d)/(total encounters on day d)

The use of such proportions may remove the unwanted effects of unexpected increases or decreases that are irrelevant to biosurveillance. For example, if the data-processing system in one hospital in a monitored hospital system is out of operation for a week for replacement, or if a large hospital is added to the system, the resulting change affects both the numerator and denominator and is thus likely to affect the proportion less than the diagnosis count alone. Figure 4.3 gives a sample comparison of time series of syndromic counts and proportions, with the effect of a small outbreak indicated. The event is clearer from the proportion plot.

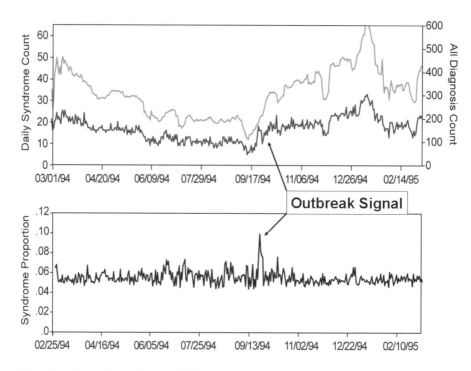

Fig. 4.3   When a denominator variable such as total diagnosis count is available, a proportion can clarify an outbreak signal.

Depending on what is available in the data records of the system, alternative proportions to consider are:

(no. syndromic diagnoses, day d)/(no. reporting clinics, day d)

  or

(no. syndromic diagnoses, day d)/(no. of reporting care providers, day d)

This approach is most effective if the denominator is large and the proportion is well under 0.5. For example, if the diagnosis group of interest includes most records in the system, the effect of an outbreak could be large in both numerator and denominator, resulting in a loss of sensitivity. Further, an unexpected change might have a differential effect on the numerator and denominator; for example, the total number of visits could rise because of the addition of a hospital, but this hospital might not have a clinic treating the syndrome of interest.

- *Modeling the size of the denominator as a function of time.* Models may include:

  - Information within the monitored data, as in the previous approach
  - Known calendar-based effects
  - Data history
  - Information from external data streams, such as daily maximum temperature for respiratory-related clinical diagnoses groups or sales discounts for OTC purchases

Calendar-based effects and the use of external data streams are discussed in Section 4.3. A well-known use of data history for denominator adjustment is the "Figure 1" approach used in the mortality and morbidity weekly reports of the Centers for Disease Control and Prevention [2]. In this approach, the count from the current 4-week interval is compared with the average of counts from the past 5 years from the same and the two immediately adjacent intervals. See Fig. 4.4 for an example.

Neither of these approaches to denominator adjustment can be expected to work well for all monitored data sources; knowledge of both the data source and the syndrome of interest should drive the choice of approach.

4.2.2 Recognizing the Unexpected

Anomalies are determined by asking statistical questions such as:

- Are the observed data sufficiently close to forecasts of an analytical model? For example, regression models of varying sophistication have been applied to represent systematic behavior such as cyclic trends. The residuals, or values of observation minus forecast, are then tested [3].

- Could the observed data reasonably belong to a theoretical or empirically observed frequency distribution? For example, count data from a homogeneous

year / 4-week interval	15 – 18	19 – 22	23 – 26
1995	95	88	85
1996	91	84	83
1997	89	86	87
1998	96	82	84
1999	85	84	79
2000		91	

Mean	86.53
Standard Deviation	4.66
UCL = mean + 2 std. dev.	95.85
LCL = mean - 2 std. dev.	77.22

Fig. 4.4   Historical limits method of Stroup et al. [2] used in CDC Figure 1 summaries.

population are often assumed to obey a Poisson distribution, with a variance equal to the mean. The classical control charts of industrial quality technology are based on data that are grouped or otherwise transformed to fit a Gaussian distribution. Under this assumption, upper and lower data thresholds are derived to test for values that are too high or too low [4].

4.2.3   Use of Data Covariates

Various adaptations and combinations of these approaches are used for prospective health monitoring. Data records used for biosurveillance commonly include covariates such as patient age, sex, and address, in addition to syndromic information. Data privacy regulations commonly limit the detail of these covariates, so that a postal code may be available instead of an exact address, or an age group instead of a birth date. Two strategies for including covariate information are:

1. Stratify records by covariate value and monitor individual stratified counts. For example, apply algorithms to monitor diagnosis counts separately for different age groups. The stratification may be imposed by the data — for example, when only age groups or postal codes are present in the records — or it may be chosen by system developers. This strategy may give added sensitivity if the strata are well chosen based on epidemiological considerations: for example, when certain age groups are of particular interest. However, if there are multiple covariates, each with several strata, the multiple-testing problem may be formidable. The count over all strata must be monitored in addition to individual stratum statistics because the outbreak effect may be distributed evenly, thus aggravating the multiple-testing issue. Approaches to managing this problem are discussed in Section 4.6 on distributed monitoring.

2. Stratify the data as in strategy 1, but keep the stratified records together and apply alerting algorithms to the distribution of covariates. For example, a change in the distribution of diagnoses among age groups may give an early warning of an outbreak affecting one particular group. The elderly are often seen as sentinels for the population at large, and seasonal influenza in cities often affects children first; however, in the pandemics of 1918 and 1968, young adults were disproportionately stricken. To establish a baseline age distribution for such a case, the historical distribution of respiratory diagnoses among m age groups can be calculated as a set of expected ratios $R_j, j = 1, \ldots, m$. The recent daily or weekly counts c_j can be compared with the expected ratios based on the well-known D^2 statistic:

$$D^2 = \Sigma_j (c_j - nR_j)^2 / nR_j \tag{4.1}$$

which can be approximated by a χ^2 distribution with $m - 1$ degrees of freedom. The χ^2 tables will then yield nominal threshold values for alerting at the desired confidence levels. In practice, as with many alerting algorithms, the underlying data conditions may fail; these thresholds can then be adjusted by empirical observation to attain the desired maximum false alarm rate.

A covariate of particular interest is the patient address. Spatial information is important because a group of records of patient encounters or customer transactions from the same time period and nearby addresses may indicate a cluster of cases caused by a common exposure. Such detailed information is extremely valuable for epidemiological investigation. For this reason, spatial and spatiotemporal scan statistics have been widely used in biosurveillance in place of overall anomaly measures such as the D^2 statistic [5]. These methods look for significant clustering without bias aa to the location or extent of the cluster, and they attempt to control for multiple testing. For each continuous set of candidate clusters, scan statistics test the hypothesis that the relationship of within-cluster data to exterior data differs from expectations based on model predictions or recent data history. Scan statistics and related issues are discussed in Section 4.5.

4.2.4   Components of an Alerting Algorithm

The following terms are used in the discussions in subsequent sections:

- *Adaptive algorithm*: an algorithms that is adjusted according to recent data behavior, as distinguished from an algorithm with unchanging parameters and thresholds.

- *Baseline period, training period*: the time interval used to calculate expected data behavior. The expectations may be based on simple statistical moments such as the mean or standard deviation, or they may require calculation of regression coefficients or covariate proportions from data in this interval.

- *Test period*: the time interval of the current data to be tested, which depends on the data source and acquisition rate. Before the year 2000, surveillance was generally applied to monthly or weekly totals. More recent methods have sought anomalies based on daily data. Advances in hospital informatics are approaching real-time capability, and this interval continues to shorten.

- *Buffer period, guardband*: a time interval between the baseline and test periods. If the baseline period covers data all the way to the test period, and if the outbreak effect on the data is spread over several days, early undetected outbreak effects may inflate the baseline data, increase the data expectation, and mask the rest of the outbreak. The buffer gives a separation between the baseline and test intervals to avoid this masking.

- *Test values*: the current or recent values derived from test period observations that will be tested for anomaly. These values may be visit counts, proportions, or model residuals from the current test period.

- *Test statistic*: value computed from the test values to be used for making alerting decisions.

- *Reset criterion*: rule for clearing the test statistic or reducing it to a moderate level after extreme data values to prevent flooding of subsequent alerts.

- *Threshold*: limiting value for the test statistic above which an alert is issued. Multiple threshold values may be used for layered alert levels.

- *Warmup period*: initial data interval that may be required to establish a minimum baseline before an algorithm may be applied prospectively.

Figure 4.5 schematically illustrates the baseline, buffer, and test periods for an adaptive algorithm. Key features of these quantities that can influence algorithm utility and performance are:

- *The length of the required warmup period.* An algorithm that needs years of data for training will not be useful if little data history is available.

- *The length of the baseline.* Is it long enough to smooth noisy fluctuations but recent enough to capture current data behavior?

- *The presence of outliers.* Are outliers removed from the baseline data to prevent training on extreme values for calculation of expected statistics?

- *Sparse data.* What does the algorithm do when the baseline data are very sparse or contain no cases? For example, suppose that the scaled test statistic must be divided by the baseline standard deviation, similar to a sliding z-score:

$$z_t = (x_t - \mu_t)/\sigma_t \tag{4.2}$$

where x_t is the recent observation, μ_t is the mean estimate, and σ_t is the standard deviation estimate. If the x_t are sparse because a rare syndrome is chosen or a small geographic area is monitored, a minimum value for σ_t is required to avoid a zero denominator. This minimum must be large enough to avoid oversensitivity, such as if system users wish to avoid alarms caused by isolated cases.

Data stream(s) to monitor in time:

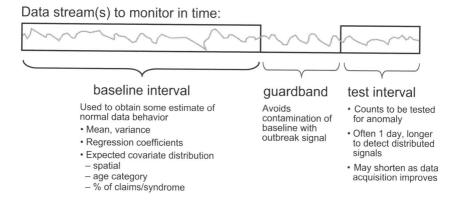

baseline interval

Used to obtain some estimate of normal data behavior
• Mean, variance
• Regression coefficients
• Expected covariate distribution
  – spatial
  – age category
  – % of claims/syndrome

guardband

Avoids contamination of baseline with outbreak signal

test interval

• Counts to be tested for anomaly
• Often 1 day, longer to detect distributed signals
• May shorten as data acquisition improves

Fig. 4.5   Adaptive strategy for aggregating data in time.

4.2.5   Steps in Algorithmic Processing

The following steps are customary parts of the algorithmic procedure, although some algorithms do not apply them all explicitly:

1. Update the computation of the expected data values for the current test period. If the algorithm is adaptive, refit any model according to recent data. This step may be as simple as updating the baseline mean and standard deviation.

2. Compute the difference between the test data and expectations.

3. Normalize this difference to account for variability inferred from the baseline data. For a z-score, this difference would be divided by the recent standard error estimate, whereas for a regression-based model, the difference would be divided by the standard error of regression.

4. Compute the detection statistic based on the normalized difference. Some algorithms use the normalized difference itself as the detection statistic, whereas others might filter it with a time window or apply a CUSUM or EWMA (Exponentially Weighted Moving Average) control chart.

5. Apply the empirical or theoretical threshold to make an alerting decision.

4.3 OUTBREAK DETECTION AS A SIGNAL-TO-NOISE PROBLEM

A disease outbreak may be seen as an event whose effect on a data stream is a detectable signal. This effect is the set of data stream elements, be they emergency department visits, physician office visits, pharmacy sales, or work absences, that are attributable to the outbreak. However, the resulting signal may be obscured by noise (i.e., by the variation of the data stream background) due to factors that are not of interest to the surveillance system. The noise background is considered the data stream behavior in the absence of signals of interest. Detection algorithms are designed to "increase the signal-to-noise ratio" by reducing background noise from the data while preserving as much as possible of the signal of interest. Designing such algorithms requires an understanding of both the background noise and the signal of interest.

4.3.1 Understanding the Noise Background

Background noise in a particular data stream will have a variety of causes. Some can be modeled because the causes are expected and any required information is available at the time of forecast; some cannot be modeled because the causes are unexpected or required information is unavailable. The former group includes:

- Natural random variability that can be measured from data history

- Day-of-week variation

- Seasonal trends

- Calendar events such as holidays or school closings

- Available climatic changes such as maximum daily temperature

All of these factors have been incorporated in models of daily syndromic data.
Causes of noise that cannot be modeled readily include:

- Informatics and data-acquisition issues, such as:
    - Changes in syndromic case definition
    - Changes in health care billing or coding practices
    - Intermittent, sometimes lasting, data dropouts resulting from system problems
    - Changes in health care eligibility: for example, a change in monitored claims from a medical care entitlement program
    - Changes in the behavior or size of the monitored population. An extreme example would be the data background from a military treatment facility on a base that experiences sudden population increases or decreases when large units are relocated.

- Changes in the participation of data providers, such as the addition of a private group of hospitals to a citywide system
- Variable and late reporting by data providers. This factor has been modeled by Brookmeyer and Gail [6], and research is ongoing on its application in syndromic data modeling, but much data history and analysis are required.

- External influences on the data streams, such as:

    - Unscheduled holidays or institutional closings
    - Inclement weather interference with usual patient or consumer behavior
    - Changes in population health care behavior
    - Sales promotions affecting OTC sales data
    - Media reports and other influences. A famous example was the "Clinton Effect" in Fall 2004, when chief complaints of chest pain peaked in several data sources after former U.S. President William Clinton underwent heart surgery.

Most of these factors can be modeled retrospectively with extensive research, but including them in prospective models would require resource-intensive auxiliary data feeds: for example, a daily capability to receive detailed information about OTC sales promotions. These factors are responsible for the gap between the statistical and epidemiological significance of algorithm results.

Note that the definition of background noise provided is flexible in its specification of factors "not of interest to the surveillance system." An event that is significant in one context may be irrelevant to another. Thus, the onset of seasonal influenza in a monitored population is a signal for a system whose goal is general public health surveillance, but it is noise to a system concerned only with detecting a bioterrorist attack.

4.3.2   Characterizing the Outbreak Signal

The appropriate choice of algorithm for routine surveillance depends on what is to be detected. Recall that the signal to be detected is the imprint of a health event of interest on the data. Beyond seeking sharp increases, if the shape of the signal is known, one can look for time-series segments with that shape.

Figure 4.6 illustrates some signal shapes, exaggerated for discussion purposes, of practical interest in surveillance data. Figure 4.6(a) shows a sustained step increase in the level of the time series. The signal shape is a simple step function that might result from an increased relative risk of incidence of a chronic disease throughout the monitored population. If the monitoring objective is to detect such an increase, control charts designed to detect a mean shift are appropriate. However, users of modern biosurveillance systems are often interested in detecting outbreaks of infectious disease, whether natural or human-made. Signals resulting from such outbreaks are likely to be transient and seasonal, and traditional alerting methods require adaptation to detect such signals.

Figure 4.6(b) illustrates the onset of influenza season in a time series of ILI data. As autumn progresses, the diagnosis counts increase as a result of normal viral infections and, in most years, accelerate when influenza rises to epidemic levels. The date and severity of influenza outbreaks vary from year to year; the double peaks in the figure are observed in some years when different viral strains have prevalence peaks weeks apart. In normal years, diagnosis counts subside after a period of days or weeks, returning to the level of the winter cold shelf and then dropping off as spring progresses. In the exceptional situation of a pandemic, the population is affected by a new or modified flu strain to which it has no immunological defense. The ILI data series might then display peaks in any season, which could occur in distinct waves [7].

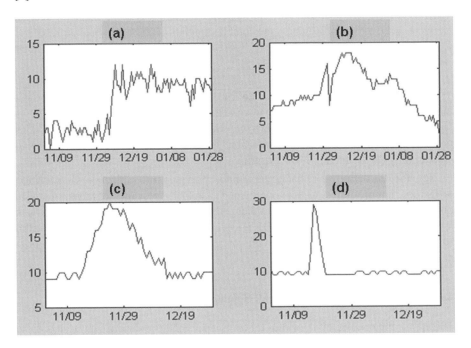

Fig. 4.6   Possible outbreak signals in surveillance data streams.

What would be a likely data signal in the event of a bioterrorist attack such as a localized, intentional release of a weaponized pathogen? The signal would depend on a number of factors, including the number infected, the dosage, and population susceptibility, and its shape would be a function of the distribution of incubation periods. Among diseases known to be weaponized, the median incubation period can range from 1–2 days to 1–2 weeks. A reasonable hypothesis is that the signal would be proportional to the number of new symptomatic cases on each day, with adjustments according to the nature of the data. For example, the effect of a serious outbreak on school absenteeism would be cumulative, with none on weekends. The signal problem is then to estimate the epidemic curve, or the number of new symptomatic cases on each day after exposure, resulting from a point-source outbreak.

For a model of the shape of such a signal, one may use the lognormal distribution first discussed by Sartwell and widely used since [8]. From analysis of incubation periods of 17 data sets that includd 12 infectious diseases, Sartwell observed that incubation periods awere well approximated by a lognormal distribution, with parameters dependent on the disease agent and route of infection [8]. In other words, the logarithm of the incubation period had a Gaussian distribution, say with mean ζ and standard deviation σ. Figure 4.7 is an example of the lognormal distribution. Figure 4.7(a) shows the cumulative distribution function for incubation periods with $\zeta = 1.3(3.7 - $ days expected incubation) and $\sigma = 0.4$. Figure 4.7(b) plots the probability density curve. The probability of symptoms occurring during day 4 may be approximated at 0.242 by integration under this continuous curve from day 4.5 to day 5.5, as shown. Given that m patients are infected, one would expect $0.242m$ of them to become symptomatic during day 4. Figure 4.7(c) shows the resulting expected epidemic curve by day for a total of 200 infected patients; the rounded values are charted at the right. This plot approximates the total epidemic curve for a noncommunicable disease, where all patients are infected at the initial exposure. For a communicable disease, the plot represents only primary cases, not those infected in subsequent waves, and one can test for signal detection based on primary cases alone.

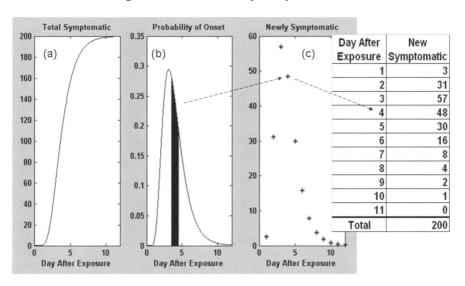

Fig. 4.7   Lognormal incubation period distribution example.

To model a specific disease, the values of lognormal parameters may be inferred from histograms of incubation period data from the medical literature (e.g., such as [9]). These parameters and a hypothetical number of total cases can be used to produce a model epicurve of primary symptomatic cases–all cases if the disease is not communicable. Figure 4.6(c) shows the signal for a disease with a long median incubation period of 25 days superimposed on a quiet data background, while Fig. 4.6(d) shows the signal for a 3.7-day incubation. Detection is more difficult against a noisier background or for a smaller number of infected, and knowledge of the signal shape may be critical.

4.3.3 Importance of Data Aggregation Decisions

The outbreak signal and the background noise are strongly affected by decisions about how to aggregate the surveillance data. There is a thematic trade-off between expanding the data window to increase structure for modeling and masking a potential outbreak signal with the additional counts. For example, to see a seasonal pattern in the background or a lognormal shape in the signal, it may be necessary to look at week-long counts of county-level data, whereas confining attention to community counts or 4-hour time intervals might mask such features. These decisions relate to how the data are grouped in:

- *Time.* Should quantities such as clinic visit counts be grouped by week, by day, or, as sample rates and analysis approach real-time capability, by 8-hour or smaller blocks?

- *Space.* The signal-to-noise background depends on whether data are monitored at state, city, or local levels. Monitoring of smaller spatial units may allow greater sensitivity to small-scale outbreaks, but only if the system is capable of controlling or managing the resulting multiple alerts and if the algorithms are effective for the scale chosen.

- *Syndrome classification.* Limiting a syndrome group to diagnoses closely related to a disease of interest should improve alerting specificity but will likely yield a sparse, unstructured data background, and many such groups may be needed for general public health surveillance. For more general signals, larger and noisier syndrome groups must be analyzed.

4.4 ALGORITHMS BASED ON TIME-SERIES DATA

4.4.1 Control Charts for Public Health Monitoring

4.4.1.1 Control Chart Concepts. For decades, graphical tools based on concepts of probability theory have been applied to industrial processes such as manufacturing. These tools, widely known as control charts, have traditionally been used to monitor time series of measurements from industrial processes to aid in understanding their variability, improving their quality, and recognizing abnormal conditions requiring correction as soon as possible. For the last of these objectives, abnormal conditions are thought to exhibit *special cause variation*, i.e., variability that control charts can help to distinguish promptly from the usual *common cause variation* of a process.

Control charts have traditionally been used to monitor time series of measurements from industrial processes. The importance of assuring quality in such processes has led to the mature discipline of statistical process control (SPC). See the text by Ryan [4], among much useful survey literature, for a detailed introduction to this field. Of the listed objectives of using control charts, the early warning feature has motivated most control chart applications in medical surveillance. The data forming the time series in industry are typically physical quantities, measured from manufactured products, whose understanding may lead to product improvements. In contrast, the time series of health monitoring are observations such as nosocomial infection counts, surgical outcomes, or in the syndromic surveillance context, counts of emergency department visits for influenza-like illness. Thus, the process underlying the time series of visit counts in a monitored population cannot be improved by understanding its background variability; it depends on the spread of endemic disease and is amenable to improved hygiene and other public health measures. Control charts have been applied in health surveillance to seek prompt alerting capability at acceptable false alarm rates.

A wide variety of control chart applications in health care were reported by Benneyan [10], and many subsequent applications have arisen [11]. Accounting for common cause variation depends on the quantity chosen for monitoring and on its underlying distribution. Several common distributions are associated with canonical chart types. For example, for continuous quantities (e.g., blood pressure, temperature) that are often considered to have a normal distribution, X-bar and S charts are used for the mean and standard deviation, respectively. P-charts, with limits derived from the binomial distribution, are used for proportions such as the fraction of total admissions with gastrointestinal chief complaints. U-charts derived from the Poisson distribution are often used for count data such as the weekly number of admissions for neurological disorders. Numerous other basic and hybrid chart types are available.

4.4.1.2   Types of Control Charts.   This section presents three chart-based methods that have been used in biosurveillance. Methods based on other types of charts should also be considered. Each method presented is applied to the time series shown in Table 4.1, which is a set of averages of weekly counts of clinic visits classified in a rash syndrome. Traditional control chart applications use subgroup averages like these 7-day means to reduce the amount of *in-control variation* and to take advantage of the *Central Limit Theorem*, which states that a series of means approaches a Gaussian distribution as the subgroup size increases.

Control charts are usually applied in two phases. Phase I is an assessment of the appropriate chart for the data and an analysis of the relevant statistical data properties based on a set of training data that represent the process in control. Working values of the mean, standard deviation, and other chart-related parameters are derived. Phase II is the prospective monitoring, which applies the chart with these parameters to monitor subsequent values for special cause variation. When this monitoring determines that the process is "out of control," the process may be interrupted for correction, which may be expensive and time-consuming in a manufacturing environment. Depending on subsequent chart findings over time, the phase I analysis may be revisited.

Table 4.1   Three Control Chart Methods Used in Biosurveillance

	Phase I Estimates:						
	μ Estimate: 3.041			Xbar Upper Limit: 5.892			
	σ_7 Estimate: 0.951			Xbar Lower Limit: 0.189			
Date	7-Day Mean	z	CUSUM Upper Sum	CUSUM Lower Sum	EWMA	EWMA stat
1/14/1997	1.429	-1.696	0.000	1.196	1.909	-2.380
1/21/1997	2.857	-0.193	0.000	0.000	2.288	-1.583
1/28/1997	2.429	-0.644	0.000	0.144	2.345	-1.465
2/4/1997	2.714	-0.343	0.000	0.000	2.492	-1.154
2/11/1997	2.429	-0.644	0.000	0.144	2.467	-1.207
2/18/1997	2.857	-0.193	0.000	0.000	2.623	-0.879
2/25/1997	2.429	-0.644	0.000	0.144	2.545	-1.042
3/4/1997	2.143	-0.945	0.000	0.445	2.384	-1.381
3/11/1997	2.429	-0.644	0.000	0.144	2.402	-1.344
3/18/1997	3.429	0.408	0.000	0.000	2.813	-0.480
3/25/1997	1.714	-1.395	0.000	0.895	2.373	-1.404
4/1/1997	2.857	-0.193	0.000	0.000	2.567	-0.997
4/8/1997	2.000	-1.095	0.000	0.595	2.340	-1.474
4/15/1997	4.143	1.160	0.660	0.000	3.061	0.043
4/22/1997	1.857	-1.245	0.000	1.405	2.580	-0.970
4/29/1997	4.571	1.610	1.110	0.000	3.376	0.706
5/6/1997	5.500	2.587	3.198	0.000	4.226	2.494
5/13/1997	4.857	1.911	3.411	0.000	4.478	3.025
5/20/1997	5.571	2.662	4.162	0.000	4.916	3.945
5/27/1997	6.143	3.264	4.764	0.000	5.406	4.978
6/3/1997	4.857	1.911	3.411	0.000	5.187	4.516
6/10/1997	3.714	0.709	2.209	0.791	4.598	3.276
6/17/1997	3.714	0.709	2.209	0.791	4.244	2.533
6/24/1997	3.571	0.558	2.058	0.942	3.975	1.966
7/1/1997	2.429	-0.644	0.856	2.144	3.357	0.665

One of the most widely used control charts is the X-bar chart, which tests the variation of the process mean. In phase I, the overall mean $\overline{X}$ and the standard deviation $\hat{s}_k$ of the subgroup mean are estimated, where k is the subgroup size (7 days in Table 4.1). The subgroup mean is considered to be in control if it lies between the lower control limit $\overline{X} - 3\hat{s}_k$ (LCL) and the upper control limit $\overline{X} + 3\hat{s}_k$ (UCL). Figure 4.8 is a plot of the chart corresponding to Table 4.1. Equivalently, the mean is in control if z_t is between -3 and 3, where

$$z_t = (\bar{x}_t - \overline{X})/\hat{s}_k \tag{4.3}$$

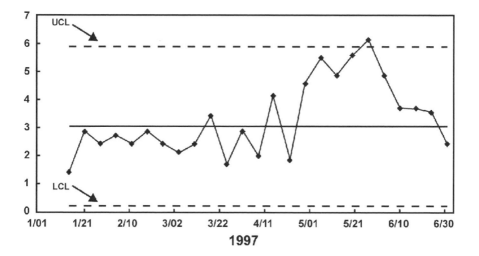

Fig. 4.8   X-bar chart created from weekly syndromic data.

Table 4.1 also includes a column of values of z, and those for which the mean is considered out of control are indicated in boldface. Note that once the control limits have been chosen, the in-control decision depends only on a single value, the subgroup mean $\bar{x}$ in question. This type of chart does not allow an early warning by giving extra weight to a local trend that may signify a problem.

Two additional charts have been shown to be timelier than the X-bar chart at detecting small mean shifts and have been applied to biosurveillance. The first is the cumulative summation, or CUSUM, chart. This chart maintains a running upper sum of differences of $\bar{x}_t$ above the overall mean estimate $\overline{X}$ and a corresponding lower sum of differences below $\overline{X}$. Furthermore, small differences are ignored; only differences at least $2k$ standard deviations above or below $\overline{X}$ are counted for a fixed multiple k. A common practice is to set k at 0.5 to detect a shift of 1 standard deviation. In terms of the statistic z, scaled formulas for these upper and lower sums are then:

$$S_{H,t} = \max(0, z_t - 0.5 + S_{H,t-1}) \tag{4.4}$$

$$S_{L,t} = \max(0, (-z_t - 0.5) + S_{H,t-1}) \qquad (4.5)$$

This formulation assures that both sums are nonnegative, with $S_{H,n}$ accumulating increases above $\overline{X}$ and $S_{L,n}$ accumulating decreases below it. The process is considered to be out of control if either sum exceeds a threshold h, selected according to the desired run length properties of the chart. For illustration here, h is set to 4, a common choice.

The CUSUM chart allows earlier detection of small shifts than the X-bar chart because multiple subgroup measurements may influence each chart value $S_{H,t}$ or $S_{L,t}$; however, this feature also has a disadvantage in that large chart values, especially if exaggerated by measurement or transcription error, may inflate subsequent ones and flood the chart with out-of-control signals. This problem may be aggravated by untreated or residual autocorrelation in the input time series. Lucas and Crosier treated this problem in their *fast initial response* (FIR) CUSUM. They obtained the desired chart behavior by starting each chart value $S_{H,0}$ and $S_{L,0}$ at $h/2$ and resetting it to $h/2$ when the threshold h was exceeded [12]. The values of S_H and S_L in Table 4.1 were calculated following this procedure with $k = 1$ and $h = 4$. Note that the out-of-control condition is signaled an observation earlier than in the X-bar chart and that the reset feature prevents further signals.

A second chart used to gain early detection of small mean shifts is the EWMA chart. For this chart, the current time-series value is replaced by a weighted average of the recent values such that the weight decreases with the age of the value. This weighted average is expressed by the recursive formula:

$$E_t = \omega \bar{x}_t + (1 - \omega)E_{t-1} \qquad (4.6)$$

where ω is a constant between 0 and 1 that expresses how weight is distributed back in time. For a value of ω near 0, the decay is slow, and more weight is given to past values; if ω is close to 1, only the most recent values influence this average. Values of ω between 0.1 and 0.3 are often used in the SPC community. The initial value E_0 is often set to $\overline{X}$; this initial value has little influence after a few observations, so E_0 may be set to $\bar{x}_1$ if a good estimate of $\overline{X}$ is unavailable. This expression is generally used for practical calculations, but it may be expanded to yield:

$$E_t = \omega \bar{x}_t + \omega(1 - \omega)\bar{x}_{t-1} + \omega(1 - \omega)^2 \bar{x}_{t-2} + \omega(1 - \omega)^3 \bar{x}_{t-3} + \cdots, \qquad (4.7)$$

thus illustrating the decreasing weighting. Because E_t is a smoothing of $\bar{x}_t$, its estimated standard deviation is smaller, depending on the number of steps t elapsed:

$$\hat{s}_{E,t} = \hat{s}_{k,t} * \sqrt{\omega/(2 - \omega)} * (1 - (1 - \omega)^{2t}) \qquad (4.8)$$

The rightmost factor in the equation, $1 - (1 - \omega)^{2t}$, is very close to 1 after four to five steps for conventional values of ω. The process is considered to be in control if E_t lies between $(\overline{X} - 3\hat{s}_{E,t})$ and $(\overline{X} + 3\hat{s}_{E,t})$, or essentially, if the statistic

$$(E_t - \overline{X})/(s_{k,t} * \sqrt{\omega/(2 - \omega)}) \tag{4.9}$$

lies between -3 and 3.

The values of this statistic are plotted in Table 4.1 for $\omega = 0.4$ and for $E_0 = \overline{X}$. Note that the out-of-control value is attained here a step before the CUSUM chart and two steps before the X-bar chart. However, as discussed above, the past values keep the statistic above the threshold for several steps after the X-bar chart signal stops. This "ringing" could devalue the statistic by causing a loss of sensitivity to subsequent problems; it can be remedied with reset procedures similar to those described for FIR CUSUM.

4.4.1.3 Challenges and Strategies for Adaptation to Biosurveillance. Why would a public health monitor use a control chart? As discussed at the beginning of this chapter, the monitor must decide when to initiate an epidemiological investigation. Beginning the investigation 1–2 days earlier than traditional monitoring might indicate could reduce the disease burden and save lives, but the investigation could be costly, and excessive false alarms could weaken the credibility of the alerting system and of the public health agency itself. Surveillance system developers seek to exploit the large body of process control research to implement biosurveillance control charts with high specificity and few false alarms.

There are several key differences between monitoring a manufacturing process and seeking public health anomalies:

- The modifier "control" applies in industrial processes because the engineer can apply physical science to change the process underlying the data. In a closed health setting such as a hospital department monitoring nosocomial infections, infection control procedures may affect the data similarly. In contrast, public health surveillance data, such as hospital or clinic visits, nurse hotline calls, and pharmaceutical purchases, cannot be influenced by the monitor.

- Unlike a mechanical or electronic out-of-control decision, a public health alerting decision is a complex function of:
  - The objectives of the monitoring agency and the resources available for investigation. The capacity and willingness for follow-up are likely to influence the acceptable false alarm rate.
  - The health alert status or degree of concern that a natural or human-made infectious disease threat exists. The degree of concern may be affected by outbreaks in neighboring populations or by political or media reports.
  - The human monitor's experience and knowledge of the population and the data. These factors will allow many signals to be explained away without further investigation.

These considerations have led to modifications of traditional charting procedures. A common modification is that lower bounds are not enforced because monitors are concerned about increases in care-seeking behavior, not decreases. Discarding out-of-control signals caused by low data values reduces the overall alert rate, and there are many causes for data reduction that are irrelevant to outbreak monitoring. However, the potential danger is that the time-series values could be low because the increased demand on health care personnel caused by an outbreak is interfering with the usual data reporting and transmission. Few health applications monitor low values; if the staff is too overburdened with emergent cases to send data, resulting in unusually low values, they know they have a problem. Depending on the data collection and transmission arrangements, this justification is debatable.

Another common modification is to apply control charts to individual observations rather than subgroup averages, mainly because most biosurveillance data sets are available only on a daily basis, and rapid alerting is a principal motivation for automated surveillance. Using individual observations has two drawbacks. First, using subgroup means reduces the variance as well as the autocorrelation between time-series elements. The variance of a time series of individual observations is k times the variance between means of subgroups of size k. To the health monitor, the added variance will mean more false alarms. Second, from the Central Limit Theorem, taking subgroup averages moves the time series toward a Gaussian distribution. Many control chart properties are derived under the assumption of a Gaussian input time series, but the unaveraged diagnosis counts of most series in syndromic surveillance have a negative binomial or overdispersed Poisson distribution. The tails of these observed distributions are longer than Gaussian, so, again, more false alarms are expected if individual observations are used. In practice, the false alarm rate depends on the background data, and both statistical and heuristic measures are applied to reduce or otherwise manage false alarms.

4.4.1.4   Effect of the Changing, Correlated Data Background.

The two-phase control chart development paradigm assumes that observations are independent and that the training data are representative of future data to be monitored. Among biosurveillance data streams, however, a changing baseline is the rule, not the exception, as illustrated by the discussion of background noise in Section 4.3. These data streams are typically nonstationary in the sense that a fixed set of baseline data is often unrepresentative of the data to come.

Biosurveillance time series also commonly violate the independence assumption underlying many control chart methods. Figure 4.9 is a plot of 200 weeks of rash syndrome diagnosis counts expanded from the data of Fig. 4.8. While the mean weekly count is clearly close to 3, individual counts appear to be correlated with recent counts. For example, values tend to stay above or below the mean; among the 19 weekly counts beginning May 25,1995, only one is below the mean. This time series does not satisfy the independence assumption of most control charts: if one observation is near a control limit, subsequent observations are more likely to be near the same limit. Thus, the overall mean is not a uniformly good measure of central tendency. Traditional subgrouping can actually worsen the correlation [4]: in the original rash data used to form the weekly averages of Fig. 4.9, the correlation coefficient of a daily count with the previous day's count was a significant 0.65; taking weekly means raised this coefficient above 0.9.

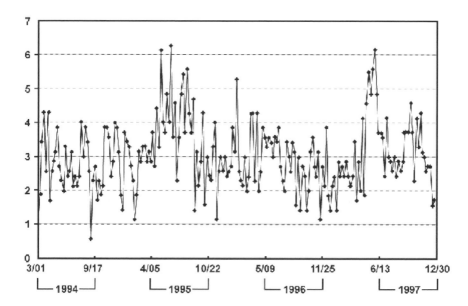

Fig. 4.9   Time series of syndromic diagnosis counts displaying serial correlation.

A practical approach to the obstacles of nonstationary and correlated data is to adjust the estimates of the mean and standard deviation with a sliding baseline, as shown in Fig. 4.5. The baseline is separated from the current value by the buffer of immediately preceding values. This adaptive procedure may be seen as a continually updated phase I. Two common implementations of this procedure that use time series of individual daily counts are:

- *Algorithms C1, C2, and C3 of CDC's Early Aberration Reporting System* [13]. A 7-day baseline is used for these algorithms, and z-scores are computed each day:

$$z_t = (x_t - \overline{x}_{7,i} - \hat{s}_{7,t})/\hat{s}_{7,t} \tag{4.10}$$

  where the mean and standard deviation of the seven preceding counts x_{t-j-1}, $x_{t-i-2}, \ldots, x_{t-i-7}$ are used as the current estimates $\overline{x}_{7,t}$ and $\hat{s}_{7,t}$. Algorithms C1 and C2 are comparable to adaptive X-bar charts, and C3 is a type of cumulative summation that can include the previous two z-scores. Specifically:

  - For algorithm C1, $j = 0$, so there is no buffer interval, and an alert is issued if $z_t > 2$. From the algebraic expression for z_t, this criterion is the X-bar chart condition that the current observation is 3 standard deviations above the mean.

- For algorithm C2, $j = 2$, so there is a 2-day buffer, and the alerting criterion is the same.
- For algorithm C3, $j = 2$, and the alerting condition is:

$$z_t + z_{t-1} + z_{t-2} > 2 \qquad (4.11)$$

where the current z_t must be positive, and a reset condition is imposed by adding z_{t-1} and z_{t-2} only if they are each less than the threshold of 2. Thus, if the C2 algorithm produces an alert, C3 must also alert, and C3 gives additional sensitivity from the past two observations. For sparse data where the short baseline may include all zeros, a minimum standard deviation of 0.02 is imposed.

The 7-day baseline makes these algorithms somewhat volatile, with an upper confidence limit $\bar{x}_{7,t} + 3\hat{s}_{7,t}$ that can fluctuate noticeably from day to day. However, their simplicity and wide distribution by CDC has made them popular among many public health departments. Local users have adopted a variety of procedures for combining and interpreting C1, C2, and C3 outputs and for coping with the resulting alert rates.

- *The adaptive EWMA algorithm of ESSENCE* (Electronic Surveillance System for Early Notification of Community-based Epidemics) *biosurveillance systems.* This algorithm uses a 28-day baseline and a 2-day buffer. Following the EWMA development, the detection statistic is:

$$(E_t - \bar{x}_{28,i})/\hat{s}_{28,t} * \sqrt{\omega/(2-\omega)} \qquad (4.12)$$

The threshold was derived for a Gaussian data series for a desired confidence level that can be expressed as a probability p. This threshold is the inverse cumulative T distribution for 27 degrees of freedom, evaluated at p. For baseline length m, the number of degrees of freedom would be $m - 1$. Thus, for a confidence level of 0.99 with the 28-day baseline, a table lookup gives the threshold of 2.427. Because the input time series of counts are not Gaussian, more recent ESSENCE systems apply a threshold correction assuming a Poisson data distribution. Two values are used for the smoothing coefficient ω. For detection of gradual or sudden signals, ω is set to 0.4 or 0.9, respectively. With the latter value, the algorithm is similar to an X-bar chart. For sparse data, a minimum $\hat{s}_{28,t}$ is calculated to avoid alerts on isolated single cases.

4.4.1.5 Role of the Outbreak Signal.   Much control chart development has been directed toward rapid detection of mean shifts. As discussed in Section 4.2, outbreak data signals expected from infectious disease outbreaks are not the lasting step increases that one would expect of a mean shift. The signals of interest are transient data effects of epidemic curves of attributable cases lasting from a few days to a month or more. Even for a given disease such as influenza, the outbreak signal may be sudden and explosive or more gradual, reflecting the annual variability in seasonal epidemics. Morton et al. applied CUSUM–Shewhart and EWMA–Shewhart charts to detect both types of signal in the monitoring of hospital infections [14]. Their EWMA–Shewhart chart was chosen for correlated background data. The ESSENCE EWMA algorithm with dual smoothing coefficients was chosen to follow this strategy.

4.4.2   Data Forecasting for Public Health Monitoring.

Much research has been devoted to forecasting public health data for surveillance. Figure 4.10 gives the motivation for this research by illustrating some natural causes of background noise (see Section 4.3). The upper plot presents 3 years of daily counts of respiratory outpatient visits from a large metropolitan area. The seasonal and day-of-week effects of these counts are evident, and the section magnified in the lower plot illustrates the reduced visits on calendar holidays, when many clinics are closed. There are obvious drawbacks to applying the chart-based methods discussed previously to such data: the natural background would give a large bias against alerting on a weekend or holiday, and Monday counts would likely be seen as "out of control." Seasonal trends provide additional bias for or against algorithm threshold crossings depending on the direction of the trend. Additional causes of bias are well known but not graphically obvious: extreme temperatures on weekdays will increase visits to certain clinics, and annual sales promotions will increase sales of OTC remedies. Forecasts can be applied to remove these known effects and thus prevent the masking of potential outbreak signals.

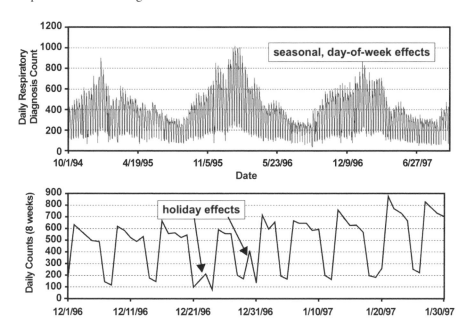

Fig. 4.10   Seasonal, weekly, and holiday effects in daily time series.

However, for outbreak detection, perfect data forecasting may be misleading. For example, if an outbreak signal is distributed over time, including early data effects in the training data can cause subsequent effects to fall within expected limits and thus mask the outbreak event. The desired forecast is the data background *as it would develop in the absence of an outbreak.* If only single-day spike signals are of interest, there is no danger in using next-day forecasts. For detection of more gradual signals, the use of a buffer period to predict several days ahead should be considered.

Sections 4.4.2.1 and 4.4.2.2 discuss data forecasting by regression modeling and by generalized exponential smoothing.

4.4.2.1 Regression Modeling of Biosurveillance Data. In epidemiological applications, regression is generally used to establish or clarify associations rather than make predictions. The typical research questions are:

- Do regression covariates such as age or sex affect the treatment outcome?

- Does treatment success differ among sites if we control for covariates?

Predictive capability is not a primary goal in such studies. These studies often use static data sets and apply careful exploratory analyses, like the phase I analysis of process control, to specify a regression model and covariate set that explain the data features of interest without bias. By contrast, the use of regression for prospective biosurveillance is more like financial applications that forecast market prices, so that model criteria are goodness-of-fit measures for out-of-sample prediction. To illustrate the principles and pitfalls of using regression modeling for biosurveillance forecasting, a traditional approach and a modified one are presented.

Traditional Use of Regression for Prediction. The loglinear model described by Brillman et al. [3] fits an ordinary least-squares loglinear model to a set of training series values to obtain regression coefficients. These coefficients are then used to forecast values beyond the training data without adjusting for subsequent changes in time-series behavior.

Defining $V(t)$ as the number of syndromic hospital visits on day t, the authors model the "started log" $S(t) = \log(V(t) + 1)$ as:

$$S(t) \sim \left[\sum_{i=1}^{7} c_i I_i(t) \right] + (c_8 + c_9 \times t)] + (c_{10} \times \cos kt + c_{11} \times \sin kt) \quad (4.13)$$

where c_1–c_7 are coefficients for day-of-week effect indicators, c_8 is a constant intercept, c_9 is the slope of a long-term trend, and c_{10} and c_{11} are coefficients for continuous harmonic terms representing seasonal trends $k = 2\pi/365.25$ to give a 1-year sinusoidal period for these terms.

For the predictors in this model, note that:

1. The six day-of-week indicators, with the seventh day used as reference, require a separate model coefficient for each day. This approach is flexible for modeling

multiple types of data that may differ in weekly proportions. For example, counts of physician or clinic visits often drop on weekends when office hours are reduced, OTC remedy sales may peak on Saturdays, emergency room visit patterns depend on staffing of a particular hospital, etc. However, if only one type of data is to be forecast, a simpler model may perform as well, such as using indicators only for weekends and weekdays. Also, indicators for calendar holidays may be used if counts are known to drop on such days, and post-holiday indicators may be added to model the surge following the drop-off.

2. The harmonic terms are often used to model an annual seasonal cycle [15]. These terms are generally used when multiple years of historic daily data are available and should not be used if the data history changes drastically from year to year or if it includes only a small fraction of a year.

3. The term to capture long-term trends should be considered carefully. If the outbreak signal is likely to be gradual, this term could effectively mask the signal, as discussed above.

This model is based on the premise that a large set of representative training data is available and desirable. It reflects the strategy of traditional retrospective studies concerned primarily with a good fit within the historical data. However, the forecast errors may be excessive if the data history does not represent the data to be monitored and if covariate relationships change, as often happens in consumer health data. As Brillman et al. [3] realistically remark, "When monitoring complaint levels over multi-year time frames, it is necessary to periodically update baseline model coefficients in order to minimize the extrapolation in forecasting. One approach . . . is to do a planned update every year, but also monitor residuals for patterns . . . to check whether additional updates are needed." Such updates require an active quality assurance effort, and separate updates may be required for different data types. An adaptive model described next does not model seasonality but uses fewer historical data and updates itself to an extent.

Adaptive Example and Result Comparison. The second forecast method is an adaptive regression model with a sliding 8-week baseline interval [16]. This model is similar in form to the traditional one:

$$S(t) \sim \left[\sum_{i=1}^{7} c_i I_i(t) \right] + (c_8 + c_9 \times t) + [c_{10} \times I_{hol}(t)] \qquad (4.14)$$

where c_1–c_7 are coefficients for day-of-week indicators, c_8 is a constant intercept, c_9 is the slope of a linear trend using a centered ramp function, and c_{10} is a coefficient for a holiday indicator. This method recomputes the regression coefficients for each forecast using only the series values from the 8 weeks before the forecast day. The short baseline is intended to capture recent seasonal and trend patterns. The sinusoidal covariates cannot be used because the baseline interval is a small portion of their 1-year period, which means that the harmonic terms would be nearly linear over some baseline intervals. The holiday indicator was added to avoid exaggerated forecasts on known holidays and the computation of spurious values for c_1 to c_7 when holidays occurred in the short baseline interval. A similar model is applied for anomaly detection in ESSENCE biosurveillance systems when an automated goodness-of-fit criterion is satisfied. In those operational implementations, a post-holiday indicator is also added to account for increases following a holiday, and a 2-day buffer is inserted between the baseline and the forecast day to enable the detection of gradual outbreaks.

Figure 4.11 shows a comparison of the performance of these methods on a syndromic time series of citywide respiratory visit counts similar to the data of Fig. 4.10. For this comparison, a holiday term was also added to the nonadaptive model to avoid bias in the results because of a small number of holidays. The curve in Fig. 4.12 shows the daily recorded visit counts, and the solid diamond and open square symbols indicate respective forecasts of the nonadaptive and adaptive regression methods just presented. Only next-day forecasts are shown, so the baseline of the adaptive model ends on the day before each test day. The nonadaptive method was applied with a fixed 1-year baseline, and the adaptive method with a sliding 8-week baseline. The baseline adaptation and continuous model refitting show both positive and negative effects. For the 3 weeks beginning September 29, 2002, the refitting clearly improves the forecast agreement, but for the next 2 weeks, the adaptive method overpredicts. The adaptive method reacts well to the 5-week drop beginning at the end of December 2002, but the high March peaks cause it to overpredict on Mondays in April. From a tabulation of forecast errors over a larger, 350-day test interval, the median of the absolute errors was 22.6 for the nonadaptive, long-baseline seasonal method and 20.0 for the adaptive method. The corresponding mean absolute percentage errors were 11.7% and 9.7%. This comparison illustrates that model decisions should reflect the behavior of the data stream to be monitored and that traditional methodologies may be worth rethinking for health surveillance.

Potential Modifications for More Reliable Forecasting. For the application of models like those just described, analytic modifications may prove helpful, depending on the data background and the additional information available:

1. *Use of external covariates.* The covariates in the models above may be seen as *internal* covariates because they use no information outside the time series being modeled. An *external covariate* would be a predictor based on additional information. For example:

    (a) If the surveillance system receives daily temperature along with health indicator data, the temperature can be added as a continuous variable in the model as a surrogate for the seasonal harmonic terms. The use of such a direct measurement might have better predictive value than a covariate based solely on the calendar in years with unusual seasonal behavior,

    (b) In the case of syndromic time series such as daily respiratory counts, suppose that daily totals of all clinic visits are available. If these totals were stored as another time series, this series could be added as another predictor of the syndromic counts. Such a predictor would help prevent forecast errors due to unscheduled clinic closings, inclement weather,

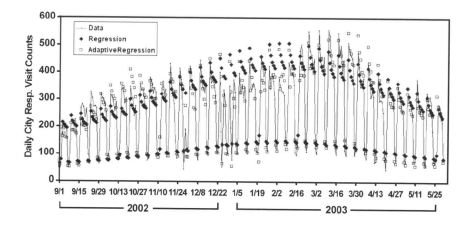

Fig. 4.11   Comparison of forecasts using non-adaptive and adaptive regression.

and other circumstances that cannot be modeled. The utility of such a predictor depends on several factors, including the relative frequency of the syndrome group.

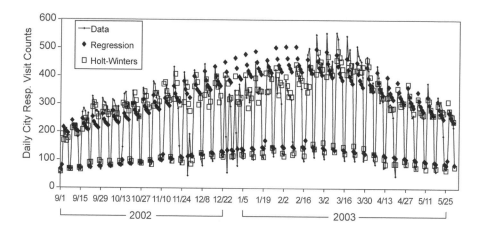

Fig. 4.12   Comparison of forecasts using non-adaptive regression and Holt–Winters exponential smoothing.

2. *Outlier removal or replacement.* For both adaptive and nonadaptive methods, forecasting may be improved if counts that are anomalous in some sense are removed from the model-fitting days or replaced with imputed values. Recall that the objective of the regression is to forecast the background data as they would appear with no disease outbreak. For example, if a daily count in the baseline exceeded the fitted value by more than 3 standard deviations, either the day could be skipped from the training, or the count could be replaced by the anomaly threshold value. However, if such a rule were automated in a model with a sliding baseline, checks must be in place to prevent the rejection of all training data because of a sudden drastic change in the time series.

3. *Avoiding model specification or convergence problems.* For adaptive methods and for nonadaptive methods applied to many regions and syndromes, the fitting of the regression model could fail because of nonsingularity of the covariate matrix or because a nonlinear model fails to converge. For example, suppose that for a sparse data syndrome, no Sunday visits were recorded. For reliable daily forecasting, the implementation should catch such situations and remove problematic covariates like the Sunday indicator from the model. If such situations occur often, a question should be raised as to whether the model is appropriate for the data.

Extended Regression Techniques

- *Nonlinear regression.* A variety of nonlinear methods have been developed; one method widely used for biosurveillance data [17] is general linear modeling (GLM), where the model may be expressed as:

$$L(y) = \beta_1 x_1 + \beta_2 x_2 + \cdots + \beta_n x_n + \varepsilon \qquad (4.15)$$

where L is a link function, and the error term ε has an assumed distribution that need not be Gaussian as assumed in ordinary least-squares regression. For example, in Poisson regression, L is a logarithm function, as in the models discussed previously, but the error distribution is assumed to be Poisson. For modeling with small-count data and with baselines of at least several months, GLM regression should be considered.

- *Autoregressive modeling.* A popular approach for forecasting time series with short-term linear trends (see Figs. 4.11 and 4.12) is to model the error term in addition to the other covariates. Chatfield warned that general ARIMA (autoregressive integrated moving average) modeling may require too much data analysis and statistical expertise for application to many types of data [18]. However, Reis and Mandl [19] investigated ARIMA modeling for biosurveillance data and found two ARMA (autoregressive moving average) models that achieved substantial forecast improvements on several syndromic hospital data streams. These models were able to adjust to data features such as the local trends that caused the obvious forecast problems for the nonadaptive model in

Fig. 4.12. These models should be considered for city-level data with counts on the scale of the examples; research is needed with authentic surveillance data to determine their usefulness on smaller data scales.

Beyond regression-based models, a number of other forecasting methods have been applied in biosurveillance. See Zhang et al. [20] for a discussion of the wavelet-based approach applied in RODS (Real-time Outbreak and Disease Surveillance) systems, and see Shmueli and Fienberg [21] for a more general discussion of wavelets and related methods. For an approach adapting LMS (Least Mean Square) filters of signal-processing technology to the forecasting of OTC sales data, see Najmi [22].

4.4.2.2 Forecasting by Generalized Exponential Smoothing.

This relatively simple approach has shown promising results. It generalizes the exponential smoothing concept to forecast time series with changing trends and cyclic effects as well as changing mean level. In industrial and financial time-series forecasting, a well-known implementation of this generalization is the Holt–Winters forecasting method [23, 24]. Along with the level L_t, the method includes two additional recursive terms, one for the trend T_t and one for a seasonal component S_t. The k-step ahead forecast is given by:

$$\hat{y}_{t+k} = (L_t + kT_t)S_{t+k-M} \qquad (4.16)$$

where M is the number of seasons in a cycle (e.g., for a monthly periodicity M=12), and L_t, T_t, and S_t are updated as follows:

$$L_t = \alpha \frac{Y_t}{S_{t-M}} + (1 - \alpha)(L_{t-1} + T_{t-1}) \qquad (4.17)$$

$$S_t = \gamma \frac{Y_t}{L_t} + (1 - \gamma)S_{t-M} \qquad (4.18)$$

$$T_t = \beta(L_t - L_{t-1}) + (1 - \beta)T_{t-1} \qquad (4.19)$$

The seasonal effects in syndromic time series are generally proportional to the level L_t, so that the relationship between S_t and L_t in these equations is multiplicative. An additive formulation is also available [25].

This method requires three smoothing constants, α, β, and γ. Note that this formulation is not a global model but an ad hoc adjustment procedure that assumes a few variation factors. The amount of ongoing adjustment for each factor is set by the smoothing constants. See Chatfield [18] for a thorough discussion of the choice of these constants. The chosen updating equations should be the simplest formulation that can capture the expected data features.

Holt–Winters forecasting requires initial values for the level, trend, and the M seasonal components. The choice of these initial values is more important than in simple exponential smoothing, especially for the cyclic behavior terms. If the cyclic behavior is consistent, and representative starting values for $c_0, c_1, \ldots, c_{M-1}$ are available, a γ value near zero may give optimal forecasts. If this behavior changes seasonally or changes fairly often as a result of artifacts in the data-acquisition chain, a larger γ value is indicated; analogous simpler guidance applies to the choice of α and β.

One forecast comparison study applied both regression models and Holt–Winters smoothing to 16 time series of daily city-level syndromic counts [26]. For the Holt–Winters implementation, the cyclic component M was set to 7 to capture the common day-of-week effects. Note that this method, like the regression method using day-of-week indicators, does not assume a particular weekly pattern but can be used for time series where weekend counts drop slightly or nearly vanish; where Saturday counts are elevated as in some OTC sales data; and where the pattern is more unusual, as in visits to clinics with fixed weekly schedules. With a positive γ value, this smoothing method can also adapt to changes in this pattern. To avoid forecasts of negative syndromic counts, a lower bound of zero was imposed for the recursively computed level L_t. To avoid zero divisors, L_t and S_t were defined as:

$$L_t = L_{t-1} + T_{t-1}, \text{ if } S_{t-M} = 0 \qquad (4.20)$$

$$S_t = S_{t-M}, \text{ if } L_t = 0. \qquad (4.21)$$

Another modification was analogous to outlier removal: the updating of the level and trend were suppressed when the forecast error was very large to avoid incorrect learning from outliers. An empirical choice for this criterion is to *update* only when the absolute forecast error is at most half the forecast value. For time series with small counts, a different criterion should be applied. This modification avoids misleading training but does not avoid large holiday forecast errors.

Figure 4.12 extends the comparison of Fig. 4.11 to traditional regression versus Holt–Winters predictions. For these data, the exponential smoothing method shows the same ability to capture local trends as the adaptive regression method but does not show the same few intervals of large errors caused by the rigid baseline. The median of the absolute errors for the Holt–Winters method was 17.5, compared with 22.6 for the traditional regression, and the corresponding median absolute percentage errors were 9.1% and 11.7%, respectively.

Table 4.2 gives a more quantitative comparison of these methods over a 350-day test interval. Recall that the forecast residual is defined as the observed value minus the forecast. Residuals from the nonadaptive and adaptive regression methods and the Holt–Winters smoothing are compared for respiratory syndrome counts for 10 cities; the column for city a gives the results for the data just discussed. For forecasts extended a full week ahead, note that even with the overall degradation in the adaptive methods, both are still superior overall to traditional regression with a long, fixed baseline. In the residual columns for city c and city j, the poor forecasts of nonadaptive regression represent situations where subsequent data behavior diverges

Table 4.2   Comparison of Predictions from Three Methods for 1 Day and 7 Days Ahead

	1-Day Ahead Residual Comparisons for 10 Respiratory Count Series										
	Forecast Method	City a	City b	City c	City d	City e	City f	City g	City h	City i	City j
Median	Nonadaptive Regression	22.6	31.7	83.1	13.3	27.3	35.6	43.9	53.7	76.7	131.1
Absolute	Adaptive Regression	20.0	29.3	25.8	16.3	27.7	22.9	28.0	47.6	68.1	39.0
Deviation	Holt-Winters	17.5	26.7	21.9	13.3	26.3	19.2	24.7	30.6	50.7	33.6
Median	Nonadaptive Regression	11.7	11.6	18.8	10.0	10.5	19.1	19.8	8.6	10.4	32.6
Absolute	Adaptive Regression	9.7	9.8	6.5	12.0	12.4	14.0	14.1	7.8	10.4	9.8
% Error	Holt-Winters	9.1	9.3	5.3	10.4	9.9	11.3	12.2	5.1	7.7	8.1
	7-Day Ahead Residual Comparisons for 10 Respiratory Count Series										
	Forecast Method	City a	City b	City c	City d	City e	City f	City g	City h	City i	City j
Median	Nonadaptive Regression	22.6	31.7	83.1	13.3	27.3	35.6	43.9	53.7	76.7	131.1
Absolute	Adaptive Regression	20.4	36.9	28.1	18.0	35.8	23.5	32.0	60.0	81.8	49.3
Deviation	Holt-Winters	21.1	28.9	26.0	15.3	28.6	22.5	24.7	39.2	63.7	35.3
Median	Nonadaptive Regression	11.7	11.6	18.8	10.0	10.5	19.1	19.8	8.6	10.4	32.6
Absolute	Adaptive Regression	11.1	11.8	7.3	15.0	14.1	15.5	16.1	9.6	12.2	13.0
% Error	Holt-Winters	9.0	9.3	6.3	12.3	11.8	13.2	12.9	6.6	9.6	10.1

sharply from the baseline. In practice, the need for refitting should be obvious soon after the start of a season showing consistent, obvious errors.

Judging from these median-based measures, which ignore the sizes of errors on all unusual days, the Holt–Winters forecasts are almost uniformly the best among the methods. However, use of the median residuals drops the effects of the 10 calendar holidays as well as the post-holiday effects from the 350-day test interval. If residuals are compared using the root-mean-squared error criterion, the inclusion of all 10 holidays degrades the Holt–Winters forecasts for most of the time series relative to the other methods, and the adaptive regression forecasts look best. A Holt–Winters treatment of calendar holidays analogous to the regression holiday indicator should be considered. The median percentage error measures, comparable in scale over the test series, averaged 16.5, 11.6, and 9.7 for the nonadaptive regression, adaptive regression, and Holt–Winters methods, respectively.

Application of Residuals for Alerting. Forecast residuals have been used for health surveillance in two ways. The first is to form a native regression detector by assuming that the residuals obey a theoretical distribution: Gaussian in ordinary least-squares regression or a preferred distribution for general linear modeling. Experience with a variety of health surveillance data streams shows that the residuals are rarely Gaussian and often have too high a variance for a Poisson distribution. A negative binomial distribution, discussed in the EWMA–Shewhart chart of suitably describes the residuals in many types of data [14]. Once such a distribution is adopted, the detector is a hypothesis test for membership in the distribution, and distribution tables may be consulted for thresholds at desired confidence levels. From the epidemiological viewpoint, such a detector tests only for 1-day data spikes.

A more general and flexible use of residuals is to incorporate them in a control chart [28]. The basic idea is to substitute the forecast for the expected value in a z-score and to scale by an estimate of the residual standard deviation:

$$z_t = (x_t - \text{forecast}_t)/\sigma_{\text{residual}} \qquad (4.22)$$

The upper confidence limit may then be the conventional 3-sigma rule, or an empirical limit may be calculated. Such a control chart may employ forecasts from regression modeling, generalized exponential smoothing, or other methods. The chart-based method may be adaptive or nonadaptive, but from the previous discussion, the use of a nonadaptive method should be accompanied with diligent inspection for the need to refit. The implementation in ESSENCE is adaptive but also automates the decision to use a regression model with daily goodness-of-fit testing with the current baseline data.

As an example of regression-based charts, Page's test [27] is a CUSUM applied to regression forecasts. Variants of X-bar, EWMA, and other chart types may be derived similarly. Brillman et al. [3] reported the plausible finding that Page's test gave better detection performance on distributed outbreak signals, while an X-bar type of chart had better sensitivity for 1-day events.

4.5   SPATIOTEMPORAL ALERTING METHODS

4.5.1   The Search for Hotspots and the Spatial Baseline

Section 4.2 described the importance of spatial information in biosurveillance data. The utility of automated surveillance for detection is to trigger investigations of possible outbreaks. Information regarding the location or extent of a possible outbreak can be extremely valuable for guiding an investigation. The concern for when and where to spend resources on investigation has stimulated research in the area of spatial cluster or *hotspot* detection, which has an extensive literature [29]. Methods intended to search for anomalous case clusters look at the data differently than the time-series methods of Section 4.4. Instead of testing for anomalous levels or patterns in a specific data stream, cluster-detection methods seek anomalies in the spatial distribution of data. Rather than baseline time-series behavior, these methods require a baseline spatial pattern in the data.

An important consideration for evaluating these methods for a given data source is how well the expected spatial data distribution can be estimated and how stable it is. This distribution is represented by a probability vector $\mathbf{p}(k)$ for subregions $k = 1$, $\ldots$, K, such that if N cases, sales, or other data items are recorded over a test period, the expected number of counts in subregion k is N $\mathbf{p}(k)$. Various methods are used to estimate this distribution:

1. If the data cover the entire monitored population and if all subregions report without bias, the set of census population estimates of the subregions may be used to derive the expected distribution. Hence, a usable estimate of $\mathbf{p}(k)$ is $c(k)/\Sigma c(k)$, where $c(k)$ is the census count for subregion k. However, for many data types, distributions are not population based. The distribution may depend on the area coverage of data providers, the locations of eligible medical plan subscribers, or unknown hospital or store catchment areas.

2. For data sets with sufficiently large counts, subregion counts may be modeled as individual time series by the methods of Section 4.4. The $c(k)$ may then be replaced by forecast values. Hierarchical modeling helps reduce the occurrence of excess clustering in subregions with few counts and/or high variance [17].

3. A popular means of estimating the vector $\mathbf{p}(k)$ is to form the sum of counts in a baseline period for each subregion. The $c(k)$ values may then be replaced by these subtotals. This approach is a simplified form of strategy 2 that can be modified depending on what is known about the data. For example, if there is a day-of-week effect and interaction between the distribution and the day of week, stratified day-of-week distributions may be used.

A driving factor in the choice of a cluster-detection approach is the quality of the spatial information in the data. Typically, electronic records are spatially sorted by address fields that denote patient or customer residence or just clinic location. Before selecting an analysis method, a system designer should ask:

- Are these address fields left blank in many records, and is there a bias in who uses them?

- Are many of the patient addresses institutional or clinic addresses?

Because of privacy and legal restrictions, this information is often limited to a five-digit zip code or postal code. If nearly all the records in the data catchment area are limited to a few postal codes, a sophisticated cluster-detection approach will not be justified.

4.5.2 Spatial Scan Statistics and Enhancements

Epidemiological interest in rapid cluster detection and localization has generated corresponding interest in scan statistics and, in particular, in the free downloadable program *SaTScan* developed by Martin Kulldorff for the National Cancer Institute [30]. The several versions have kept pace with user needs in a variety of applications; see the site bibliography for their range. The underlying concepts and application issues are discussed in Sections 4.5.2.1 and 4.5.2.2.

4.5.2.1   Scan Statistics Concept.   Assume a set of public health data records, each
of which is mapped to a subregion of a monitored region, as discussed previously.
The objective is to find the clusters of these subregions whose current record counts
are most significant relative to the rest of the region, given the expected distribution
of cases. Some definitions are required:

- *Current record counts* refers to counts within the period being tested, which
  may be a day, a week, or longer.

- Theoretically, a *most significant cluster* could be one whose counts are most
  anomalously high or low compared with expectation. SaTScan allows the user
  to look for high values, low values, or both. Most biosurveillance users restrict
  attention to anomalously high counts.

- In purely spatial scan statistics, a *cluster* is a connected set of subregions within
  the monitored region. In spatiotemporal scan statistics, a cluster may be seen as
  a three-dimensional cylinder–a set of subregions and a set of contiguous time
  intervals over which the cases occur. In most applications, the cases in the
  cylinder end at the current date, so that only *active clusters* are considered.

To find purely spatial clusters, a set of grid points is taken as possible centers of case
clusters; often, the centroids of all of the data subregions are used for this purpose.
For one of the grid points, candidate clusters are formed by testing the case counts of
each member of a family of circles centered on that point, as shown in Fig. 4.13. Such
a circle may contain a single subregion or many subregions up to a preset fraction of
the total number of cases or total region area. A likelihood ratio statistic is computed
and stored for each such circle. These statistics are then computed and stored for
families of circles centered at the other grid points as well. The most commonly used
formulation of this statistic is Kulldorff's *likelihood ratio* (LR) [31]:

$$LR(J) \equiv [O(J)/E(J)]^{O(J)} \cdot [(N - O(J))/(N - E(J))]^{(N-O(J))} \qquad (4.23)$$

where J is the set of subregions whose centroids lie in a candidate circle, $O(J)$ is the
sum of the counts observed in the subregions included in J, $E(J)$ is the sum of the
counts expected in the subregions included in J, and N is the total number of cases in
the region. The cluster J^* whose LR is largest over the sets J obtained from all grid
centers and all radii up to a fixed limit is then the maximum likelihood cluster.

For every data set and each test period monitored, a maximum likelihood cluster
may always be found, but when is this cluster statistically significant? Unfortunately,
the likelihood ratios do not satisfy a known distribution, so there is no lookup table for
significance at a given confidence level. SaTScan determines a p-value estimate for
the statistical significance of this cluster empirically by ranking the value of $LR(J^*)$
against a set of other maximum likelihood ratios. Each of these trial maxima is
calculated similarly from another sample of the N cases chosen randomly from the

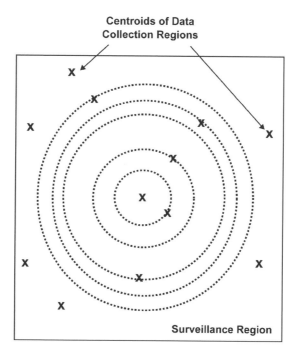

Fig. 4.13 Geometric search method for significant clusters.

expected spatial distribution. If M additional trial case distributions are chosen and tested, a p-value for the maximum observed cluster J^* is:

$$p(J^*) = \mathrm{rank}(J^*)/(M+1) \qquad (4.24)$$

In practice, the number of trials M is usually at least 999, so that the lowest possible p-value is 1/1000. The p-value is then compared with a preset significance threshold to determine significance. Experience is often required to determine an appropriate threshold for a given data type.

Following the determination of the maximal cluster, the remaining ordered likelihood ratios may be examined with the same significance test. The usual practice is to find disjoint clusters of decreasing significance by dropping clusters with subregions that belong in a more significant cluster.

The extension of this procedure to the spatiotemporal scan statistic adds the dimension of time (i.e., the number of time intervals for aggregating test cases in each candidate set of regions). In common practice, likelihood ratios for the candidate regions are stored and compared for cases from the current day, from the current and previous day, and so on, back to some limit. Because of both epidemiological and run-time constraints, this limit is typically a week at most or a small number of intervals. The Monte Carlo significance determination must also be modified for an added dimension of multiple testing bias; see Kulldorff [5] for details.

The map in Fig. 4.14 illustrates a cluster of ILI cases found using authentic clinic and physician visit data as part of a simulation in which cases attributable to a hypothetical aerosol attack were injected. The sizes of the solid circular symbols on the map correspond to case counts, and the cluster illustrates the ability of scan statistics to control for the usual spatial case distribution.

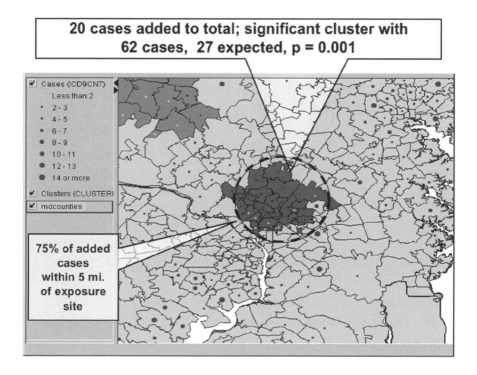

Fig. 4.14   Significant ILI cluster found in bioterrorist attack simulation, with 20 cases added to a total daily count of 739.

4.5.2.2   Scan Statistics Application.

There are practical issues to be considered in the application of SaTScan or similar cluster detection methods. First, some common data issues:

1. *Spatial data organization.* The patient or customer location in biosurveillance data is often limited to a patient residence postal code. Point-pattern methods such as SaTScan require an exact location for each subregion and, when possible, the postal code population centroid should be used. When hospital, clinic, or store locations are used to find the desired clusters, the exact addresses are usually available and can be geocoded to derive latitude and longitude coordinates.

2. *Classification bias.* Data records should be examined for classification bias across subregions. For example, recent analysis of a county data set revealed that some school nurses were using a "respiratory distress" category very broadly, whereas others used it only for asthma-related problems. If not corrected, this inconsistency would badly bias detection of spatial respiratory distress clusters. Simple histograms of data across subregions should be used to check for such problems before surveillance is implemented.

3. *Inconsistent reporting.* The consistency of data reporting should be checked for the region overall and for individual subregions. If certain clinics or other data providers report intermittently or characteristically late compared with other providers, cluster detection will be biased away from the late reporting subregions, and the clusters may reveal more about reporting practice than about disease incidence. The best solution is to correct the problem data reporting, but it is often more feasible to omit the problem subregions from the analysis. See Kulldorff [32] for a fuller discussion.

Surveillance system designers should also consider the population and data distributions, the subregion shapes, and the epidemiology of diseases of interest in decisions affecting the clusters of interest:

1. *Noncircular clusters.* Several factors may suggest that likely geographic disease clusters may be elongated in one direction or even disconnected. For example, in a coastal city, the population may be heavily concentrated near the water and increasingly sparse inland. Therefore, residences in a large school district may be concentrated along a main highway. In such situations, a search for circular clusters is not optimal. SaTScan has an option to seek elliptical clusters, and other approaches have been developed for clustering of arbitrary shapes. However, such enhancements impose a cost in computation time–computation time for the elliptical option is proportional to the number of aspect ratios and orientations to be considered–and this cost must be included in system design. For the capability to test for disconnected or multiple clusters, designers should consider the p-value threshold and the number of secondary clusters to present to health monitors.

2. *Selection of the test period.* When purely spatial scan statistics are used, the choice of test period is important. If the emphasis in on single-day clusters, the analysis should be applied only to data that are usually available within a day. Although the recent emphasis in outbreak detection has been on early detection, longer test periods of 3–4 days or a week give more stable results, and this trade-off should be weighed in system design. Spatiotemporal scan statistics are used to seek clusters of varying duration, and one must decide how far back to look. A practical problem is that an extremely unusual case distribution recorded 6 days ago may cause a week-long cluster to appear more significant than a current-day event of interest. Again, there is a trade-off between comprehensive monitoring and efficiency.

4.5.3 Global Clustering Methods and Adaptations

Scan statistics are popular in part because they can be used to determine both the location and the extent of clusters of interest. There is also a large literature of methods for determining global clustering, some of which make more detailed use of spatial information and the matrix of distances between subregions than do scan statistics. These methods are usually applied to historical data sets to test the null hypothesis of no clustering. Recent research efforts have attempted to adapt and, in some studies, localize these methods for prospective surveillance. A few of these adaptations are cited here:

1. If **p** is the vector of expected spatial probabilities (as in Section 4.5.2) and **r** is the corresponding vector of spatial proportions observed, Tango's measure [33] of the clustering of a data set is

$$C_G = (\mathbf{r} - \mathbf{p})^t \mathbf{A}(\mathbf{r} - \mathbf{p}) \qquad (4.25)$$

   where the matrix **A** is obtained by applying an exponential kernel to the distance matrix for a damping constant τ:

$$a_{kj} = \exp(-d_{kj}/\tau) \text{ if } k \neq j; a_{jj} = 1 \qquad (4.26)$$

   and d_{kj} is the distance between subregions k and j. Rogerson presented a cumulative sum statistic based on this measure for early cluster detection and applied it in a prospective fashion [34].

2. Drawing on a large data set of patient records containin g anexact patient address, Olson et al. [35] used the distance matrix (d_{kj}) intensively by sorting all pairwise distances between record residences into a discrete set of bins. They then applied the M-point statistic to form a prospective test for an anomalous distribution of paired-distance counts in these bins. The M-statistic is an algebraic expression similar to Tango's statistic, with the matrix **A** replaced by the variance–covariance matrix **M** of the bin proportions calculated for a large baseline period. This statistic helps to control for the variability within the distribution of distances. The authors applied the method to several years of hospital data with simulated outbreaks of various spatial concentration, with promising results. Efforts are ongoing to identify local disease clusters based on this approach.

3. The Knox test for space–time interaction was applied by Theophilides et al. to use a database of reported dead bird locations as a sentinel for human cases of West Nile virus [36]. Because ertain mosquito species function as vectors for this virus and carry it between human and avian hosts, timely knowledge of the spread of the virus can guide strategies for mosquito control. Among localization methods for global clustering statistics, this one is noteworthy because it used the ecology of the mosquito vector to choose temporal and

spatial grid limits, and the statistic was applied in each grid cell. The clusters identified were significantly associated with the regions where human cases occurred.

4.6   METHODS CONSIDERING MULTIPLE DATA SOURCES

4.6.1   Decision Making with Multiple Data Sources

The growing availability of data streams for biosurveillance requires corresponding growth in the methodology to analyze them. Both full- and part-time monitors examine these data on a daily basis at state and local health departments. Investigation of statistical anomalies beyond the database level is labor intensive and time consuming. A multiplicity of data sources is appealing because a combination of evidence types suggests additional sensitivity and corroboration for a prospective outbreak with enhanced characterization of the spatial and temporal spread of disease, more accurate identification of the population at risk, and an improved capability to specify effective interventions.

In practice, however, multiple data sources can give contradictory findings. Figure 4.15 shows time-series plots of syndromic data taken from a large Maryland county leading into the influenza season of 2004. The data sources represented are counts of respiratory diagnoses from visits to civilian physician offices, military clinic visits, hospital emergency departments, and sales of related OTC remedies. Retrospectively, there is a sharp rise in respiratory illness, confirmed by positive laboratory influenza tests, beginning in late November 2003. Public health status in the preceding weeks is less clear. The September increase in OTC sales and in civilian office visits is not reflected in the other data streams. Sporadic influenza cases were documented in October and early November, but the plot shows only gradual increases in the clinical data streams for those weeks. The dilemma of the prospective data monitor is when and how extensively to investigate and when to issue alarms. Unambiguous, corroborated data spikes are the exception rather than the rule. For single data streams, univariate algorithms can use data modeling and hypothesis tests to provide systematic alerting protocols. In the multivariate data environment, the statistical decision requirements of the data monitor include which combinations of data sources to test, which algorithms to use according to the correlation characteristics of the data background, how to achieve distributed sensitivity over many locations with manageable alert rates, and how much corroboration among data streams is required for a credible alert. The remainder of this section describe an approach for adapting multivariate testing methodologies from other disciplines to meet these requirements.

In a classical hypothesis test, values of an observed quantity are treated as realizations of a random variable, and the null hypothesis is that this variable satisfies an assumed distribution. A test statistic is computed from the observed values. The mean or some other property of the assumed distribution is used to calculate the probability, or p-value, that randomly chosen values are at least as unlikely as those observed. The

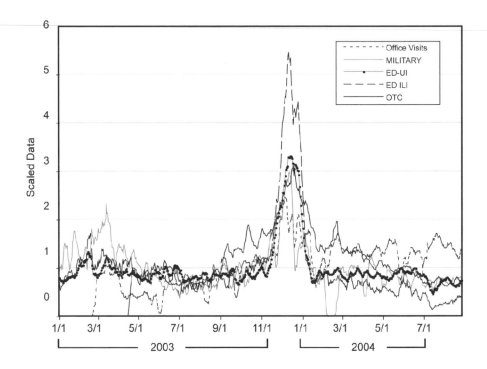

Fig. 4.15   Scaled daily data from multiple sources during influenza season in a large county.

null hypothesis is rejected if this p-value falls below a predetermined threshold α. In the biosurveillance context, the null hypothesis is an assumed data distribution in the absence of a disease outbreak affecting the data streams monitored. An alert is issued if the null hypothesis is rejected. However, an outbreak is not a necessary condition but only one possible cause for an alert. Other possible causes include changes or errors in diagnosis coding, increases in participating data providers, and database problems. However, if a single data stream represents the care-seeking behavior of the monitored population for a given syndrome group, an outbreak may be a sufficient condition for an alert. Thus, alerts may be used to focus the attention of health monitors on potential outbreaks if they occur at a reasonable rate. The question is how to extend hypothesis testing to the multisource, distributed surveillance context.

Two prototype monitoring problems are considered for the multivariate context [37]. The *parallel monitoring problem* pertains to time series representing distributed locations, such as counties or treatment facilities, possibly stratified by other covariates, such as syndrome type or age group. The statistical challenge is to maintain sensitivity while limiting the number of alerts arising from testing the resulting time series. The second problem, the *consensus monitoring problem*, entails testing a single hypothesis using multiple sources of evidence. For example, the combination of syndromic counts of emergency department visits, outpatient clinic office appointments, and sales of OTC remedies may be used to test the hypothesis that there is no current outbreak of gastrointestinal disease in the monitored population.

4.6.1.1 The Parallel Monitoring Problem.

Multiple testing can lead to uncontrolled alert rates as the number of data streams increases. For example, suppose that a hypothesis test is conducted on a time series of daily diagnoses of influenza-like illness. In a one-sided test, this test results in a statistic whose value in some distribution yields a probability p that the current count is as large as observed. For a desired type I error probability of α, the probability is then $1 - \alpha$ that an alert will not occur in the distribution assumed for background data. Thus, for the parallel monitoring problem of interest here, if such tests are applied to n independent data streams, the probability that no background alerts occur is $(1 - \alpha)^n$, which decreases quickly for practical error rates α. For a single-test error rate of $\alpha = 0.05$, for example, the probability of at least one background alert exceeds 0.5 if more than 13 independent tests are applied.

A common method of controlling this multiple testing problem is to replace the probability threshold α with the Bonferroni bound α/N, where N is the number of monitored data streams. The resulting criterion is sufficient but usually not necessary to ensure an overall type I error rate of at most α, and it often results in an increased type II error, or loss of sensitivity. Several published modifications of the Bonferroni procedure maintain the error rate of α with less stringent rejection criteria. Let $P_{(1)}$, ..., $P_{(N)}$ be the p-values sorted in ascending order. Hommel's method [38] was to reject the combined null hypothesis if for any j, $j = 1, \ldots, N$:

$$P_{(j)} < j \cdot \alpha/C \cdot N \qquad (4.27)$$

where $C = \Sigma 1/j$.

This criterion gives an overall error rate of α or $C = 1$ if the tests are independent and this relaxed Simes criterion has been shown to maintain this error rate for many common multivariate data sets with positive correlation [39]. These improvements gained wide application when it was shown that they control the false discovery rate (FDR) or expected ratio of false alerts to the total alert count [40]. For example, FDR methods have been used to monitor CUSUM results of hospital data streams from numerous districts in the National Health Service of the United Kingdom [41]. For a large number of data streams and a well-defined signal, Bonferroni modifications may improve detection performance significantly. However, for a relatively small number of data streams–say a few dozen counties or treatment facilities–these criteria differ little in practice from the pure Bonferroni bound unless the data are highly correlated. The combination methods control the increase in alert rates with the number of data streams, and for nearly independent streams, Simes-based alert rates are only slightly above the Bonferroni-based rates. This difference grows as additional data streams are added, as the correlation among them increases, and as the alerting threshold α is raised. These factors should be considered in the choice of a parallel monitoring method intended to control alert rates.

Several practical considerations should be noted regarding the Simes method. In view of the sorting, only those p-values that are below the nominal threshold α affect the result. There is no consensus effect (see Section 4.6.1.2)–the method applied to 10 p-values of 0.06 returns 0.06. The Simes criterion does not specify which of the data streams is anomalous; a popular procedure is to reject the null hypothesis for all streams with p-values below the largest one that satisfies the Simes method inequality.

4.6.1.2   The Consensus Monitoring Problem.

Multiple Univariate Consensus Monitoring Methods. The multiple univariate methods resemble those of Section 4.6.1.1 except that the p-values are combined to produce a single p-value $p^* = f(p_1, \ldots, p_n)$ with the consensus property that several near-critical values can produce a critical value. Many such functions are possible; two methods are considered here, adapted from use in independent, sequential clinical trials. The first is *Fisher's rule* [42], a function of the product of the p-values. The statistic is:

$$F = 2 \sum_j \ln(p_j) \tag{4.28}$$

For independent tests, values of this quantity form a χ^2 distribution with $2n$ degrees of freedom. As a multiplicative method, it is more sensitive to a few small p-values than to a broader number of moderate values. It is recommended if the objective is to extract a single decision on whether to reject the overall null hypothesis and to avoid considering the individual p_j.

An alternative combination statistic is *Edgington's method* [43]. This additive method is more sensitive to multiple near-critical values. For more than a few dozen data streams, this formula cannot be computed accurately. In such cases, the expression:

$$[\text{mean}(p) - 0.5]/(0.2887/\sqrt{n}) \tag{4.29}$$

gives a z-score whose Gaussian probability is a close approximation to this formula [44].

If the data streams are independent, Edgington's method gives fewer alerts than Fisher's at nominal thresholds, but is more sensitive to data correlation. Edgington's method is recommended if the number of data streams is modest — say, less than a dozen — and the user wishes a sensitive consensus indicator in addition to the individual test results. The desire for such an indicator has been expressed by epidemiologist users of the ESSENCE biosurveillance systems and is common among large system users who require some summarization but are skeptical of bottom-line results that hide the contributions of individual sources of evidence. In experiments with syndromic data collections, both the Fisher and Edgington methods control the alert rate growth with the number of data streams. Edgington's method gives smaller alert rates if the data streams are independent, and most of the alerts found with Fisher's method are also individual stream alerts. However, the alert rate produced by the Edgington method grows quickly with the number of data streams if they are correlated. Furthermore, very small single p-values do not necessarily cause alerts in the additive Edgington, so if the system is not also monitoring single streams, the use of Fisher's method or both methods is recommended.

Multivariate Statistical Process Control Charts. Alerting algorithms that combine values from separate time series in a single computation have the potential to detect distributed faint outbreak evidence that may be lost in individual hypothesis tests. Although strong correlation among data sources tends to dilute the benefit of FDR-like methods, prospective multivariate algorithms can exploit consistent correlation. Published work on multivariate methods, based on weekly data from large regions, has focused on multivariate statistical process control (MSPC) because of the long usage of control charts for hospital surveillance. Little published research deals with more complex multivariate hypothesis tests based on wavelets, Bayesian statistics, etc., partly because of the lack of availability of health surveillance data. Most MSPC methods are based on Hotelling's T^2 as applied in monitoring efforts in related fields [45]. The T^2 statistic may be written as:

$$(X - \mu)^T \mathbf{S}^{-1}(X - \mu) \tag{4.30}$$

where X is the multivariate data from the test interval, μ is the vector mean estimated from the baseline interval, and S is an estimate of the covariance matrix calculated from the baseline interval.

Although Hotelling's T^2 may be viewed as a multidimensional z-score, this method has been generalized to obtain other multivariate control charts. A multivariate EWMA chart (MEWMA) has shown improved run-length characteristics and has yielded promising results with health surveillance data [46]. In Lowry's MEWMA, the data vector is replaced by the exponentially weighted moving average:

$$\mathbf{Z}_j = \mathbf{RX} + (1 - \mathbf{R})\mathbf{Z}_{j-1} \tag{4.31}$$

where $\mathbf{R}$ is a diagonal matrix of smoothing coefficients, and the covariance matrix is a scalar multiple of the data covariance matrix $\mathbf{S}$ in the usual application where equal smoothing coefficients are used. Analogous multivariate CUSUMs have also been applied to surveillance data, with Pignatiello's MCUSUM applied to yearly spatially distributed counts of breast cancer incidence [47]. While the attraction of these multivariate methods is their signal sensitivity, they are also sensitive to noise background changes. Rogerson notes that combined univariate methods are directional in that they may be quick to detect shifts in just a few data sources but less sensitive to shifts in more general directions [47]. These methods are omnidirectional–a property that can be useful in detecting an earlier signal but can also cause false alerts if there is a change in the covariance matrix that is irrelevant to any outbreak signal of interest. Figure 4.16 illustrates this problem with applications of three MSPC methods — Hotelling's T^2 [4], Lowry's MEWMA [48], and Crosier's MCUSUM [49] — to two syndromic time series that are highly correlated. The spikes in the algorithm outputs are in general agreement and are plausible alerts except for the sharp spikes seen for

August 7, which are purely the result of a change in day-of-week behavior for one of the two data streams. For practical monitoring to take advantage of the added sensitivity of these MSPC methods, robust methods must be developed and proven to avoid irrelevant alerts.

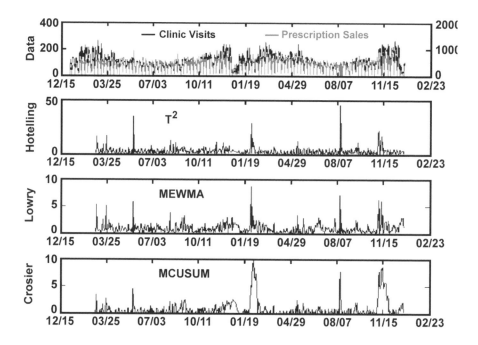

Fig. 4.16 Application of multiple statistical process control-based methods to two correlated data streams.

4.7   STUDY QUESTIONS

4.1 A major question in the design and implementation of any automated surveillance systems is how much to trust the system with decision making. Few public
health officials would initiate an investigation based solely on indications from
a "black-box" algorithm suite. On the other hand, the coordination of many data
sources can be highly labor intensive. *Q: What do you see as the required role
of the man-in-the-loop in the operation of a surveillance system? How should
algorithmic alerts be used in routine monitoring? What data visualization tools
would be important for verification?*

4.2 *Q: Aside from pure count or proportion levels, what covariate distributions or
other quantities could be monitored (certain age groups, demographic groups,
clinics, etc.)? As the number of quantities to monitor increases, so does the*

chance of a random alert. What are some schemes for combining results from these quantities to reduce the number of algorithm outputs that must be weighed?

4.3 A concern for the utility of health surveillance systems is the effect of media reports and rumors on consumer and patient behavior. Such effects could change background data levels drastically. *Q: Would time series of counts or proportions be more robust to such effects? For what syndrome groups and other data aggregation strategies would you expect the use of proportions to be effective? What other alerting methods might be less sensitive to changes in mass health care-seeking behavior?*

4.4 *Q: For each of the control charts discussed, give a type of data signal for which the chart would be an optimal detector. For each of these signals, can you hypothesize a public health event and/or data collection feature that would result in such a signal? As a health department assigned definite surveillance objectives, how would you devise a minimal set of detectors to get sensitivity to all outbreak types of interest?*

4.5 *Q: What data sources would lend themselves to the effective use of spatiotemporal scan statistics? What would be an obstacle to using scan statistics to detect the start of the influenza season in a large city with complex commuter patterns? For this situation, what data features or data filtering strategies might make scan statistics more useful?*

4.6 *Q: If multiple data sources divided into syndrome groups are available, how could the knowledge of disease symptomatology reduce the number of data stream combinations to test? What visualization methods could be used to make the monitoring of many data combinations understandable to a skilled user? How should nonclinical data sources such as work or school absenteeism be combined with clinical data for decision making?*

REFERENCES

1. Gordis L. Epidemiology. 2nd ed. Philadelphia, PA: WB Saunders; 2000.

2. Stroup DF, Wharton M, Kafadar K, Dean AG. Evaluation of a method for detecting aberrations in public health surveillance data. Am J Epidemiol. 1993; 137: 373-379.

3. Brillman JC, Burr T, Forslund D, Joyce E, Picard R, Umland E. Modeling emergency department visit patterns for infectious disease complaints: results and application to disease surveillance. BMC Med Inf Decision Making. 2005; 5(4): 1-14. Available at http://www.biomedcentral.com/content/pdf/1472-6947-5-4.pdf.

4. Ryan TP. Statistical Methods for Quality Improvement. New York: Wiley; 1989.

5. Kulldorff M. Prospective time-periodic geographical disease surveillance using scan statistic. J R Stat Soc. 2001; A164: 61-72.

6. Brookmeyer R, Gail MH. AIDS Epidemiology: A Quantitative Approach. New York: Oxford University Press; 1994, Chap 7.

7. Taubenberger JK, Morens DM. 1918 influenza: the mother of all pandemics. Emerg Infect Dis. January 2006; Available at http://www.cdc.gov/ncidod/EID/vol12no01/05-0979.htm.

8. Sartwell, PE. The distribution of incubation periods of infectious disease. Am J Hyg. 1950; 51: 310–318.

9. US Army Medical Research Institute of Infectious Diseases. Medical management of biological casualties. Fort Detrick, MD; Sepember 2000.

10. Benneyan JC. Statistical quality control methods in infection control and hospital epidemiology, infection and hospital epidemiology. Part I: Introduction and basic theory; Part II: Chart use, statistical properties, and research issues. Infect Control Hosp Epidemiol. 1998; 19(3): 194-214.

11. Woodall WH. The use of control charts in health care monitoring and public health surveillance. J Qual Technol. 2006; 38(V2): 89-104.

12. Lucas JM, Crosier RB. Fast initial response for CUSUM quality control schemes: give your CUSUM a head start. Technometrics. 1982; 24: 199-205.

13. Hutwagner LC. The bioterrorism preparedness and response Early Aberration Reporting System (EARS). J Urban Health. 2003; 80: i89-i96.

14. Morton AP, Whitby M, McLaws M-L, et al. The application of statistical process control charts to the detection and monitoring of hospital-acquired infections. J Qual Clin Pract. 2001; 21: 112-117.

15. Serfling RE. Methods for current statistical analysis of excess pneumonia–influenza deaths. Public Health Rep. 1963; 78: 494-506.

16. Burkom HS. Development, adaptation, and assessment of alerting algorithms for biosurveillance. Johns Hopkins APL Tech Dig. 2003; 24(4): 335-342.

17. Kleinman K, Lazarus R, Platt R. A generalized linear mixed models approach for detecting incident clusters of disease in small areas, with an application to biological terrorism. Am J Epidemiol. 2004; 159: 217-24.

18. Chatfield C. The Holt–Winters forecasting procedure. Appl Stat. 1978; 27: 264-279.

19. Reis BY, Mandl KD. Time series modeling for syndromic surveillance. BMC Med Inf Decision Making. 2003; 3:2.

20. Zhang J, Tsui FC, Wagner MM, Hogan WR. Detection of outbreaks from time series data using wavelet transform. AMIA Annu Symp Proc. 2003:748-752.

21. Shmueli G, Fienberg SE. Current and potential statistical methods for monitoring multiple data streams for bio-surveillance. In: Wilson A, Olwell D, eds. Statistical Methods in Counter-terrorism. New York: Springer; 2006: in press.

22. Najmi AH. Estimation of hospital emergency room data using OTC pharmaceutical sales using normalized LMS filters. In: Proceedings of the 7th International Conference on Signal Processing, ICSP'04; Beijing, China, August 31 – September 4, 2004. Beijing.

23. Holt CC. Forecasting seasonals and trends by exponentially weighted averages. ONR Memorandum 52/1957. Carnegie Institute of Technology, 1957.

24. Winters PR. Forecasting sales by exponentially weighted moving averages. Manage Sci. 1960;6:324 - 342.

25. Chatfield C, Yar M. Holt–Winters forecasting: some practical issues. Statistician. 1988;37:129 - 140.

26. Burkom HS, Murphy SP, Shmueli G. Automated time series forecasting for bio-surveillance. Stat Med. 2006;submitted.

27. Page ES. Continuous inspection schemes. Biometrika. 1954;41:10 - 115.

28. Mandel BH. The regression control chart. J Qual Technol. 1969;1(1):1 -9.

29. Patil GP, Taillie C. Upper level set scan statistic for detecting arbitrarily shaped hotspots. Environl and Ecol Stat. 2004; 11: 183 -197.

30. Kulldorff M. SaTScan v4.0: Software for the Spatial and Space-Time Scan Statistics. Information Management Services, Inc. 2004. Available at http://www.satscan.org/.

31. Kulldorff M. 1999. A spatial scan statistic. Commun Stat.–Theory Methods. 1999; 26: 1481 - 1496.

32. Kulldorff M, Heffernan R, Hartman J, Assunção R, Mostashari F. A space–time permutation scan statistic for disease outbreak detection. PLoS Med. 2005; 2(3): e59. Available at http://medicine.plosjournals.org.

33. Tango T. A class of tests for detecting 'general' and 'focused' clustering of rare diseases. Stat. Med. 1995; 14: 2323 - 2334.

34. Rogerson PA. Surveillance systems for monitoring the development of spatial patterns. Stat Med. 1997;16:2081 - 2093.

35. Olson KL, Bonetti M, Pagano M, Mandl KD. Real time spatial cluster detection using interpoint distances among precise patient locations. BMC Med Inf Decision Making. 2005;5(1):19 -30.

36. Theophilides CN, Ahearn SC, Grady S, Merlino M. Identifying West Nile virus risk areas: the dynamic continuous-area space-time system. Am J Epidemiol. 2003;157:843 - 854.

37. Burkom HS, Elbert, YA. Feldman A, Lin J. Role of data aggregation in biosurveillance detection strategies with applications from the Electronic Surveillance System for the Early Notification of Community-based Epidemics. MMWR. 2004;53(SU01):67 - 73.

38. Hommel G. A stagewise rejective multiple test procedure based on a modified Bonferroni test. Biometrika. 1988;75:383 - 386.

39. Simes RJ. An improved Bonferroni procedure for multiple tests of significance. Biometrika 1986;73:751 - 754.

40. Benjamini Y, Hochberg Y. Controlling the false discovery rate: a practical and powerful approach to multiple testing. J R Statl Soc B. 1995;57:289 - 300.

41. Marshall C, Best N, Bottle A, Aylin P. Statistical issues in prospective monitoring of health outcomes across multiple units. J R Stat Soc A. 2004;167(pt 3):541 - 559.

42. Bauer P, Kohne K. Evaluation of experiments with adaptive interim analyses. Biometrics. 1994;50:1029 -1041.

43. Edgington ES. An additive method for combining probability values from independent experiments. J Psychol. 1972;80:351 - 363.

44. Edgington ES. A normal curve method for combining probability values from independent experiments. J Psychol. 1972;82:85 - 89.

45. Ye N, Cheng Q, Emran S, Vilbert S. Hotelling's T^2 multivariate profiling for anomaly detection. In: Proceedings of the 2000 IEEE Workshop on Information Assurance and Security, West Point, NY, June 2002.

46. Hong B, Hardin M. A study of the properties of the multivariate forecast-based processing scheme. Presented at the Joint Statistical Meetings, Toronto, August 2004.

47. Rogerson PA, Yamada I. Monitoring change in spatial patterns of disease: comparing univariate and multivariate cumulative sum approaches. Stat in Med. 2004;23(14):2195 - 2214.

48. Lowry CA, Woodall WH. A multivariate exponentially weighted moving average control chart. Technometrics. 1992;34(1):46 - 53.

49. Crosier RB. Multivariate generalizations of cumulative sum quality-control schemes. Technometrics. 1988;30(3):291 - 303.

5 Putting It Together: The Biosurveillance Information System

Logan Hauenstein, Richard Wojcik, Wayne Loschen, Raj Ashar, Carol Sniegoski, Nathaniel Tabernero

Chapter 4 examined analytic processes that can be applied to data streams that are acquired and archived automatically for disease surveillance. It included a survey of algorithms chosen based on the characteristics of the data and the performance metrics required to achieve timely recognition of abnormalities.

This chapter describes the processes and tools needed to present data and information to the users of the surveillance system. The chapter begins with a discussion of the various system architectures and how they influence the operation and scalability of a surveillance system. Web-based applications are discussed because they permit easy access to a system, which is important for usability. Also addressed are approaches to grouping data into syndromes and parsing free text into a structured format for use in the analytic processes (described in Chapter 4). Visualization techniques for conveying large amounts of data to users and interfaces that permit users to customize a system are described. The chapter ends with a discussion of skills needed to operate and maintain a surveillance system. The chapter is arranged so that readers can skip directly to topics of interest if they do not want to read the entire chapter.

5.1 INTRODUCTION

Chapter 3 introduced a few of the fundamental technologies commonly used to build data-driven surveillance applications. This chapter expands on these concepts and provides practical considerations for building disease surveillance systems. It also introduces some important Information Technology (IT) tools and technical information that is useful in the planning and decision-making process.

The cornerstone of a robust and effective electronic information system is a carefully designed architecture that meets the needs of its users for reliability, performance, and usability and the requirements of the development team for cost, scalability, security, and maintainability. Decisions made early in the design process will have a significant impact on the future of the system.

One of the first issues to consider when building an information system is the software architecture. A system's software architecture provides a plan that separates the system into logical parts and defines the relationships between those parts. Subtle differences between various architecture choices can greatly affect how the system is used and how it performs under different conditions.

Designing the software architecture for an information system is much like designing the architecture for a house. Many decisions must be made along the way, and these small choices dictate many aspects of how the resulting system is used. Figure 5.1 shows two example architectures: a client-server architecture that enables a system to share data simultaneously with multiple clients, and a simple stand-alone system that limits data access to a single user.

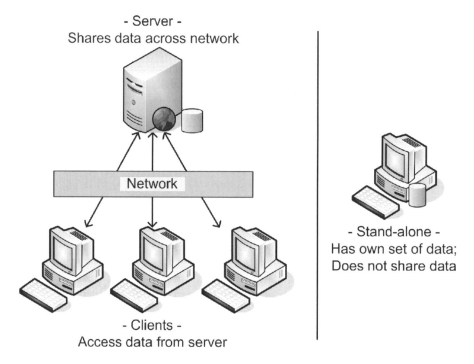

Fig. 5.1   A client-server architecture shares data with its clients; a stand-alone system stores its own data.

Software architecture choices will affect the cost, scalability, performance, and maintainability of the overall system. A web-based system could potentially use several web servers and several database servers to help handle very high volumes of user traffic, but the startup and system maintenance costs will be high. On the other hand, a stand-alone system would be comparatively easy to maintain.

After a general software architecture direction is chosen, decisions must be made about computer hardware and software. In many cases the selection of hardware and software may be constrained by budget and an organization's IT system configuration and maintenance policies. Designing systems to meet the project's goals within these constraints can be challenging. Inappropriate choices can affect the system's overall performance adversely.

Documents on the World Wide Web evolved from a simple set of unchanging interlinked pages into today's dynamic, interactive, widespread, and interconnected collection of sites. The universal connectivity provided by the Internet, combined with the ease of data exchange provided by web applications, has fundamentally changed the ways in which we share data. Because of this flexibility, many current disease surveillance systems use web applications to access information for their users.

Mapping software makes it possible to situate certain types of data into a geographical context, providing additional insights about the data collected. Geographers and software engineers have collaborated to produce tools that make it easier to combine geographical data from a multitude of sources and display the results in interactive maps.

When combined, web-based, mapping and other technologies enable the development of powerful disease surveillance systems.

5.2 SYSTEM ARCHITECTURES FOR DISEASE SURVEILLANCE

Disease surveillance systems contain three major components, corresponding to the functional areas of the system: ingestion, detection, and visualization. Ingestion is responsible for reading in the data from the data providers; detection runs anomaly detection algorithms on the health data; and visualization enables a user to interact with the system through data querying, graphing, and geographic map displays.

The architecture of the system defines how these components operate and interact with each other and the user of the system. Several types of system architecture designs can be used to implement a disease surveillance system, ranging from a single-user stand-alone application to a multiuser client-server application. Ultimately, the architecture implemented is defined by the amount and frequency of the data ingested into the system, the computational requirements of the detection algorithms, the availability of data to the end user, and the budget. Sections 5.2.1 through 5.2.3 cover some common architecture design concepts and their impact on the development of a disease surveillance system.

5.2.1 Stand-Alone System Application Design

Before the explosion of the Internet and web applications, most applications were designed to execute on stand-alone systems. Although such a system may be connected to a network, all data input, algorithm processing, and user interaction takes place on a single computer. Commonly, this design requires user intervention to input data and start the analysis algorithms. This design is usually intended for applications that accommodate one user at a time and are developed for a specific operating system, such as Microsoft Windows or Unix variants. Examples of stand-alone system applications are a desktop word processor or spreadsheet. A disease surveillance application that can be considered a stand-alone application is the CDC's early aberration reporting system (EARS) surveillance application [1].

The benefit of this type of design is that all the functional components of the application reside on one computer, making the application easier to install. In most cases, the cost to maintain the application is usually low for the user. However, new releases to the application can be difficult to distribute and install.

The decision to deploy a stand-alone application depends primarily on the budget available to implement and operate the disease surveillance system. For a modest-sized public health jurisdiction, a stand-alone application may be sufficient or appropriate for the amount of data that it receives, processes, and monitors.

5.2.2 Thick Client vs. Thin Client Application Design for client-server Architectures

Client-server architectures separate the system into two components, the client and the server. The client communicates with the server over a network connection. All user interactions with the server application are performed through a client program residing on the user's computer. The server commonly stores the data needed by the client in a central repository, processes data requests by the client, and returns data to the client. Other server-side functions, such as data gathering, ingestion, and detection, are performed by applications that operate behind the scenes. This architecture is usually implemented to accommodate multiple clients or users simultaneously. The primary benefit of this architecture is increased performance and reduced system response time because the processing load is distributed across multiple computers.

For client-server applications, the user interacts with the system through a client program. The client may be deployed as a thick desktop application or a thin (often web-based) application. A thick desktop client is similar to a stand-alone application in that it relies on the user's computer resources to perform analysis and processing. However, thick clients still rely on the server for the bulk of their data storage. An example of a thick client desktop application is an e-mail application such as Microsoft Outlook. Thick clients typically are more complex and allow developers tighter control over the application, enabling the developer to deploy a more customized and richer user interface than with a thin client. However, the tighter control usually requires longer development time because of the increased code complexity and imposes higher performance requirements on the user's computer. In many cases, thick clients are distributed through a one-time download from a server and installed on the user's computer. Ensuring that users are using the latest version of the user interface may be problematic. A common method used to address this issue is to prompt the user to update the application through a built-in update feature or by manual retrieval and installation of the application when a new version of the client becomes available.

Users access thin client applications using a tool such as a web browser. An online search engine is an example of a thin client application. Although the web browser itself is a thick client, the actual web application accessed through the web browser, i.e., the user interface to the search engine, is considered a thin client. Thin web client applications use minimal processor and data storage resources on the user's computer. The majority of the application logic resides on the server, as does most, if not all, data processing. The client is used primarily for visualization of the data. Thin clients are typically easily installed and maintained on the user's computer. In the case of a web browser client, the code to control the user interface is downloaded from the server every time the server is accessed, which guarantees that users are accessing the latest version of the user interface. The underlying design benefit of deploying a thin client is that the application usually places loose or minimal performance requirements on the user's computer to perform its function. It assumes that users will have varying hardware capabilities.

In the past, only stand-alone and thick client applications could provide content-rich user interfaces. Now, thin client applications can produce equally rich user interfaces by using advanced web-based technologies such as the Document Object Model (DOM) [2], JavaScript, and Asynchronous JavaScript and eXtensible Markup Language (AJAX) [3, 4]. These technologies allow both thick and thin clients to implement maps, graphs, and other useful user interface components with the same functionality and interactivity as stand-alone desktop applications.

Aside from budget, which is always of concern to public health jurisdictions, the decision to deploy a client-server system application depends primarily on the number of simultaneous users that it needs to reach. Large jurisdictions with multiple users will probably choose to implement a client-server system.

5.2.3   Three-Tier and Multitier Architectures

Client-server systems are commonly implemented as a three-tier architecture (Fig. 5.2) where the functions of the client-server are defined in three separate tiers or layers: presentation, business logic, and data [5]. These layers exist as separate software modules and are often installed on separate servers.

The three disease surveillance functions discussed earlier fit into these three tiers. The top tier corresponds to the visualization or presentation layer, detection fits into the logic tier, and ingestion fits into the data tier.

One of the benefits of this architecture is that each layer may be upgraded or replaced independently. For example, if a new detection algorithm is developed, only the detection layer and the detection server are affected. Or, if new ingestion methods are developed, only the ingestion layer and ingestion server are affected. Assigning each layer to a separate server distributes the processing load, increasing performance and system response.

Client-server systems are not limited to three tiers. The architecture may be further segmented into additional tiers to form an *n*-tier system. Additional tiers or servers may need to be added to increase security, isolate computationally intensive functions,

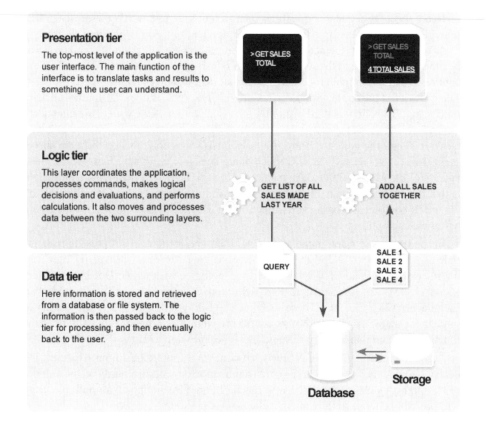

Presentation tier

The top-most level of the application is the user interface. The main function of the interface is to translate tasks and results to something the user can understand.

> GET SALES TOTAL

> GET SALES TOTAL

4 TOTAL SALES

Logic tier

This layer coordinates the application, processes commands, makes logical decisions and evaluations, and performs calculations. It also moves and processes data between the two surrounding layers.

GET LIST OF ALL SALES MADE LAST YEAR

ADD ALL SALES TOGETHER

Data tier

Here information is stored and retrieved from a database or file system. The information is then passed back to the logic tier for processing, and then eventually back to the user.

QUERY

SALE 1
SALE 2
SALE 3
SALE 4

Storage

Database

Fig. 5.2   Three-tier architecture (*Source:* Wikipedia).

and increase performance. For example, the data tier usually maintains a database as a data repository. However, it may be necessary to split the database into multiple databases, such as when a disease surveillance system is collecting patient-identifiable information as part of its data stream. Because of privacy or confidentiality policies, the patient-identifiable information may be required to be stored in a database that is physically separate from the web-accessible database. The system would use network firewalls to prevent unauthorized users from gaining inappropriate access to the sensitive data.

Another important reason to separate the databases in the data layer is to optimize performance. In many cases, detection algorithms can consume most of a server's processing resources. It is likely the algorithms will retrieve and process data from a database. If the same database is used by the user interface, the interface may be adversely affected every time a detection algorithm is run. Ideally the detection and user interface layers will access their own independent database in order to solve this problem.

Partitioning the database into different layers also results in greater independence between the application layers. For example, consider a disease surveillance system in which the data ingestion server is unavailable because of maintenance. If the data ingestion server contains the same database that is used for the user interface, the user interface will be inoperable. However, if the data layer is split to create a database specifically for the user interface, the user interface could remain operational during the maintenance.

5.3 DATABASES

Nearly all disease surveillance systems include one or more database servers as part of their overall architecture. In Chapter 3, fundamental concepts relevant to databases were discussed. This section introduces high-level database design considerations, along with practical issues concerning database hardware and software choices.

5.3.1 Database Design

Hundreds of books have been devoted entirely to database design considerations. The primary concern with the design of a relational database is the degree of normalization. *Normalization* is the process of organizing data and breaking it into smaller tables that are easier to manage. The primary reason to normalize a database is to prevent redundant data.

A database design can achieve a number of different levels of normalization. At the lowest level, pieces of data are defined in multiple places in the database. For example, imagine that a company with a partly normalized database stores copies of a customer's current billing address in two tables: CustomerInfo and BillingInfo. When a customer wishes to update a billing address, the software needs to update two separate tables to keep the database state consistent. If, instead, the database stores the customer billing addresses in a single table, the database content becomes more normalized and generally easier to maintain. Higher levels of database normalization reduce redundant data and optimize data dependencies.

In theory, a more normalized database is easier to maintain than a less normalized database. However, it is quite impractical (and nearly impossible) for databases to achieve the highest levels of normalization. Higher levels of normalization usually mean that data are spread across a greater number of tables. As a result, data manipulation language (DML) queries are often more complicated, and the database management systems (DBMSs) must work harder to retrieve data from the tables. Designers must carefully balance the requirements for database maintainability and performance when designing a database.

Another important task for database designers is developing indexes for the tables in a database. A table index works in much the same way as the index at the back of, for example, a cookbook. The index contains an ordered list of items (recipe names) along with a link (a page number) to the item's associated row (the recipe itself).

Imagine querying a cookbook to find all of the recipes that contain the ingredient "paprika". Normally, a DBMS performing a search like this would need to scan each recipe's ingredients, but if the DBMS maintained an "ingredient" index, it would be able to quickly look up "paprika" and return a list of the associated recipes.

Computers use methods to track down individual pieces of data in an ordered list that are usually much faster than scanning every single entry in the table. As a result, rejoining data that are spread across multiple tables can be surprisingly efficient if the tables are indexed in an optimal manner. The way in which these indexes are used and maintained is typically transparent to the users of the system. Some structured query language (SQL) variants have options for providing the DBMS with hints about which indexes to use, but modern systems usually do a very good job of deciding which indexes will result in optimal overall performance.

5.3.2 Database Server Software

Many software vendors provide DBMS solutions. Some database solutions, such as Microsoft Access [6], Corel Paradox [7], and dBase [8], are well suited for small-scale applications. Generally, these databases are small in size and portable compared with their full-scale counterparts; many of the features in the larger systems have been stripped away to provide a simpler database experience. They tend to cost less and can be geared toward beginners so that little or no programming language experience is required to use them. These databases usually do not scale upward well because they are tuned for small-scale usage. The level of control over these databases is usually limited, and data access from multiple concurrent users is often not well supported. These types of databases are generally used in situations where a robust database solution is not necessary.

Larger scale database server software packages, such as Oracle Database [9], IBM DB2 [10], Microsoft SQL Server [6], MySQL [11], and PostgreSQL [12], provide a finer level of control over the database and scale upward well as the demands on the database increase. Their software is designed to be used by multiple concurrent users in a networked environment. Generally, they offer wider support of the SQL language standard, tighter control over database tuning, and special considerations for database maintenance (e.g., performing data backups, executing routine maintenance). They also tend to offer better security than their smaller counterparts. Of course, these added benefits usually come along with added complexity and cost. Keeping the larger database running smoothly and securely is more complicated in all cases. The software tends to cost more (although not in the case of the open-source solutions), with vendors often charging per user or per processor. These large-scale solutions are used where robust, high performance is required.

5.3.3 Database Server Hardware

Because most large-scale database software scales well with increasing demands, the main limitation on database performance is server hardware. Databases are resource intensive, requiring high levels of performance from the server's processors, hard drives, and network connection. DBMS software solutions take advantage of multiple processors if they are available and if the software is licensed to run on those processors. Most DBMS vendors provide support for a variety of processor architectures, and many support the newest architectures, such as the 64-bit x86 processors offered by AMD [13] and Intel [14] among others.

In an effort to boost overall performance, database servers use a great deal of random access memory (RAM). Hard disk operations are very slow, and physical memory is (comparatively) much faster. Databases often read large amounts of data from the disk into physical memory so that they can perform operations on the data quickly. Physical memory, while fast, is very expensive compared with hard drive space. Ideally, the amount of physical memory installed in a database server should be maximized.

One of the major performance hindrances for the DBMS is the hard disk input/output. High-performance database servers must find and retrieve large amounts of data quickly from the hard disk, a traditionally slow-to-respond technology. Data integrity is also an important aspect of data storage. The server still needs to respond if a disk drive starts to malfunction or stops working completely.

The main objectives for hard disk storage performance are to maximize data throughput and to ensure high levels of data integrity. A very popular way to meet these criteria is to use a redundant array of independent disks (RAID) configuration [15]. A RAID setup allows a server to use multiple disks together in a flexible configuration to maximize data integrity and performance. When a server needs to write data to physical storage, the RAID can perform a number of operations transparently. First, in a "mirrored" configuration, the RAID can write a copy of the data to two or more sets of disks. Because each disk runs independently, the data write operation occurs simultaneously on all of the mirrored disks. Second, the RAID system can perform "parity" checks on the data written to the drives to ensure that the disk actually writes the requested data to the drive. Finally, the RAID system can "stripe" the data across multiple drives to improve disk throughput dramatically. For example, if the RAID were asked to write the bits "123456" to a system with three disks in this configuration, it could write "1" to the first disk, "2" to the second disk, and "3" to the third disk — all simultaneously. In the next time slice, the bits "4," "5," and "6" could be written to the first, second, and third disks, respectively. This RAID setup takes two steps to perform what would take a regular disk six steps to perform. The RAID system is highly configurable — different "levels" of RAID provide customizable sets of functionality.

Two relatively new solutions to the storage problem involve moving the disk storage away from the server. In the storage area network (SAN) and network attached storage (NAS) models, disk storage operations are sent over a network to machines that are dedicated to performing storage operations using large arrays of hard disks. The network can be either a part of the server's regular network connection or a separate network dedicated to the storage subsystem. These approaches enable multiple servers to access the same storage space in a relatively efficient and easy-to-administer manner.

The final hardware consideration relating to database servers concerns power usage. Most server-oriented machines come with multiple redundant power supplies in case one of the power supplies fails. If the power to the server goes out, however, uninterruptible power supply (UPS) systems will use their rechargeable batteries to keep everything running. Smaller UPS units will keep the server powered only long enough for everything to shut down safely. Larger UPS units are designed to keep everything working until the power comes back on.

5.3.4 Database Server Costs

The startup cost for a database server is higher than the cost of a typical personal computer. Major computer vendors offer help with customizing hardware and software when a server is ordered. In addition, they will help determine the kinds of software licenses required for the setup and offer warranty-related support for the server if technical issues arise.

In general, servers incur ongoing maintenance costs. Database data need to be backed up regularly in case of a catastrophic system failure. The server's software needs to be upgraded regularly with the latest security releases to minimize the security risks associated with connecting to the Internet. As discussed previously, the cost of a database server is a key consideration when jurisdictions are deciding how best to establish a disease surveillance capability within their health department.

5.3.5 DBMS Vendor Overview

Many DBMS software solutions are available, all of which vary in terms of cost, hardware support, operating system support, and overall performance. Table 5.1 provides a simple overview of some of the different vendor options available for database software, which are also described here.

Microsoft's most recent database solution is called Microsoft SQL Server 2005 [6]. A variety of editions of the DBMS are available, from a stripped-down workgroup edition to the full-blown enterprise edition. Microsoft offers flexible licensing options, including individual user licensing and processor licensing. The software is supported only in the Windows operating system and on x86 processor architectures, including the newer 64-bit processors.

The Oracle Database 10g software [9] offers much of the same functionality as Microsoft's database family. Like Microsoft, Oracle offers flexible licensing options that scale upward as more growth is required. Oracle's software will run on many different operating systems, such as Windows and Linux, and also supports a number of different processor architectures.

IBM offers the last of the big three commercial database solutions with their latest software version, DB2 version 8.2 [10]. Their software is supported on Windows, Linux, and many other Unix variants, such as AIX, HP-UX, and Solaris. Correspondingly, their software supports a very wide variety of processor architectures, making it a very flexible solution for different hardware configurations.

The open-source software movement has resulted in several strong and popular database solutions. MySQL [11] and PostgreSQL [12] both offer high-performance solutions that will run on many operating systems across many different kinds of processors. MySQL is licensed under the GNU public license (GPL) [16], which allows users to download and use MySQL for a software project but restricts the distribution of the resulting software. PostgreSQL is licensed under the more liberal Berkeley software distribution (BSD) [17] license, which allows software to be redistributed regardless of how it is used.

In response to the popularity of open-source databases, Microsoft, Oracle, and IBM have all released free stripped-down versions of their database solutions. All three offer free downloadable "Express" (or for IBM, "Express-C") variants of their latest databases. The Express versions usually limit the number of processors the software will use, the amount of memory it can use, and the physical size of the database. These solutions work well for small-scale development and prototyping, but must be upgraded to the costly database versions if higher performance is required.

There are many benchmark performance tests available for all of these popular database solutions. Often, though, database performance relies greatly on how the database itself is designed. The open-source solutions can offer results that meet or exceed the performance of their commercial counterparts. Before choosing database software, consider how the database will be used. Will it be easy to find developers to design and maintain the database? What tools are available to support database-related tasks? Databases have become an important part of the IT infrastructure. Fortunately, this means that support is widely available for most database solutions.

5.4   WEB APPLICATIONS

Web applications can be accessed by any network-enabled device with a web browser. Web browsers exist for almost every operating system and platform, including smaller devices such as personal digital assistants (PDAs) and cell phones. As a result, users can access web applications using a variety of devices almost anywhere that network connectivity is available. In contrast, thick client applications will usually run only on a specific device (such as a personal computer or PDA) and operating system (such as Windows or Mac OS X). These applications must also be installed on every potential user's device, whereas web applications can usually be accessed immediately without any initial setup.

Web applications offer a strong advantage over thick client applications when software needs to be updated. Users who access a web application always see the latest version of the application that resides on the web server. The software developers need to update the software only on the web server to deploy application updates. Thick client applications, on the other hand, reside on the user's computer. Software updates must be deployed to each individual computer through an installation program run manually by the user or possibly by an update mechanism built into the application itself.

Table 5.1   General Comparison of Database Vendor Software

Vendor/ Product Name	Operating Systems Supported	Licensing Options	Processors Supported
Microsoft SQL Server	Windows	Per processor, per user, and per device; multiple editions	x86 and x64 variants
Oracle database	Windows, Linux, Unix	Per processor, per user; multiple editions	Wide variety, including 64-bit variants
IBM DB2	Windows, Linux, Unix	Per processor, per user; multiple editions	Wide variety, including 64-bit variants
MySQL	Windows, Linux, Unix	Open source under GPL license; support packages available	Wide variety, including 64-bit variants
PostgreSQL	Windows, Linux, Unix	Open source under Berkeley license; community and corporate support available	Wide variety, including 64-bit variants

In designing a website, the developer must make some initial decisions to ensure a well-functioning end product. The first step is to decide how the site will work. Will the pages all be static, or will the content be dynamic and driven by data retrieved from a database? On what external resources will the server rely? How will users interact with the web page? Today's large websites are typically quite dynamic and offer much in terms of user interaction. For example, users of Amazon's website can search through thousands of products, read user-entered recommendations, and even participate in online auctions.

Web applications do, however, have limitations. Traditionally, web applications tend to be restrictive in terms of user interaction, although this is a small trade-off for universal availability. Security continues to be an important issue for websites, especially as the incidence of identity theft increases. Web server software must be patched regularly to maintain tight security.

5.4.1   Web Servers

Web servers listen for hypertext transfer protocol (HTTP) requests on the network from client computers. At the most basic level, these client requests specify the name of the page to be accessed. The web server maps this page name request to a particular file on the computer and performs different actions based on the contents of the file and the configuration of the server. Essentially, the web server acts as an interpreter between the client and the content of the files on the web server's disk drive. The most basic operation for a server is simply to return an unchanged copy of the file to the client. Alternatively, the web server can interpret the requested file as a scripted set of commands to execute, in which case it returns the resulting output of the script to the client. Essentially, this output is a webpage that is written on the fly. The script can pull data from other sources (such as a database) and dynamically generate the content displayed to the user. In this way, web servers act as a very powerful tool for information exchange.

Web servers have a big responsibility, especially if the data they distribute are sensitive. Even the most basic web server software can be configured with basic levels of security, but it is the responsibility of the developers and system administrator to ensure that the web content is secured properly. The information sent between the web server and the client can be encrypted using the secure HTTPS protocol to prevent others on the Internet from eavesdropping. Conversely, steps must be taken to ensure that the data being served by the web server are available when needed. Browsing through an unresponsive website can be a very frustrating experience.

Much like database servers, web servers benefit from faster and more numerous processors, more memory, and faster disk access. Larger, more complicated, and busy websites will require faster hardware to keep up with their demands. Luckily, it is very easy for the software to run web page requests in parallel, so many different clients can make simultaneous page requests to the web server with few bottlenecks.

Two major web server software solutions are used by virtually all major websites: Apache HTTP server [18] and Microsoft's Internet Information Service (IIS) [6]. The Apache package, the most popular, is free, open source, fast, widely supported, extendable, and reliable. It runs on a very wide array of operating systems, such as Windows, Linux, and the Unix variants, and on all sorts of processor architectures. Microsoft's IIS is available only for Windows, but it has become popular because it is tightly integrated with the Windows server set of tools. IIS and Apache are comparable in performance.

Other web server variants are available for more specialized applications. For example, Jakarta's Tomcat application server [18] can serve up dynamic web pages created by Java servlets, which can be executed on most operating systems and processor architectures. Table 5.2 highlights some of the differences between these three web server applications.

Table 5.2   Feature Comparison of Popular Web Server Applications

Vendor/ Product Name	Operating Systems Supported	Licensing Options	Processors Supported
Microsoft IIS	Windows	Per user/device license; multiple editions	x86 and x64 variants
Apache HTTP server	Windows, Linux, Unix, etc.	Open source, released under Apache license	Wide variety, including 64-bit variants
Apache Tomcat	Windows, Linux, Unix, etc.	Open source, released under Apache license	Wide variety, including 64-bit variants

5.4.2   Web Applications and Browsers

A web browser is a popular and useful platform-independent tool used to support information exchange. Browsers help users make requests to a web server, translating their actions into HTTP requests that web servers understand. Web servers send an HTTP response back to the browser, where the information is again translated into a human-readable format. Browsers are responsible for formatting the hypertext markup language (HTML) data supplied by a web server in a form that is meaningful for end users. Some of the popular browsers in use today include Internet Explorer, Netscape, Mozilla Firefox, Apple Safari, and Opera. Although most browsers are designed to function in a large graphical desktop environment, portable Internet-enabled devices such as cell phones and PDAs have their own specialized browsers that display web pages on small and occasionally text-only screens.

On the web server side, web applications are the software packages that create the content and implement the elements of user interaction for the users of a web page. As mentioned previously, web servers often assemble web pages dynamically to deal with constantly changing data and to provide a rich and customized interactive experience for the users.

In the past, web applications often used a very simplistic (and error-prone) common gateway interface (CGI) technology to pass data between users and web servers. As tools were developed to simplify the process of creating a web application, it became much easier to create secure web pages that responded to user-entered information in an interactive environment. One example is Java's introduction of Applets into a web page. Applets are essentially self-contained Java programs that are embedded into web pages, complete with all of the highly interactive graphical user interface (GUI) components available in the Java library. These tools make it easier for developers to maintain large-scale, high-volume, data-driven websites.

Specifications developed by the W3C organization define standards for the HTML data that browsers are expected to display to the user. These standards, however, can be interpreted somewhat differently by different browser applications, which can result in odd differences in the layout created by different browsers. Sometimes, a page that works perfectly in one browser will not function at all in another browser.

Web applications provide data and analysis results to the end user as either static or dynamic content. Web pages with static content have pregenerated and predefined data, analysis results, maps, and other visualization elements that are recreated at scheduled intervals. These static web pages are usually delivered to the client very quickly because the web server does not need to perform any advanced processing.However, users are unable to perform ad hoc analysis through this type of web application.

Web pages with dynamic content provide the user with data, analysis results, maps, and other visualization elements that are generated on-demand by either server- or user-defined queries. These web pages need to access data from the surveillance system's data repository as needed. Users of these dynamic web pages are free to explore and analyze the data however they see fit. Becauses the web server needs to perform much more work to deliver this dynamic content, the query response time can increase, potentially up to tens of seconds or even several minutes, for very large systems.

A website with dynamic content will need to use a programming language. Popular choices include the open-source PHP (PHP hypertext processor) language, Java, and Microsoft's ASP.NET (application server pages in .NET). The choice of the language should be driven by the availability of developers who understand the language and by the support in the language for the development tools required, such as database drivers. The good news is that most languages are quite functional in terms of the external libraries available for software development.

Deciding on a web application language depends on just a few factors. How portable does the application need to be? If the application needs to run on only a single operating system, nearly any language will work. Most popular languages offer a large library of extensions. If the user interaction provided by the HTML language is too limited for the application, solutions such as Java Applets or Macromedia Flash applications running on the client's computer will provide a more expansive environment for interaction. However, using these client-side solutions can cause compatibility problems. For example, Flash applications require users to download and install a plug-in from Macromedia's website.

Website developers do not generally get to choose a web browser — they must, instead, try to make their pages compatible with all of the browsers available. It is nearly impossible to account for every single version of every single browser in the world, but the developer should at least ensure compatibility with the current, most popular browsers. It may also be worthwhile to think about how the pages load on alternative browsers, such as those used by PDAs and cell phones.

5.4.3 Web Applications and Geographic Information Systems

It is often very useful in data analysis to project the data onto a geographical map. Several factors must be considered for displaying a map. Where can one get the map data, such as the shapes of the counties or the layout of the streets? What kinds of data can be projected onto a map? How can map data, which represent real-world physical objects, be associated with the user's own data? How will users interact with the map?

Geographic information systems (GIS) software solutions offer answers to all of these questions. They manage and associate pieces of spatial data, provide data-querying functions with a map-oriented interface, and offer customized data displays on maps through the interactive use of layers, navigation, item selection, etc. Most important, they provide a way to load different kinds of data onto a map from a variety of sources.

GIS data can appear in a variety of ways. They can be either discrete or continuous and can be stored in either vector or raster format. An example of discrete data would be an object in the real world, such as a hospital. Continuous data, on the other hand, can hold a value: for example, the annual count of emergency department visits at a hospital. Vector data are described as a shape, such as a polygon, line, or point. Raster data are described as a multidimensional array of values, like a satellite picture of rainfall data, where each pixel in the picture represents the annual rainfall amount of a square area of land below. The data are registered with a physical landmark, such as latitude/longitude coordinates, global positioning satellite (GPS) coordinates, or a road intersection. GIS applications read in map information and associated map features, allowing users to interact with those maps and features.

Traditionally, GIS applications were implemented entirely as client-side applications, which meant that heavyweight software had to be installed on client computers to allow users to interact with the map data. This setup allowed for a tight feedback loop between the user and the GIS program, resulting in a high-quality interactive experience.

More recently, web-based GIS solutions are gaining in popularity. The lower level elements of user interaction, such as pressing a button and selecting an object, happen on the client's computer. These solutions typically retrieve maps and map features from systems running GIS server software. The Open Geospatial Consortium [19] — a consensus standards organization — has defined the architecture for two service-oriented systems for retrieving map and feature data from online sources. The first architecture, called *web map service* (WMS), acts as a server that responds to requests for maps. Clients request a particular kind of map centered around a certain location on the earth using a certain scale, and the WMS returns an appropriately formatted map. Multiple types of maps can be requested and layered on top of each other. The second defined architecture, called *Web Feature Service* (WFS), responds to requests for map features. A client can query a WFS for certain map features, such as a list of regional hospitals or a set of shapes representing zip code boundaries for a state, and the WFS will return an appropriate set of map objects using a specialized geography markup language (GML).

Three important issues to consider in the selection of a GIS software package are accessibility, data import flexibility, and security. Map data can come in a variety of formats, but fortunately, a number of standards are becoming popular, such as the ShapeFile format for vector data and the Geotiff format for raster data. The final important issue for GIS systems concerns security. Mapping applications occasionally must display sensitive data. Special consideration must be given to ensure that sensitive data are viewed only by authorized users.

The Environmental Systems Research Institute (ESRI) [20] has developed one of the most used GIS solutions in the industry. They provide a family of applications, including desktop and server-oriented options. Although licenses must be purchased to use this software, it is very popular and enjoys widespread use among the GIS community.

Another example is the free geographic resources analysis support system (GRASS) GIS solution [21], originally developed by the U.S. Army Construction Engineering Research Laboratories (USA-CERL). GRASS GIS is currently the most popular open-source GIS solution. Like the ESRI products, it supports a wide variety of data importation formats. Several extra tools are available as extensions to the GRASS GIS software. Currently, the system is supported primarily in Unix-like environments (including Linux and MacOS X). Support for Windows is offered via the Cygwin Linux emulation software.

5.4.4   Web-Based Application Integration and Automation

There are various web-based disease surveillance systems with varying levels of product integration and automation. They range from fully integrated and automated to loosely coupled and manually intensive. In many cases the commercial products used in the system influence the ability to integrate and automate the system easily.

Some systems use a single programming environment, such as SAS [22], to implement all functions of the system. Other systems use several different products that perform specific functions. For example, the data store may be in a relational database management system (RDMS) from Microsoft [6], Oracle [9], or others, data analysis may use SAS, and mapping may be performed using products by Environmental Systems Research Institute [20], Microsoft, or MapInfo [23]. Most of these products have application programming interfaces (APIs) that allow developers to access their functions and integrate them into larger systems.

Some systems, such as BioSense [24], Electronic Surveillance System for Early Notification of Community-based Epidemics (ESSENCE) [25], and real-time outbreak disease surveillance (RODS) [26], have automated input streams, detection algorithm schedules, end-user graphics generation, and tightly integrated processes. Other non-web-based applications, such as the EARS surveillance application, have tightly integrated processes in one application that is not necessarily designed or intended to input data or analyze the data automatically. Still other systems, such as the New York City syndromic surveillance system [27], are a mixture of manual and automated inputs, with the processing, analytics, and visualizations integrated in SAS.

5.5   IMPLEMENTING SYNDROMIC GROUPING

Most types of health indicator data used for surveillance are binned into syndromic categories before analysis and visualization. Some systems require data providers to categorize their data, often by hand, before the data reach the surveillance system. More commonly, however, the data are categorized within the system by automated methods. Using automated approaches offers several advantages. It shifts the processing burden onto the computerized surveillance system and away from busy data providers. It helps ensure that categories are assigned in an objective, standardized manner. It makes updating syndrome mapping schemes simpler because editing computer code is generally easier than retraining staff. The technical complexity of grouping surveillance data varies according to their type. Fixed vocabulary data can be handled in a straightforward manner, while free-text data pose a greater challenge. This section provides a brief overview of the technical aspects of implementing automated processes for assigning syndrome categories to both fixed vocabulary and free-text data.

5.5.1   Fixed Vocabulary Data

The values in fixed vocabulary data belong to a finite set of defined terms. Terms may be alphanumeric, such as the set of approximately 15,000 International Classification of Disease, Ninth Edition, Clinical Modification (ICD-9-CM) codes used for reporting medical services and diagnoses, or they may be English words and phrases, such as the variety of locally defined pick lists often used for nurse triage or EMS data.

From a technical standpoint, categorizing a record containing fixed vocabulary data consists of identifying the term that appears in the record and tagging the record with the appropriate syndrome. Database techniques make this mapping from terms to syndromes straightforward. If the surveillance data are kept in a relational database, a good approach is to set up a static reference table to represent the mapping. The table contains two columns, one listing the standard terms and the other listing the names of the syndromes to which they map. A database *join* function is used to link terms appearing in surveillance data records with the corresponding entries in the reference table, thus mapping data records to syndromes.

Several common technical issues arise when fixed vocabulary data are grouped syndromically:

- **Messy data**

  Problem: Frequently, the field containing a fixed vocabulary term in the surveillance data records also contains extra characters or multiple codes, preventing clean joins.

  Approach: Write preprocessing steps to clean the data beforehand. Alternatively, perform the join using wildcard matches instead of exact matches. Decide how to handle records containing multiple terms. A system may choose to use only the first term, under the assumption that it is the most important. Others use all terms, even though each record will likely map to multiple syndromes.

- **Code updates**

  Problem: Standard vocabularies commonly undergo periodic revision. The updates may introduce new terms, render old terms obsolete, or even cause coding conflicts in which a term has different interpretations under the old and new versions.

  Approach: Check vocabulary standards on a regular basis for updates, and add new terms to the mapping reference tables as appropriate. Allowing old terms to remain in the reference table is advisable because, in practice, they may continue to be used for some time. Coding conflicts are more difficult to address. To handle them correctly, one must know which vocabulary version each data provider uses and implement mappings accordingly — sometimes an impossible task.

- **Syndrome mapping updates**

  Problem: If the surveillance system's syndrome mapping scheme is updated, some terms may map to different syndromes in the old and new schemes. Updates to the syndrome mapping may therefore alter the behavior of the system significantly by changing the total daily counts in syndrome groups, which can affect detection algorithm baselines, the timing and numbers of alerts, and the appearance of time-series graphs.

  Approach: Consult with users and algorithm designers on how to introduce the mapping changes. To smooth the transition to the new mapping scheme, consider remapping a few months or weeks of recent data using the new definitions. Otherwise, the transition may disrupt detection algorithm baselines and throw off alerting for days, weeks, or even months afterward. Inform users in advance when syndrome mappings are being changed to prepare them for temporary unusual behavior in the system.

- **Multiple mappings**

  Problem: Although syndrome mappings are most often mutually exclusive, some terms may map into multiple syndromes. For example, in the CDC's syndrome definitions for bioterrorism-associated agents, ICD-9 code 786.3, *Hemoptysis*, belongs to both the respiratory and hemorrhagic illness syndromes [28].

Approach: Database tables can be designed so that each record contains multiple syndrome fields, some of which may be empty. This approach has a number of disadvantages. It wastes database space, it artificially limits the number of syndromes per record to the number of extra syndrome fields, and it requires special processing that checks all syndrome fields when records are counted or retrieved by syndrome. An alternative is to create duplicate records, one for each syndrome into which a given record maps. This approach requires special handling that adjusts for the presence of duplicates when counting and retrieving records. Another approach is to use relational table design to link each record to multiple syndrome assignment records that are stored in a separate table. Although this design is technically the cleanest, care must be taken not to introduce database design features that hurt performance. The join operations that are needed to relink each record with its syndrome assignments are expensive on the large data sets typical of surveillance systems and are likely to be performed frequently.

- **The "other" syndrome**

  Problem: How should the system handle records that do not map into any syndromes?

  Approach: One possibility is to simply eliminate records that do not map to any syndrome besides the default "other" category. The resulting space savings can be significant in a surveillance system, where typically over half the data map to "other." Preserving all records, however, offers other advantages. It enables users to access and view all records, even those not assigned to a syndrome group. It can also more readily support the calculation of denominators to use in epidemiological algorithms and statistics.

5.5.2   Free-Text Data

Free-text data consist of unstructured textual data composed without reference to pick lists, codes, or other fixed vocabularies. In surveillance data, free text most commonly appears in patient medical records, such as the chief complaint in hospital emergency department records.

Working with free-text data can be challenging. There is no single best method for grouping data, although many approaches have been implemented and appear to work adequately [29]. The methods used are generally adopted from the related fields of natural language processing, text classification, machine learning, and similar areas [30]–[32]. Two fundamental approaches should be understood: trained and untrained.

5.5.2.1   *Trained Approaches*   In trained approaches, sometimes referred to as *supervised learning*, the algorithm uses a labeled training set to learn automatically how

to classify data. Labeling refers to examples of free text data provided by public health officials that map into various syndromes. After the algorithm has been trained, it can be used to classify new records whose syndrome assignments are unknown. Basic issues to consider when generating a trained classifier include:

- *Establishing a good training set.* The training set must be reasonably representative of the data to which the final, trained algorithm will be applied. It must be sufficiently large, contain sufficient instances of each syndrome, and have accurate and consistent labels.

- *Selecting the right data representation.* The input data supply the raw material from which the learning algorithm must induce meaningful patterns. Text data may be represented as word vectors, sets, or bags in which individual terms may be stemmed, spell-checked, converted to a standard vocabulary, or weighted by topical relevance or frequency of occurrence. Good results can depend on finding a data representation able to support effective learning.

- *Selecting the right learning algorithm.* Every learning algorithm makes assumptions about the nature of the patterns to be found in the data. If the algorithm's assumptions are well suited to the data, the patterns it learns are more likely to be true and meaningful ones that generalize beyond the training set. Trained approaches that have been used on textual data include Bayesian learning, support vector machines, entropy maximization, and neural networks.

- *Trained algorithms offer a significant advantage.* Given a properly labeled and formatted training set, the algorithm iteratively refines and optimizes itself. However, a number of disadvantages arise as well. Labeling an adequate training set can be tedious and time consuming. Any labeling errors or inconsistencies may be learned by the algorithm. Training sets for surveillance data must be sufficiently large to represent even the rarer syndromes. Further, when syndromes need to be redefined, the training set must be relabeled and the algorithm retrained. In addition, algorithms trained to perform well on data from one hospital system or region may not be as successful on data from other sources.

Despite being well understood and established in other domains, trained algorithms are not currently widely used in syndromic surveillance. A notable exception is the RODS "CoCo" algorithm, a Bayesian classifier [33].

5.5.2.2 Untrained Approaches
With untrained algorithms, all knowledge about data classification must be explicitly encoded by the developer. Untrained algorithms do not require a training set, although labeled data sets may be used for testing. To classify complex textual data, untrained algorithms might employ relatively sophisticated techniques for understanding syntax and parsing sentences ([34]–[36]). Simpler keyword-matching approaches may suffice to classify the briefer, less structured text that appears in chief complaint data.

The major advantages of untrained algorithms are control and comprehensibility. The algorithm developers can explicitly fine-tune all aspects of classification. Unlike with trained methods, the reasons behind a particular classification are fully transparent. Syndrome definitions can be updated by editing code or reference tables rather than relabeling and retraining. The major disadvantage of untrained algorithms is the amount of labor required to develop and test them iteratively. In addition, like trained algorithms, an untrained algorithm proven to perform well on one data set may not perform well on data sets from other sources.

In practice, untrained keywording approaches predominate. The New York City Department of Health and Mental Hygiene's chief complaint classifier uses a keyword-matching algorithm implemented using the SAS data analysis platform [37]. The ESSENCE chief complaint classifier employs a weighted keywording approach implemented in custom software [38].

5.5.2.3 *Technical Issues*   In addition to the issues associated with fixed vocabulary data, free text introduces its own challenges:

- **Extraneous characters**

  Problem: The extraneous punctuation and alphanumeric codes frequently found in medical records can make it difficult for classification algorithms to identify individual words.

  Approach: Preprocess data to remove extraneous characters and standardize white space. Preprocessing may need to be data provider-specific.

- **Misspellings**

  Problem: Medical records are notorious for idiosyncratic misspellings and truncations, creating challenges for automated algorithms that need to recognize key words or phrases [38]. A study has found that common words such as *diarrhea*, *nausea*, and *vomiting* are misspelled in chief complaint data 11.0-18.8% of the time [39].

  Approach: Three major approaches for handling misspellings are edit distance, wildcard matching, and phonetic spelling correction [39]. Each introduces its own brand of errors, however, and should be implemented with care:

  – Edit-distance algorithms allow a certain number of character insertions, deletions, or substitutions to differentiate matching word variants. An edit-distance algorithm might recognize *vomitting* as a variant of *vomiting*, but it would also erroneously consider *head* a variant of *dead*. Check edit-distance matches against a dictionary to ensure that a valid English word is not being treated as a misspelling of another.

  – Wildcard algorithms attempt to match on an invariant word root. Wildcard matches on the root *pneum**, for example, may pick up some misspellings of *pneumonia*. Choose roots carefully, however, to avoid triggering unexpected false positives — for example, *pneum** also matches *pneumothorax*.

caused by substitution of phonetic representations of parts of words, such as the substitution of *nemonya* for *pneumonia*. A relatively small proportion of spelling errors in chief complaint data, however, is due to phonetic spelling errors. Far more are due to typographical errors and truncations [39].

— Phonetic spelling correction methods attempt to recognize variant spellings

Overall, a judicious combination of all three methods may be required to obtain best performance.

• Abbreviations

Problem: Medical records are laced with abbreviations, many of which are idiosyncratic or have multiple meanings. A recent study found that approximately 20% of all words in chief complaints were nonstandard abbreviations or acronyms whose use varied according to data source [39].

Approach: Abbreviations pose all the challenges of word misspellings without allowing as many opportunities for correcting them. The edit distance, word root, and phonetics approaches to misspelling corrections cannot be readily applied to abbreviations. Abbreviation use often varies by data provider. In some cases, a single term is abbreviated differently by different providers — *abdominal* may be abbreviated *ab*, *abd*, or *abdo*, depending on the source. In other cases, different providers interpret a single abbreviation differently— *ab* may mean *abdominal* in one provider's data but *abortion* in another's. If feasible, screen the data from new sources for new abbreviations or novel uses of existing ones. Although screening is currently a laborious manual process, methods to semiautomate it are being explored [39]. Because of substantial variation in abbreviation usage, it may be necessary to introduce contextual abbreviation interpretation, in which an abbreviation is interpreted differently depending on the words that occur along with it. The abbreviation *ab* might be interpreted as *abdominal*, for example, except in complaints that mention the eye or cornea, in which case it should be interpreted as *abrasion*.

• Negatives

Problem: Negative terms in medical records, such as "no fever present," can confuse algorithms looking for straightforward keyword matches.

Approach: For a simple approach, configure the algorithm to ignore terms that appear within a set word window (e.g., five or six terms) around or following a negative term [40]. Other more sophisticated approaches can be used if desired [41]. Although relatively rare in chief complaint data, negative terms occur frequently in longer narrative medical records. The most common include "no," "not," "denies," and "without"[42].

5.6 IMPLEMENTING DETECTORS

The anomaly detection component is an important part of disease surveillance systems. Detection algorithms are used to determine where statistical abnormalities occur in the data and, hopefully, to alert users to potential epidemiologically significant outbreaks. This section discusses how to implement detectors in the surveillance system architecture. The type of detection component implemented depends on the answers to two primary questions: (1) When will the detection component be used? (2) What will the detector interfaces look like? The design of a detector interface (i.e., the means by which detection algorithms receive data from the system and return results to the system) can make a big difference in the evolution of the disease surveillance system over time. Multiple detectors with different detection types may easily be integrated into a surveillance system if they all make use of a single well-designed detector interface.

5.6.1 When Will Detectors Be Used?

The anomaly detection component can be categorized into two types: data-driven and user-driven. Both types can run in real-time modes, and the data-driven type can also run in a more batched mode. Data-driven detection algorithms will run after the data arrive into the database. If data are arriving in batches, the detectors need to run only after the data have arrived; if the data are arriving in real time or in very frequent batches, the user must choose how often to run the detectors. The detection component can be designed to remain constantly active, pulling in new data as they arrive and producing results in near-real time. It may also be sufficient to run detectors on a batched schedule, producing results during regular intervals. Either choice is acceptable and will depend on the incoming data rate and user requirement, as defined by each health jurisdiction.

The second type of detection component is user-driven invoking of algorithms. With this type, the user can query an interactive disease surveillance system such as a website for a particular set of data and run the detection algorithms dynamically on the data requested. The results of the algorithm are returned to the system and published to the user. This type of detection component allows the user to run detectors on any subset of data the system supports.

Both data- and user-driven detectors can be used in the same system in a complementary fashion. Normally, a user-driven detection component will process one data set at a time, whereas the data-driven detection system will process an entire set of system-defined slices of data each time it runs. When the two types are used in one system, the user can view the results of a data-driven run through a large number of data slices without having to wait for the entire set of runs but will also have the flexibility to look for something that was not predefined.

5.6.2 Designing the Detector Interface

The same detector algorithms can be used for both a data- or a user-driven detection component as long as they implement a standard interface. Defining the input and output parameters of the detectors is very important for the future of a disease surveillance system. If a consistent detector interface is maintained over time, internal tools will need to be developed only once, algorithm upgrades will be easy, users can control or input data, and third-party developers will be able to add their own detector algorithms to the system. A detector interface plan must be designed not only for the input and output parameters of current detectors but also for expandability and future growth. It is best to design a detector interface that is generic enough for each detector to gather the information it will need in a consistent manner. Each of these concepts will help the detection component of a disease surveillance system to evolve gracefully as the system changes over time.

A detector interface must be generic enough for every possible detector to have access to the data it needs without the need for interface modifications each time something new is desired. For example, if the algorithm used initially in a detection component required only an array of counts as input, an interface that was hard-coded to require only an array of counts as input would cause problems later if a new detector were designed that took into account day-of-the-week or holiday effects and thus required a start date or array of dates. The detector interface would need to be modified, and the goal would not be met. Making the modification would entail not just upgrading a detector but also the interface and every piece of code that references that interface. If, however, a more generic interface were used in the beginning, only the detectors themselves would need to be upgraded.

Another benefit to keeping a consistent interface is internal tool compatibility. Many times, the algorithm developers will use internal tools to help design, build, test, and compare detector algorithms. These tools will utilize the standard detector interface and sometimes can be written in many languages or by many people with different skill levels.

A benefit of having consistent interfaces is that they allow user-created information to pass into the detectors to support real-time analysis. User-inputted parameters, such as dates, holidays, or weather information, can be used to modify an algorithm's outputs. Not surprisingly, this user-provided information can be more beneficial than any other parameter because it makes the detector results more useful to the user. The ability to tailor a detection result to a particular user's needs gives the system a higher acceptance level and makes it more user friendly.

As another benefit, a standard detector interface will allow third-party developers to contribute additional detector algorithms to the system. If the users of a disease surveillance system have a detector algorithm they prefer, being able to adjust their algorithm to the system's standard interface so that it can be used in the surveillance system can greatly influence user acceptance. This adaptability will also attract others to contribute to a disease surveillance system. If a standard interface is general enough to support almost any input and output, there is a good chance third-party developers may license, sell, or donate algorithms for use in the system.

The exact details on how to design this generic standard interface will be different for each situation. However, the general concept is to design an interface that can pass objects into and out of detectors. These objects can hold hash tables or arrays of values that can allow for new parameters to be added in without actual changes to the input and output parameters. Old detectors would just ignore these new keys and request only those it needs. New detectors could request the new data using keys that are now supported. A standard algorithm interface provides stability to give the disease surveillance system a solid, reliable foundation for upgrading and expansion.

5.7   VISUALIZATION IN A DISEASE SURVEILLANCE APPLICATION

All disease surveillance systems must be able to communicate information to their users. Time-series graphs, maps, and data tables are just some of the many visualization components that a system may contain. Deciding which components to include in a system will be determined by what type of disease surveillance system is being built. Some disease surveillance systems are detection systems only, alerting system users when either a statistical anomaly in the data has been detected, or the system believes that it has found something of interest to the user. Certain visualization components would be useful in this type of system, such as alert lists and maps of current anomalies. Disease surveillance systems may also be information systems that allow users to investigate data in many ways. Many information-based disease surveillance systems can create new case definitions, select different processing options, and customize the presentation to meet the needs of individual users. For users who rely on a surveillance system to support investigations, visualization components such as time-series graphs, GIS maps, data tables, query wizards, and real-time displays may be useful. It is also possible to build a surveillance system that combines aspects of both a detection and an information system. Such systems could include an entire suite of visualization components.

System designers must determine how much flexibility and user control each visualization or analysis component should have. Advanced users will require many different options to support their investigations. Flexible components allow users to design their own queries, modify graphic presentations, and adjust the sensitivity levels of detection algorithms. However, for some users, having too many options is confusing; these users want limited flexibility. Understanding user requirements is critical before selection of the visualization components.

5.7.1   Detection-Focused Visualizations

A disease surveillance system with a detection focus usually has visualization components that are static. This type of system will typically have a predefined set of visualization components it displays to the user. The focus is not on data displays, but on finding anomalies or patterns. A detection system can be designed with interactive features, such as allowing the user to set sensitivity levels on detection algorithms, but more often, it is designed so that little input is needed from the user. A detection component will normally have a defined set of syndromes or diseases that it is looking for and will display only those results it is set up to analyze. Because of this consistency, users become very familiar with the visualizations and can analyze them rapidly and with little interaction.

Detection-focused disease surveillance systems can function well in both real-time and non-real-time modes. In a real-time data environment, visualization components can be built to display the output of detector algorithms on the fly. In non-real-time data environments, the visualizations can be completely static. Background processes create HTML pages and images instead of the server-side technologies generating them on demand.

Detector algorithms are a major component of most disease surveillance systems. However, even the best detector will not be used to its fullest potential unless its alerts and warnings are easily accessible to users. Detection results may be shown as line listings, maps, graphs, and other more inventive displays. Each of these types of displays serves some purpose; having the right display or combination of displays creates a more useful system.

Detection algorithms may be very sensitive to anomalies and produce a large number of false alerts, or they may be specific and produce few false alerts. However, specific algorithms that are run across many different data stratifications can still produce a large number of alerts.

Because the detection algorithms are usually run across many different permutations of days, geographic regions, age groups, sex, medical groupings, and data sets, the system may need to provide visualization capabilities for a large number of alerts. Although time-series graphs are very useful for allowing users to visualize the data that caused an alert, visualizing a large number of different graphs may be impractical for most users. Maps are useful for displaying alert information, but it may be difficult to display multiple stratifications of alerts on a small number of maps. Instead, it may be more useful to show these stratifications of alerts in table format. Although not as immediately informative as maps and graphs, tables allow the user to see all of the alerts in a single view. Sorting and filtering through the alerts in these tables can also help the user discern patterns about the information. For other users, localized maps and graphs may be more useful than tables.

Users who have limited time might find it useful to see alerts at a higher "summary" level. By running a second level of detection above all the individual stratifications, the system can produce a much smaller number of alerts for users to visualize. Giving users the capability to drill down from the summary level to the more detailed levels of alerts benefits users who want to conduct further investigations. Interested users can see summary-level alerts and determine how they were formed and why. Users not interested in extra investigation have the summary-level alerts to identify a potential health event.

Interactive control of alert thresholds permits additional customization for the user. However, the option can complicate communication between users because each user may be looking at different alerts on their individual displays.

The amount of data a disease surveillance system receives typically increases over time. The visualization component should be designed with expandability and scalability to accommodate the additional data. If another data set is added, the visualization should expand down the page, not across, because it's easier for users to scroll vertically. The visualization component should allocate space for additional algorithm parameters or data sources.

5.7.1.1 *Individual Alert Listings*

Displaying detection algorithm alerts as a table or line listing is the simplest visualization technique; examples from ESSENCE are provided in Figs. 5.3 and 5.4. An example from BioSense is provided in Fig. 5.5. Detection algorithms using a large matrix of input parameters can produce many alerts, making it difficult for the user to analyze them. Sortable columns and filtering options help users to organize the table to better understand the data elements that are causing the alerting. Color coding certain sections of the table to separate normal data from alerts or warnings also helps users to see quickly if there are issues requiring further investigation.

Individual alert listings can also provide information other than a detector result. The examples in Figs. 5.3 and 5.4 provide not only the level of the detector output, but also the count of cases, how many were expected, and the rarity of this type of alert. Figure 5.5 shows the count of observed cases, how many were expected, and the ratio of the two, in addition to the detector rate. This extra information can be valuable to users for deciding if an anomaly warrants further investigation. It is also possible to overwhelm users by putting too many statistics on an alert listing page. Enabling customization of fields in alert listings can go a long way toward satisfying the needs of a diverse set of users.

The alert line listing component is a simple, effective way of displaying alerts to users. A surveillance system can aggregate data by several different parameters. Syndromes by facility, region, age, or sex are just a few of the combinations. Multiple alert listing pages may be needed to describe all the ways that detection algorithms can be used with the data. Figure 5.3 is a list of detector outputs that passed the threshold for alerting based on geographic region versus syndrome. Figure 5.4 is a list of alerts based on geographic region versus OTC drug categories. Each page has different columns, depending on the parameters used to group data for analysis by the detectors.

5.7.1.2 *Summary Alerts*

As systems grow larger and the number of alerts grows beyond what users consider to be a manageable number, the need for summary-level alerts becomes apparent. Summary alert pages give users a concise view of the detection results across the entire system or in more manageable sections. Figure 5.6 provides an example of a summary alert presentation from ESSENCE. The presentation shows a large amount of information in a small, easy-to-understand view. The

							Region/Syndrome Based Temporal Alerts						
Links	Date	Data Source	Region	Age Group	Sex	Syndrome	Detector	Level	Count	Expected	RareColor	RareLevel	NonZero
Time Series	03May05	Military Outpatient Visits	MONTGOMERY	18-44	All	UnspecifiedInfection	Regression/EWMA	0.016	3	0.964	26	15	60.822
Time Series	03May05	Military Outpatient Visits	OTHER_REGION	18-44	All	UnspecifiedInfection	Regression/EWMA	0.017	12	4	37	23	93.973
Time Series	03May05	Military Outpatient Visits	ALEXANDRIA	45-64	All	UnspecifiedInfection	Regression/EWMA	0.012	1	0.179	6	4	15.342
Time Series	03May05	Military Outpatient Visits	MONTGOMERY	45-64	All	UnspecifiedInfection	Regression/EWMA	0.035	2	0.464	27	25	34.247
Time Series	03May05	Military Outpatient Visits	PRINCE GEORGES	5-17	All	UnspecifiedInfection	Regression/EWMA	0.029	1	0.357	34	28	70.685
Time Series	03May05	Military Outpatient Visits	ALEXANDRIA	All	All	UnspecifiedInfection	Regression/EWMA	0.008	2	0.643	31	9	60
Time Series	03May05	Military Outpatient Visits	FAIRFAX	All	All	Rash	Regression/EWMA	0.044	6	1.435	32	30	69.315
Time Series	03May05	Military Outpatient Visits	LOUDOUN	All	All	UnspecifiedInfection	Regression/EWMA	0.029	1	0.357	28	20	41.918
Time Series	03May05	Military Outpatient Visits	MONTGOMERY	All	All	UnspecifiedInfection	Regression/EWMA	0.007	9	3.4	40	11	94.521
Time Series	03May05	ER by Patient	OTHER_REGION	0-4	All	Respiratory	Regression/EWMA	0.02	70	58.536	58	43	100
Time Series	03May05	ER by Patient	WASHINGTON	0-4	All	Respiratory	Regression/EWMA	0.024	16	11.821	52	32	100
Time Series	03May05	ER by Patient	ALEXANDRIA	18-44	All	Neurological	Regression/EWMA	0.001	2	0.179	21	4	23.836
Time Series	03May05	ER by Patient	MONTGOMERY	18-44	All	Rash	Regression/EWMA	0.016	8	3.607	24	8	96.164
Time Series	03May05	ER by Patient	WASHINGTON	18-44	All	Respiratory	Regression/EWMA	0.048	36	27.571	44	42	100
Time Series	03May05	ER by Patient	ARLINGTON	45-64	All	Respiratory	Regression/EWMA	0.025	6	4.393	31	18	98.082
Time Series	03May05	ER by Patient	LOUDOUN	45-64	All	Respiratory	Regression/EWMA	0.023	4	2.286	23	15	87.671
Time Series	03May05	ER by Patient	MONTGOMERY	45-64	All	GastroIntestinal	Regression/EWMA	0.008	25	19.5	29	8	100

Fig. 5.3 Simulated region/symptom-based temporal alerts from the ESSENCE disease surveillance system.

						Region/OTC Category Based Temporal Alerts						
Links	Date	Data Source	Region	Product Type	Target User	Category	Detector	Level	Count	Expected	RareColor	RareLevel
Time Series	03May05	Over-the-Counter Chain 3	WASHINGTON	All	All	COUGH/COLD	Regression/EWMA	0.028	243	190.76	41	27
Time Series	03May05	Over-the-Counter Chain 3	WASHINGTON	All	All	FEVER	Regression/EWMA	0.001	305	202.582	41	8
Time Series	03May05	Over-the-Counter Chain 3	PRINCE GEORGES	All	All	COLD/SINUS	Regression/EWMA	0.026	46	38.786	45	33
Time Series	03May05	Over-the-Counter Chain 3	PRINCE GEORGES	All	All	FEVER	Regression/EWMA	0.001	265	218.214	44	12
Time Series	03May05	Over-the-Counter Chain 3	MONTGOMERY	All	All	COLD/SINUS	Regression/EWMA	0.023	50	34.357	47	26
Time Series	03May05	Over-the-Counter Chain 3	MONTGOMERY	All	All	FEVER	Regression/EWMA	0.014	271	233.893	50	31
Time Series	03May05	Over-the-Counter Chain 3	LOUDOUN	All	All	NA	Regression/EWMA	0.044	63	45.5	30	28
Time Series	03May05	Over-the-Counter Chain 3	FAIRFAX	All	All	COLD/SINUS	Regression/EWMA	0.015	49	38.357	56	21
Time Series	03May05	Over-the-Counter Chain 3	ARLINGTON	All	All	COLD/SINUS	Regression/EWMA	0.007	31	15.929	36	9
Time Series	03May05	Over-the-Counter Chain 3	LOUDOUN	All	INFANT	COUGH/COLD	Regression/EWMA	0.001	3	0.643	26	5
Time Series	03May05	Over-the-Counter Chain 3	PRINCE WILLIAM	All	INFANT	COUGH/COLD	Regression/EWMA	0.027	5	2.107	40	29
Time Series	03May05	Over-the-Counter Chain 3	WASHINGTON	All	INFANT	COUGH/COLD	Regression/EWMA	0.028	7	3.286	32	25
Time Series	03May05	Over-the-Counter Chain 3	WASHINGTON	All	INFANT	FEVER	Regression/EWMA	0.005	56	36.036	38	6
Time Series	03May05	Over-the-Counter Chain 3	LOUDOUN	All	NA	NA	Regression/EWMA	0.044	63	45.5	30	28
Time Series	03May05	Over-the-Counter Chain 3	ALEXANDRIA	All	INFANT	COLD	Regression/EWMA	0.008	10	5.571	28	12
Time Series	03May05	Over-the-Counter Chain 3	WASHINGTON	All	CHILD	FEVER	Regression/EWMA	0.001	213	110.214	40	15
Time Series	03May05	Over-the-Counter Chain 3	PRINCE GEORGES	All	CHILD	FEVER	Regression/EWMA	0.001	187	136.464	51	20

Fig. 5.4 Simulated region/OTC category-based temporal alerts from the ESSENCE disease surveillance system.

example is a display that collapses all the alerts by data source, syndrome, and region into a single summary alert level for a day. An asterisk represents a single day, and the shading represents the summary alert level as determined by the p-value. This figure provides a week of detector output data for several syndrome groupings from emergency departments, office visits, and OTC medication sales for three geographic regions (Maryland, District of Columbia, and Virginia), all in a single screen.

It is useful to be able quickly navigate from the summary-level view into a more detailed line listing to gather more detailed information. This feature allows users to drill down into an alert line listing that has been filtered by a particular region, syndrome group, data source, etc. It might also be possible to navigate directly to a time series of data or line listings of the data that made up the alert. The user has the ability to continue investigating data of interest easily by clicking on the links provided on the display.

Statistical Anomalies

State: **Florida**

Patient Class: **ALL**

Time Period: **2 Days** Date Range: **07/19/2006 - 07/20/2006**

CuSum Analysis: **C2** Std. Dev. Threshold: **4**

Print

Data Type	Syndrome ↓	Date	Anomaly Location	Observed	Expected*	Obs./Exp.	Rate#	CuSum Anomaly
Discharge ICD-9 Diagnosis	Specific Infection	07/19/2006	Hospital - Hospital Grp A -East	1	0.000	999.00	1.12	C1 C2 C3
Chief Complaint	Respiratory	07/19/2006	Hospital - Hospital Grp D -Satellite	5	3.290	1.52	24.27	C2 C3
Chief Complaint	Respiratory	07/19/2006	State - Florida	20	9.430	2.12	7.92	C2 C3
Chief Complaint	Respiratory	07/19/2006	Hospital - Hospital Grp A -East	8	1.430	5.60	9.00	C1 C2 C3
Chief Complaint	Respiratory	07/20/2006	Hospital - Hospital Grp A -East	7	2.570	2.72	19.66	C2 C3
Chief Complaint	Rash	07/19/2006	State - Florida	1	0.430	2.33	0.39	C2 C3
Chief Complaint	Rash	07/19/2006	Hospital - Hospital Grp D -Satellite	1	0.000	999.00	4.85	C1 C2 C3
Chief Complaint	Neurological	07/20/2006	Hospital - Hospital Grp A -East	2	0.140	14.00	5.61	C1 C2 C3
Discharge ICD-9 Diagnosis	Lymphadenitis	07/20/2006	Hospital - Hospital Grp A -West	1	0.290	3.50	4.11	C1 C2 C3
Chief Complaint	Lymphadenitis	07/20/2006	Hospital - Hospital Grp D -Central	1	0.140	7.00	2.82	C1 C2 C3
Chief Complaint	Lymphadenitis	07/20/2006	State - Florida	1	0.140	7.00	0.99	C1 C2 C3
Discharge ICD-9 Diagnosis	Localized Cutaneous Lesion	07/19/2006	Hospital - Hospital Grp A -West	1	0.140	7.00	1.82	C2 C3
Chief Complaint	Localized Cutaneous Lesion	07/19/2006	Hospital - Hospital Grp A -East	2	0.000	999.00	2.25	C1 C2 C3
Chief Complaint	Hemorrhagic Illness	07/19/2006	Hospital - Hospital Grp D -Satellite	3	0.710	4.20	14.56	C2 C3
Chief Complaint	Hemorrhagic Illness	07/19/2006	Hospital - Hospital Grp A -East	4	0.570	7.00	4.50	C1 C2 C3
Discharge ICD-9 Diagnosis	Hemorrhagic Illness	07/19/2006	Hospital - Hospital Grp A -East	2	0.140	14.00	2.25	C1 C2 C3
Chief Complaint	Gastrointestinal	07/19/2006	Hospital - Hospital Grp D -Central	16	5.290	3.03	18.14	C2 C3
Chief Complaint	Gastrointestinal	07/19/2006	State - Florida	25	7.290	3.43	9.90	C2 C3
Chief Complaint	Gastrointestinal	07/19/2006	Hospital - Hospital Grp A -East	7	0.710	9.80	7.88	C1 C2 C3
Chief Complaint	Gastrointestinal	07/20/2006	Hospital - Hospital Grp A -East	9	1.710	5.25	25.28	C1 C2 C3
Chief Complaint	Gastrointestinal	07/20/2006	Hospital - Hospital Grp A -West	3	0.290	10.50	12.34	C1 C2 C3
Chief Complaint	Gastrointestinal	07/20/2006	Hospital - Hospital Grp A -South	5	0.430	11.67	20.83	C1 C2 C3
Discharge ICD-9 Diagnosis	Fever	07/20/2006	Hospital - Hospital Grp A -South	1	0.570	1.75	4.16	C1 C2 C3
Chief Complaint	Fever	07/20/2006	Hospital - Hospital Grp A -East	3	0.290	10.50	8.42	C1 C2 C3
Discharge ICD-9 Diagnosis	Botulism-like	07/19/2006	Hospital - Hospital Grp A -West	7	1.570	4.45	12.75	C2 C3

Fig. 5.5 Simulated statistical anomalies in state hospital data from the BioSense disease surveillance system.

The data depicted in Fig. 5.6 reflect a simulated outbreak. The red and yellow asterisks (here, gray and white) make it easy to identify the region and syndrome combinations with the most warnings and alerts, and thus recognize outbreaks. Another benefit of this presentation is that the user can easily see patterns over time and across data sources. For example, there were many OTC drug alerts earlier in the week, followed by a set of alerts in the emergency departments, indicating a possible relationship. The concise presentation of information provides users with a clear overview of all regions, syndromes, and data sources simultaneously, thus aiding in the discovery of data trends.

An important issue is how to calculate the summary alert levels. The simple approach would be to take the maximum levels of the alerts that fall in specific day/region/syndrome/data source combinations. However, that approach is not as effective as using a specifically designed algorithm that takes into account the underlying alert's detection levels but removes the multiple testing issues. These types of algorithms are discussed in Chapter 4, but from a visualization point of view it is important to know only if the system will allow more than one type of detector to be used. If so, that component must allow users to modify the screen and choose a different type of summary alerting algorithm.

[⊟ View Detection-Based Alerts | ⊞ View User-Based Events]

ER							
Region Group	Death	GastroIntestinal	Neurological	Rash	Respiratory	Sepsis	UnspecifiedInfection
NCR	✳✳✳ ✳✳☆	✳✳ ✳✳✳✳✳✳	✳✳✳✳	✳ ✳✳✳✳ ☆✳	✳✳✳✳☆☆☆☆✳	✳ ✳✳✳✳ ✳✳	✳✳✳✳☆☆☆✳✳
DC	✳✳✳✳✳✳✳☆	✳✳✳✳✳✳✳✳	✳✳✳✳✳☆✳✳	✳✳✳✳✳✳✳✳	✳✳✳✳✳ ☆	✳✳✳✳✳✳✳✳	✳✳✳✳☆☆☆✳✳
MD	✳✳✳✳ ✳✳✳✳	✳✳✳✳✳ ✳ ☆	✳✳✳✳✳✳✳✳	✳☆✳✳✳ ☆☆	✳✳✳✳☆☆☆☆✳	✳✳✳✳✳✳✳✳	✳✳✳✳☆☆☆✳✳
VA	☆ ✳✳✳ ✳✳✳	✳✳ ✳✳✳✳ ✳	✳ ✳✳	✳✳✳✳ ✳ ✳✳	✳✳✳✳☆☆☆☆✳	✳ ✳✳✳✳ ✳✳	✳✳✳✳☆☆☆✳✳

OV							
Region Group	Death	GastroIntestinal	Neurological	Rash	Respiratory	Sepsis	UnspecifiedInfection
NCR	✳✳✳✳✳✳✳✳	✳✳✳ ✳✳✳✳	✳✳✳✳ ✳✳✳	✳ ✳✳✳✳✳✳	✳✳✳✳ ✳✳✳✳	✳✳✳✳✳✳✳✳	✳✳✳✳ ✳✳
DC	✳✳✳✳✳✳✳✳	✳ ✳ ☆✳✳✳	✳✳✳✳✳✳✳✳	✳✳✳✳✳✳✳✳	✳ ✳✳✳✳✳	✳✳✳✳✳✳✳✳	✳✳✳✳✳✳✳✳
MD	✳✳✳✳✳✳✳✳	✳✳✳✳✳✳✳✳	✳✳✳ ☆✳ ✳	✳✳✳☆✳✳✳✳	✳✳✳✳✳ ✳	✳✳✳✳✳✳✳✳	✳ ✳✳☆☆☆☆
VA	✳✳✳✳✳✳✳✳	✳✳✳✳✳✳✳✳	✳✳✳✳✳✳✳✳	✳ ✳✳✳✳✳	✳✳✳✳ ✳✳✳✳	✳✳✳✳✳✳✳✳	✳✳✳✳ ☆

OTC							
Region Group	Death	GastroIntestinal	Neurological	Rash	Respiratory	Sepsis	UnspecifiedInfection
NCR	✳✳✳✳✳✳✳✳	✳✳✳✳✳✳✳✳	✳✳✳✳✳✳✳✳	✳✳✳✳✳✳✳✳	✳✳ ✳✳✳✳	✳✳✳✳✳✳✳✳	✳✳✳☆☆☆✳✳✳
DC	✳✳✳✳✳✳✳✳	✳✳✳✳✳✳✳✳	✳✳✳✳✳✳✳✳	✳✳✳✳✳✳✳✳	✳ ✳✳✳✳✳	✳✳✳✳✳✳✳✳	✳✳✳ ✳✳✳✳
MD	✳✳✳✳✳✳✳✳	✳✳✳✳✳✳✳✳	✳✳✳✳✳✳✳✳	✳✳✳✳✳✳✳✳	✳☆☆☆✳✳✳✳	✳✳✳✳✳✳✳✳	✳✳✳☆☆☆ ✳✳
VA	✳✳✳✳✳✳✳✳	✳✳✳✳✳✳✳✳	✳✳✳✳✳✳✳✳	✳✳✳✳✳✳✳✳	☆☆ ☆ ✳✳✳✳	✳✳✳✳✳✳✳✳	✳✳✳☆☆☆✳✳✳

Fig. 5.6   Temporal alert summary for a simulated outbreak.

In addition to the view in Fig. 5.6, summary alert pages can incorporate GIS maps or a series of graphs and plots. There is no standard view for a summary of a day's or week's worth of alerts. The main consideration is to make the page easy to understand and concise and to allow further investigation of items of interest.

5.7.1.3 Alerts in Time-Series Graphs
Displaying alerts directly in time-series graphs is a useful visualization technique. Figure 5.7 gives an example of a time-series graph. Red and yellow alerts (black concentric circles and light-gray circles) are displayed directly on the data count that produced the alert. This display permits users to view the rise and fall of the data trends simultaneously along with the anomaly detection results.

Besides colored lines and dots, a mouse-over link provide more detailed information about the underlying data that generated the alert. The link also provides the actual detection level, the expected count, and other values of interest to the user. Any textual explanation information available that helps users understand why that data count generated an alert could also be displayed.

It is useful to provide data in a tabular form on the same page as the time-series graph. A table format allows the inclusion of additional values that cannot easily be shown on a time-series plot itself. The detection values in the table can be color-coded to correspond to the color-coding on the graph so that users can easily line up alerts in the table with the graph. Users can copy and paste the data into their own analysis tools.

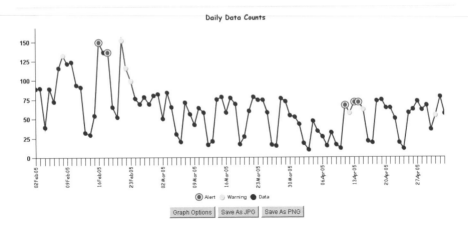

Fig. 5.7   Simulated time series of alerts from the ESSENCE disease biosurveillance system.

If the system allows for user-defined queries, the detection system must be able to run on-demand so that it can display alerts on time-series graphs. If the detection system cannot be run while it is responding to a query, the time-series page will have to differentiate between queries that it has detection results for and those it does not. Allowing a user to query dynamically for a set of data and immediately view a time series with detection results is a very valuable feature for the users of the system.

Many disease surveillance systems use more than one detection algorithm. It is useful to be able to compare the outputs for different algorithms available within the surveillance system. Figure 5.8 provides a detection algorithm comparison graphic from the ESSENCE surveillance system. The top trace is a time series of the data input into the algorithms. The second two traces compare the outputs of two different algorithms. Each detector graph shows the detector's alert and warning thresholds. This type of presentation is useful when users are trying to verify that multiple detectors are alerting on the same event. It is also useful to help determine which detector provides the best performance for a particular data stream.

5.7.1.4 Mapping Alerts   The ability to geographically locate clusters is a powerful feature of a disease surveillance system. To be mapped, the data causing an alert must have a geographical component, such as a zip code, census track, region, county, or latitude and longitude. Figure 5.9 shows a map of zip code clusters found by a spatial detector (see Chapter 4). The map shows the jurisdictions that comprise the National Capital Region along with clusters formed using the zip codes of residence for patients presenting in emergency departments with the unspecified infection syndrome.

Figure 5.10 shows a map of regions that contain alerts generated by a temporal detector. This detector determines if a county or region has an elevated number of cases, and the display color-codes that county or region appropriately. The temporal

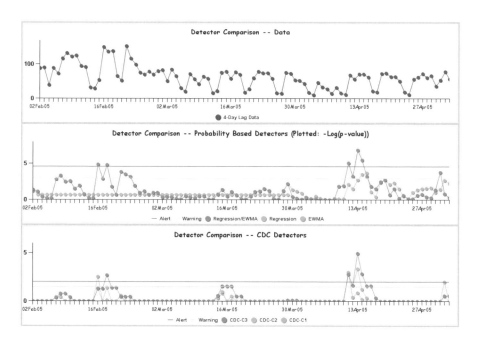

Fig. 5.8   Detection algorithm comparison graph.

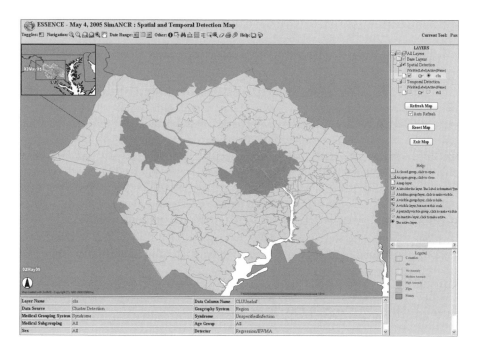

Fig. 5.9   Map displaying simulated clusters formed from a spatial detector in ESSENCE.

detector map assumes that the jurisdictions are broken down further into subregions for the purposes of aggregating data for inputting into the detection algorithms.

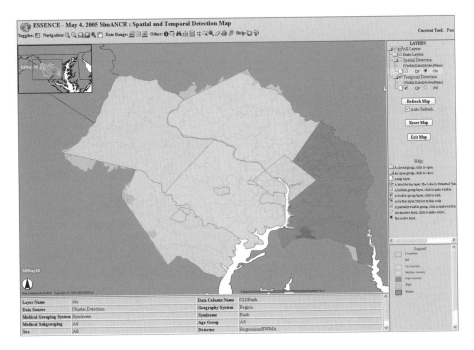

Fig. 5.10 Map displaying simulated regions alerted from a temporal detector in ESSENCE.

Placing alerts on a map allows users to determine quickly the location of potential public health issues and allows visual integration with other information available to the user. Mapping can also be used to overlay multiple layers of information from within the system and alerts to create a fused or complete picture. Multiple alerts in the same location can be distinguished by instructing the GIS display tool to overlay slightly transparent layers, which keeps the topmost layers from obscuring the bottom layers. Alternatively, the data can be fused outside the GIS display system and then displayed on a single map. If the GIS is able to overlay the alerts on the data, users may be able to visually correlate information from different sources.

Many mapping displays permit direct linking from the features on the map to the data details. Enabling the user to see an alert on a map and immediately drill down into the data is a convenient feature.

5.7.2   Information System Interfaces

A disease surveillance system should be interactive and responsive to user requests allowing users to query and visualize data in a variety of formats. Query wizards and free-text search capabilities can facilitate access to all data elements in the system.

Time-series graphs, pie charts, maps, and tables of data are all typical visualization components of a surveillance system. In static systems, which generate output in advance of user requests, the designer must create labels for the graphs. In dynamic systems, however, the users can define what they wish to view, and graphs, charts, and maps must be labeled dynamically. The more data elements that the user can query, the more complex the labeling process and the more detailed the labels. One solution to the complexity of labeling is to consider collapsible displays that allow users to see the complete information about the graph, but to hide detail if desired. Another possibility is to allow components to be customized by the user outside the surveillance system. This approach would enable users to create descriptive labels before they save, print, or export the labeled graphs or maps for further use.

The learning curve for surveillance systems can be steep. New users may feel overwhelmed by choices when they first use the system, and they should be provided with default settings while learning to customized displays.

Bookmarks can also be helpful allowing users to return to analysis sessions, for future use, or for sharing results with others. Bookmarking also allows users to perform the same analysis protocol repeatedly.

Dynamic information systems are preferred when users are knowledgeable and require additional details on the data. For example, a proactive user who is aware of an outbreak in another jurisdiction may want to specify a case definition to determine the likelihood of similar cases in their jurisdiction.

Users of surveillance systems will have different levels of skill, time commitment, and responsibilities. A user responsible for surveillance at the city level has a different level of responsibility than one tasked with monitoring a larger region. Users monitoring a particular county may be interested in anything inside that county. They may want to view multiple strata of various data elements, and if there is something of interest, they then may want to view additional details about the particular stratum. A user monitoring an entire state, region, or country may have neither time nor the need to view detailed data across an entire geographic region.

One solution to the need to view data at differing resolutions may be to create a visualization component that can view everything at the highest level of detail but also offers filtering capabilities and additional summary-level information screens. Users at the lowest geographic levels would be able to filter the entire system to view only their regions of interest. Users at higher geographic levels would be able to first view summary information to guide them to anomalies and then view the detailed information for further investigation. A benefit to this solution is that users on the smaller geographic levels will still have access to information from of the surrounding regions, if needed.

5.7.3 Visualizing Data and Information

A fundamental feature of any surveillance system is to support data visualization. There are several common ways to view the data, and each display technique has advantages and disadvantages.

5.7.3.1 Data Query A disease surveillance system should permit users to query the available data sources in a variety of ways. The data query feature should support very simple queries, such as retrieving all of the hospital records from a particular week. The query function should also support complex queries, such as retrieving all of the hospital records where patients exhibited respiratory-related illnesses and presented to a hospital twice in the same day. The query feature may also allow the user to search only a small number of fields or every field collected. The decision to implement a complex query function should consider both user experience and development complexity.

Developers must also consider how a user will perform these queries. A very complicated data query function will probably require a similarly complicated user query interface. A surveillance system may use a simple query form, such as a wizard or multipage form or a powerful but more complex SQL query-building form. If the system's users all know SQL and want to query data in complex ways, a query-building form that allows them to write raw SQL queries would be a useful tool. Users who do not know SQL, however, would probably find the interface complicated and frustrating.

A simple approach is to use a single-query configuration form. The form could have controls, such as text fields, list boxes, date selectors, and others, that would allow the user to select values for query parameters. Each parameter that the user can query on would need to be selectable on the form. Query choices may be dependent on previous user selected parameters. A dynamic client could be used to assist in selecting the remaining query choices based on the prior parameters selected. Because dynamic clients are typically more complicated to develop, another option is to design a single large form that has all possible parameter selections for all types of possible queries. This static type of form building can become complicated. Building simple and uncluttered forms that query across multiple data sources can be difficult because different data sources often have different data characteristics. It is worthwhile, however, to design the query interface carefully to provide users with an effective tool.

A "wizard"-style user interface has a series of query configuration pages, each of which represents a step in the query process. This approach allows dependent query parameters to be separated and presented cleanly. Each subsequent step presents query controls consistent with previous choices. In addition, the number of query parameters presented at any one time can be controlled. The wizard approach also allows for context-related help for each step. However, a drawback is that advanced users may find it tedious to traverse each step. A possible solution is to allow users to save routinely performed queries.

Figure 5.11 presents a query page from the ESSENCE surveillance system. On the upper part of the display, the parameters that have previously been selected are shown. On the lower part of the display, the user is presented with the next set of options. This specific query is being used to create a new syndrome category for emergency department encounters with the words *fever* and *chills* in the chief complaint text string. Males in the age groups of 0-17 years have been selected from the period March 10, 2001 – June 08, 2001.

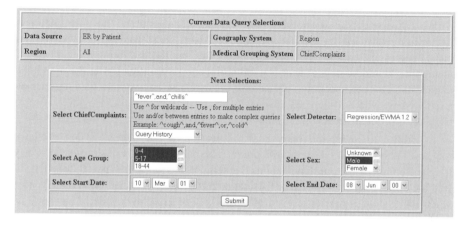

Fig. 5.11   Example of a query selection feature from ESSENCE.

The last approach to a query user interface is a query builder, which allows users to construct the actual SQL query statement. This interface may allow the user to type in the query statement or may provide sophisticated controls to build it. It thus provides the most powerful querying capability. It also requires users to have some basic knowledge of SQL. If given access to certain reference information, such as a list of hospitals, zip codes, or counties, this type of interface allows users to query for every possible combination of data, which can then be joined with other combinations of data to create even more complicated query results.

The disadvantage to a query builder approach, other than its requirement for knowledge of SQL, is that the resulting query does not follow any standard form. A user may use the query to return 1 or 100 different fields. The resulting visualization tools will therefore need to be complicated.

5.7.3.2 *Data Stratifications*   Users can be frustrated by query interfaces that contain many options for data stratifications. If, for example, the user wants to choose the hospital, age group, sex, medical grouping, discharge diagnosis, date range, and patient's home zip code, the user interface must allow all of these choices and more. A problem might also arise if a variable offers a user many choices: for example, the thousands of zip codes in a large region.

When there are many options for defining data to be viewed, the interface should present the selection process in an easy-to-understand format. A wizard-style querying screen with limited choices per screen is an option. The user can then focus on answering a small number of related questions.

Another possible solution is to separate query choices into "basic" and "advanced" sections. Commonly used choices can be placed in the basic view, whereas the less frequent query options can be placed in a separate advanced section. This solution is suitable if most of the users have similar requirements, and a large percentage of users can agree on what to include in the basic and advanced sections. If, however, the user base is very diverse, this solution may be inappropriate.

For a diverse user base, another option is to include user preference information in determining what options to make available to a user. Users would be allowed to view basic choices and components throughout the site, but those wanting more advanced techniques would be able to access them at the site level instead of at the individual page level. This method would be useful if the user base has set roles they perform on a daily basis, where some need advanced tools and others do not. However, if most users need different levels on different days, other options may be preferable.

In addition to having too many data stratifications to consider, users can also have too many choices in a single stratification. This problem generally results in overly long and cumbersome pulldown menus that require users to wade through long lists to find the options they want. These lists can sometimes be designed to be manageable when the system is first developed but are likely to grow over time. Lists such as geographic boundaries will expand if the system increases in scope, as will lists of hospitals, schools, or pharmacies as new facilities are collected by the system. There are techniques to combat this proliferation and make the system scalable.

The first technique involves pulldown list filters. Filter objects can be placed next to a long pulldown list on one of the visualization components in the system. The user would then be able to select a filter that would shorten the original list to a manageable number of entries. These filters can be useful when the pulldown list can be broken up into manageable chunks or there are metadata on which to filter.

Another technique is to carve out sections of the website via a site selection or site navigation step. The user would select a predefined subset of a particular stratification when logging into the site, and all pages from that point on would reference the selected set. For example, in a national system, a user could select a section of the country at login instead of trying to work with the entire country. In a local system, the user could select a county or smaller geographic region instead of working with all the geographic elements that the system can handle. As a further enhancement, users could select from a predefined subset of items or create user-defined subsets that could be stored and used every time they logged in. They would thus be able to create specialized views in the system without having to mix and match from predefined sets or wade through lists.

5.7.3.3   *Time-Series Graphs*   Visualizing data though graphs is a powerful and fundamental tool of a disease surveillance system. A common type of graph is the time-series graph, like the ones shown in Figs. 5.7 and 5.12, which provide examples from both the ESSENCE and BioSense surveillance systems. A time-series graph is a line graph that plots data over time. Time-series graphs allow users to distinguish trends and sudden changes. (All figures in this section use simulated data.)

Displaying alerts on the time-series graph of the data is useful. Colored dots or markers allow the user to see where a detector has found an anomaly and to locate abnormal data points quickly and easily. It may also help distinguish anomalies that are not readily visible just by visual inspection of the graph, such as data numbers that look normal but are actually high because of the day of the week, a holiday effect, or a hard-to-see seasonal trend.

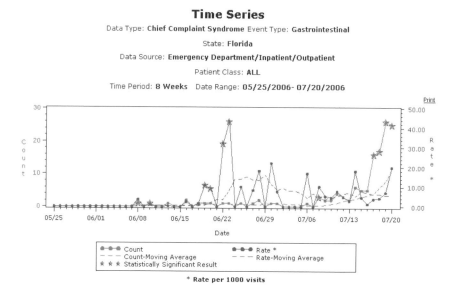

Fig. 5.12   Time-series graph of simulated gastrointestinal syndrome data from emergency departments in BioSense.

Other charts that display data over time, such as bar charts and stacked bar charts, are also useful tools for information visualization. The views from these charts are similar to line graphs, but they allow multiple series of data to be displayed simultaneously so that the user can see which stratum is most responsible for a change in variable. Figure 5.13 shows an example of a stacked bar chart displaying time-series data broken down by age group.

Several considerations must be addressed when graphs are to be incorporated into a user interface. The first is whether the graphs should be static or dynamic. There are also implementation issues that can cause problems for a system. Other considerations include the amount of customization that will be allowed, and whether graphs can be exported or saved.

Static graphs are images that have no interactive capabilities. They are normally pre-generated and are visible to the user, but users are unable to edit or modify the look and feel of the graph. The user cannot click on the graph to drill down to a more detailed view of the data, nor can they mouse-over on a point to get additional information from the data sample. These images are, however, very easy to develop and tend to load fast in a web-based application.

Dynamic graphs are more feature-rich components that not only display information, but that also allow users to gather more information, link to additional informa-

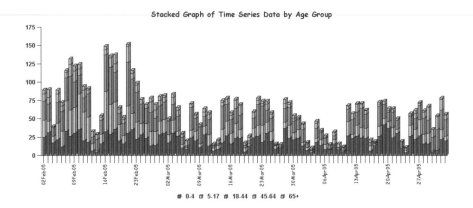

Fig. 5.13   Stacked graph of simulated data separated by age group in ESSENCE.

tion, and control the presentation of the information. Mouse-over effects and dynamic highlighting on graphs facilitate understanding of what is being viewed and selected. The user can access information about a data point on the graph, select a data point for further investigation, and immediately pop up or link to additional viewing components, thus enabling rapid investigation. The final dynamic function is the ability to modify the look and feel of the graphs. Static graphs may also support this function, but instead of dynamically changing the graph immediately, a new set of static graphs would be generated.

The look and feel of a graph may not seem important at first, but when users are required to generate reports or presentations based on what they have viewed in the system, they can save time if they are able to alter the title, adjust the axis, rename legend items, change color schemes, and change line patterns. Figure 5.14 shows a graphical options pane that allows users to change some of these features.

One issue involving time-series data is how to title and label graphs. Users want graphs to be labeled explicitly so that they are self-explanatory in reports and presentations. Graphs developed from a static list of queries can be titled easily. However, if users have the ability to create complex queries, setting graph titles can become extremely difficult. If a user queries for data using 10 or 20 different parameters, it will be impossible to fit all that information into the title of the graph. Instead, most labels are as descriptive as they can be in a limited amount of space on the graph, and the complete query parameters are described elsewhere on the page. One useful combination for labeling is to have the system define a small, uncomplicated graph title but allow the user to generate a more descriptive title for a report or presentation.

5.7.3.4 Data Line Listings   A data line listing is a display that allows the user to browse the record-level information of a data source. Figure 5.15 from ESSENCE and Fig. 5.16 from BioSense depict data line listings. The visualization component for line listings can be a very simple table. Also, similar to the alert line listing, the

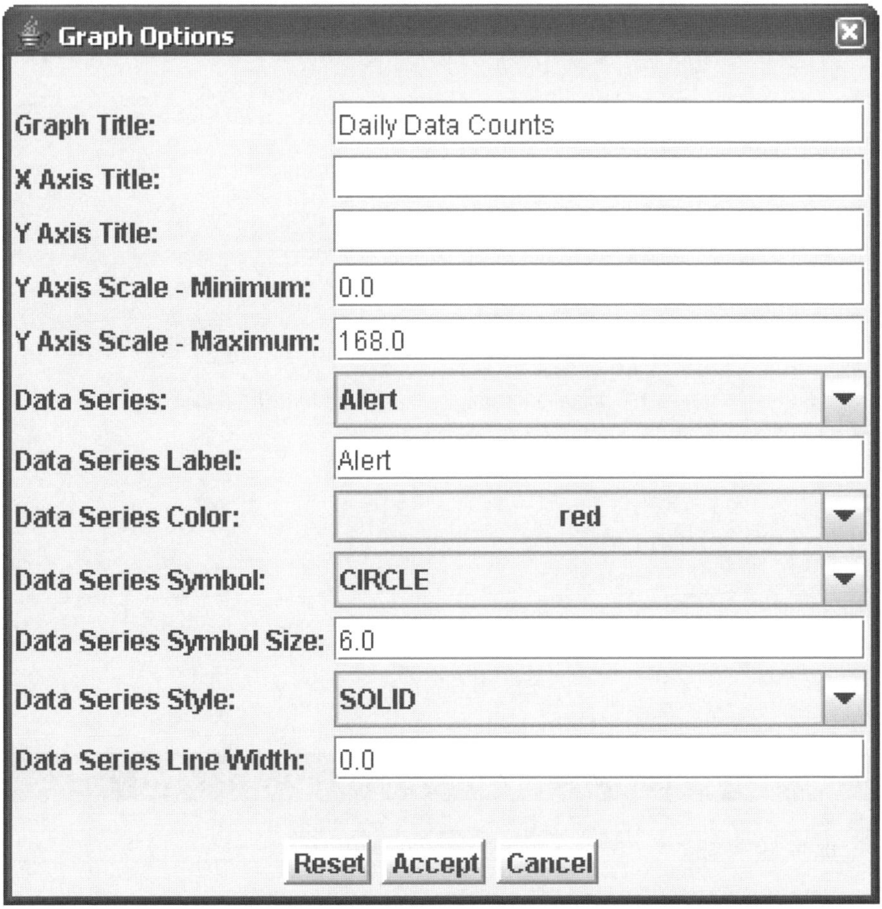

Graph Options	☒

Graph Title:	Daily Data Counts
X Axis Title:	
Y Axis Title:	
Y Axis Scale - Minimum:	0.0
Y Axis Scale - Maximum:	168.0
Data Series:	Alert ▼
Data Series Label:	Alert
Data Series Color:	red ▼
Data Series Symbol:	CIRCLE ▼
Data Series Symbol Size:	6.0
Data Series Style:	SOLID ▼
Data Series Line Width:	0.0

Reset Accept Cancel

Fig. 5.14   Options pane for changing graphical viewing parameters in ESSENCE.

data can be sorted and filtered to organize them for the user in an easy-to-understand way. The filtering capability can also allow the system to provide drilldown pages from other components. The other components can link directly to a prefiltered data line listing page, with the specific parameters filtered for easier investigating.

Beyond just a simple data table, displays of summary information might also be useful. For example, summaries could include a breakdown of the number of records from each region, syndrome, age group, and sex. The information could be presented as another line listing or as a data table or as pie or bar charts, as in Figs. 5.17 and 5.18. However, when pie charts are to be used, care must be taken not to include items that contain duplicate information. For instance, each record can be given only one sex attribute: male, female, or unknown. So if 50 records are being displayed, the pie chart will show a breakdown that adds up to 50. However, if each record allows for up to four ICD-9 codes, a breakdown of ICD-9 codes for the same 50 people could add

Date	Time	HospitalName	Zipcode	Orig Zipcode	Region	AgeGroup	Sex	ChiefComplaintOrig
30Apr05	05:22 AM	GBMCERCC	OTHER	21221	OTHER_REGION	45-64	Female	Chest Pain
30Apr05	01:01 AM	JHBVERCC	OTHER	21224	OTHER_REGION	65+	Female	Ha,chills,r Ear Ache
30Apr05	05:04 PM	HoCoERCC	OTHER	21043	OTHER_REGION	65+	Male	FEVER
30Apr05	03:42 AM	STJERCC	OTHER	21207	OTHER_REGION	65+	Male	COUGH/FEVER
30Apr05	07:56 AM	HoCoERCC	OTHER	21227	OTHER_REGION	45-64	Female	Right Leg Red,hot,fever,chills
30Apr05	10:26 AM	JHBVERCC	OTHER	21224	OTHER_REGION	45-64	Male	Fever/cough
30Apr05	01:44 PM	FSHERCC	OTHER	21220	OTHER_REGION	45-64	Male	FEVER, IRREGULAR HEART BEAT
30Apr05	06:20 PM	NWERCC	OTHER	21229	OTHER_REGION	18-44	Male	FEVER/SORE THROAT/CHEST

Fig. 5.15   Data line listings of simulated ESSENCE data.

Patient Zip	Patient State	Facility	Patient ID	Age	Gender	Chief complaint* ↓	Physician Working Diagnosis	Discharge ICD-9 Diagnosis
32218	FL	Hospital Grp A -East	135860^9991	5 Y	F	WEAK,FEVER,VOMITING,DIARHEA;		
33549	FL	Hospital Grp D -Central	71979^99925	23 M	M	VOMITING/DIARRHEA;VOMITING/DIARRHEA;VOMITING/DIARRHEA;		
32063	FL	Hospital Grp A -East	131397^9991	73 Y	M	VOMITING,FEVER,SWELLING,WEAK;		
32209	FL	Hospital Grp A -East	135878^9991	60 Y	F	VOMITING,DIZZY;		
32216	FL	Hospital Grp A -East	135893^9991	24 Y	F	VOMITING, DIARRHEA, 12 WK PREG;		
32205	FL	Hospital Grp A -East	141409^9991	70 Y	M	SMALL BOWEL OBSTRUCTION VOMITING;		
33612	FL	Hospital Grp D -Central	71995^99925	34 Y	M	NAUSEA/VOMITING/DIARRHEA;NAUSEA/VOMITING/DIARRHEA;		
32087	FL	Hospital Grp A -West	169269^9991	67 Y	F	NAUSEA,VOMITING,DIARRHEA;		
32212	FL	Hospital Grp A -West	135770^9991	67 Y	M	NAUSEA,VOMITING,ABDOMINAL PAIN;		
32084	FL	Hospital Grp A -South	53130^9991	1 Y	F	NAUSEA VOMITING DIARRHEA;		
32227	FL	Hospital Grp A -West	135690^9991	42 Y	F	NAUSEA VOMITING DIARRHEA;		
33624	FL	Hospital Grp D -Central	72347^99925	89 Y	M	N/V/D;N/V/D;		
33569	FL	Hospital Grp D -Central	72118^99925	14 M	M	N/V/D X 3 DAYS;N/V/D X 3 DAYS;		
32087	FL	Hospital Grp A -South	136044^9991	19 Y	F	LLQ PAIN NAUSEA;		

Fig. 5.16   Data line listings depicted in the BioSense system.

up to 142. Because of the potential confusion, some data may be better represented by bar charts than by pie charts.

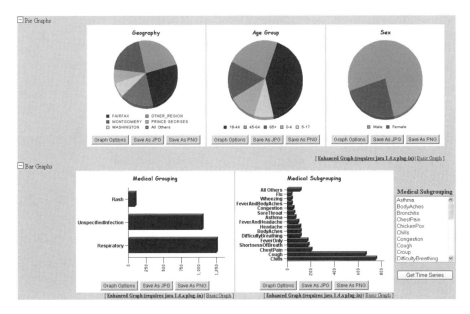

Fig. 5.17   Variety of charts displayed by the ESSENCE system.

After the user has sorted, filtered, and viewed the data available, the last operation is usually to export the data. In most situations, the data of interest on the page can be highlighted, copied, and pasted to a report or presentation. However, users may also want to export data to programs such as Microsoft Excel. Copying and pasting data may be sufficient, but with some data, such as ICD-9 codes, leading and trailing zeros are removed by programs like Excel. Hence, giving users the ability to download or export preconfigured Excel documents and comma-separated text files can be very useful.

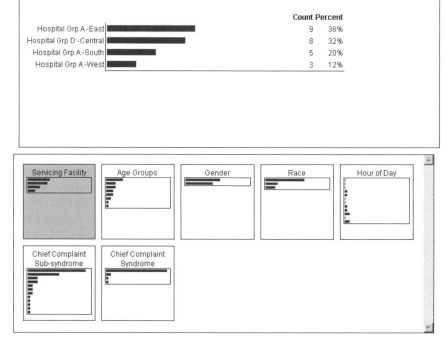

Fig. 5.18   Summary bar charts for simulated gastrointestinal patients in BioSense.

5.7.3.5   Matrix Portal   In addition to viewing time-series plots, there are occasions when users may want to create graphs with fully customizable axes. For these situations, displays can be built that give users greater control over the elements contained in a graph.

Figure 5.19 shows a sample entry screen for defining a custom data 'matrix'. This display allows the user to choose which specific data sources, syndromes, regions, age groups, and date ranges will be contained in a data set. Additionally, the user is able to choose which variable should be shown in the columns of the matrix and which variables should be shown in the rows.

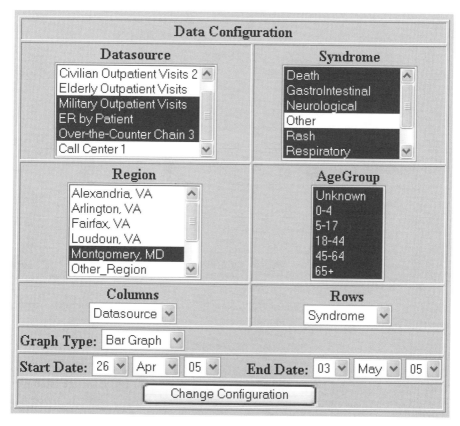

Fig. 5.19   Customizable data matrix builder in ESSENCE.

Once the user chooses the variables for the data query and matrix layout, the data matrix and resultant graph are generated. Figure 5.20 shows an example that contains the data matrix and a bar chart that corresponds to the query screen shown in Figure 5.19. This example shows multiple data sources and syndromes on the same graph. Because this type of flexible display allows all data sources or syndromes to be visible at the same time, users may be able to see patterns in the data that are not dependent on time or are obscured in multiple time-series plots. Flexible visualization components such as this matrix portal also allow users to create complex graphs and data summaries for presentations and reports without exporting data and manually creating graphs using other applications.

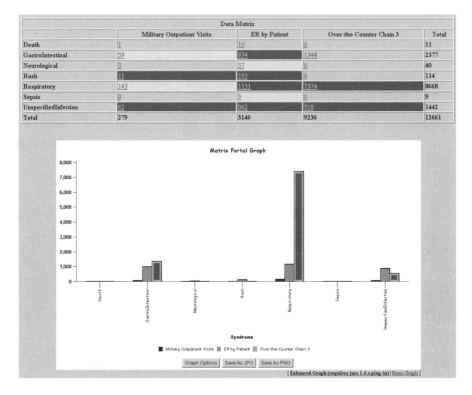

Data Matrix			
	Military Outpatient Visits	ER by Patient	Over-the-Counter Chain 3	Total
Death	1	10	0	11
GastroIntestinal	59	974	1344	2377
Neurological	3	37	0	40
Rash	11	103	0	114
Respiratory	143	1151	7374	8668
Sepsis	0	9	0	9
UnspecifiedInfection	62	362	518	1442
Total	279	3146	9236	12661

Fig. 5.20 Bar graph with generated data counts separated by syndrome and data source, generated from the query in Fig. 5.19

5.7.3.6 Mapping
Maps provide a powerful way to visualize spatially referenced health data. Figure 5.21 from ESSENCE and Fig. 5.22 from BioSense are examples of map displays in modern surveillance systems that can help users to recognize spatial patterns or clusters in health data. These data may be combined with other information, such as zip code boundries, streets, rivers, and county boundaries, to provide a comprehensive view of geographic areas. Maps enable users to superimpose additional information about water sources, environmental factors, or demographics on top of the illness layers, to explore hypotheses about regions for observed disease clusters.

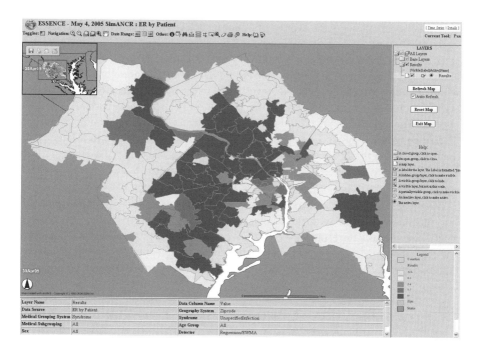

Fig. 5.21   ESSENCE example of health data mapped onto the zip codes of the National Capital Region.

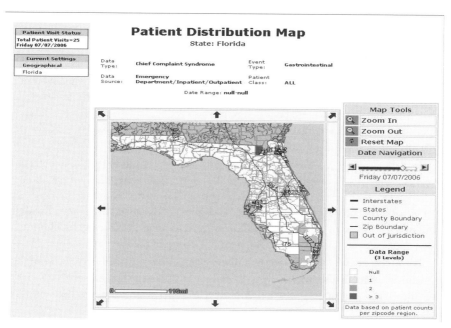

Fig. 5.22   BioSense example of road information superimposed on patient data in Florida.

In addition to allowing the overlay of multiple data layers, interactive maps can also support data investigation. Interactive displays permit users to highlight geographic areas and drill down into other parts of the system to extract information. Other useful interactive features include panning and zooming to focus attention on different areas within a map. Users are likely to investigate maps more closely if they have the ability to change perspective and the magnification to highlight a particular area of interest. The importance of zooming and paning are especially apparent in areas with diverse geographic units. Large rural zip codes may be easy to see in a large scale map, but smaller urban zip codes can be very difficult to see unless the user zooms in to particular areas of interest. Most Geographic Information System (GIS) software solutions provide these sorts of interactive features for dynamic maps.

Maps are also a powerful tools for communicating high-level community health information to nonsystem users. Whether the mapping system is interactive or static, it will become more useful to users if they can export the images into presentations and reports. Being able to view data on a map and then generate a report that includes that map quickly is convenient feature for a user of a disease surveillance system.

5.8   COMMUNICATION AMONG SURVEILLANCE USERS

The incorporation of a communication capability within a disease surveillance system will allow users to share information about events occurring in their jurisdictions. If a surveillance system supports multiple users, sharing notes helps to support collaborative investigations. Even if the system supports only a single user, tracking the history of what that user viewed as an anomaly or wanted to investigate more thoroughly can be very useful.

User communication not only helps users share information but can help to improve the system's overall performance. An electronic log of when users investigated an alert or communication among users during an investigation can help algorithm developers and system designers to build better components. A developer can fine-tune detection algorithms to produce more meaningful alerts by analyzing which alerts were (or were not) investigated by the system's users.

System designers can use the data from a user communication feature to determine how and why a user investigated a particular alert. By noting what information the users tend to investigate, the system designer can focus users' attention on those parts of the system. For example, if 9 out of 10 comments discussed anomalies involving children, a summary alert page could be designed to focus specifically on children so that all users could quickly investigate that age group in the system.

The user communications tool in a disease surveillance system may be combined with other components, such as event-tracking tools or case management tools. Users can then track ongoing events and comment to other users in the system on those events.

5.8.1   User Comments

The user comment feature in a surveillance system can be anything from an online chat room to an integrated message board system. The primary requirement is to enable users to share information about what they are currently viewing. The best design may be multiple techniques connected throughout the system, each of which is useful for certain situations.

Chat rooms work well during a crisis event or situation that demands real-time responses with many users. They are not well designed for viewing historical information (e.g., reviewing how a certain type of anomaly compares with a similar earlier one). Message board-style components are excellent for communicating asynchronously, but if they are used heavily, it is time consuming to keep current. In-page notations are good for viewing what other users discovered during similar investigations, but they do not provide an overall summary of what users are interested in.

In addition to the types of communication components used, there is also the question of what information to track. The information about a comment allows other users to filter and sort by what interests them. For example, information such as the geography, age group, or disease referred to in the comment allows users to find similar comments. Information such as the severity of an outbreak, the user's confidence in the data, or the desirability of further investigative measures allows others to filter down to just the important events.

Algorithm developers and system designers can also use the information about comments to improve the system. By keeping track of users perceptions of outbreak severity and their confidence in the data, an algorithm developer can match patterns of user behavior with algorithm behavior to provide the system with better detectors. Similarly, system designers can follow which geographies, age groups, or diseases are of most interest to users and promote those parts of the system.

As with all components, access control is a large part of the security of a disease surveillance system. User communication features are no exception. Users sometimes want to make comments that are to be viewed only by a specific subset of other users. Access control can be especially challenging if users are adding cached items in comments. Figure 5.23 presents an example of a communications function within ESSENCE, showing notes being passed between two epidemiologists monitoring a gastrointestinal event.

5.8.2   Embedding User Comments into System Components

A benefit of a user comment feature is that other parts of the system can embed relevant information from user comments. Alert information pages can note anomalies that produced both mathematical/statistical alarms and user comments with a high threshold of confidence or high severity of alarm. Thus, users can see the comments of other users for alerts that are considered to be significant. Alert summary pages

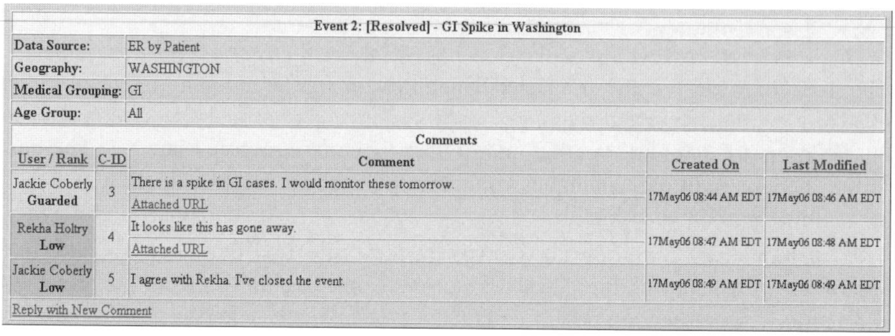

Event 2: [Resolved] - GI Spike in Washington				
Data Source:	ER by Patient			
Geography:	WASHINGTON			
Medical Grouping:	GI			
Age Group:	All			
Comments				
User / Rank	C-ID	Comment	Created On	Last Modified
Jackie Coberly Guarded	3	There is a spike in GI cases. I would monitor these tomorrow. Attached URL	17May06 08:44 AM EDT	17May06 08:46 AM EDT
Rekha Holtry Low	4	It looks like this has gone away. Attached URL	17May06 08:47 AM EDT	17May06 08:48 AM EDT
Jackie Coberly Low	5	I agree with Rekha. I've closed the event.	17May06 08:49 AM EDT	17May06 08:49 AM EDT
Reply with New Comment				

Fig. 5.23   Example of the communications function in ESSENCE.

can be designed to show these alerts that both detectors and users consider to be significant.

Presentations of time-series graphs or data tables can direct viewers to evaluations already performed by other users. Whether these pages embed the actual comment, display meta-information, or just let users know there are comments available, the user is aware of previous efforts related to the information or data being viewed.

5.9   SECURITY

Handling health data carries both legal and ethical responsibilities to preserve the confidentiality of patients, providers, and public health authorities. Those who violate that trust, deliberately or inadvertently, risk significant financial liabilities, legal sanctions, and damage to their public reputations. Electronic health data, or e-health data, offer all entities in health care and public health the benefits of faster and more in-depth access to health information, but also the greater likelihood of an unauthorized release of sensitive information and the potential for system unavailability. Mitigating the risks and overhead costs associated with using e-health data requires an understanding of the privacy and availability goals that a surveillance system must satisfy. Solutions must be identified to meet these goals:

- *Ensuring that data remain confidential.* Not only must data be safeguarded from outsiders, but access to specific data must be granted only to those personnel within an organization who have a need-to-know.

- *Ensuring data integrity.* No unauthorized party may alter the health data in any way.

- *Ensuring that the system remains available to all authorized persons.* A system should remain online for a high percentage of the times when users expect access and the system must provide results quickly enough to aid and not hinder the job performance of the requestor. Additionally, the system should be able to scale or continue functioning when there is a sudden increase in system usage [43, 44].

The system security and maintenance issues discussed here should be considered an introduction to the problems that must be addressed and not a final list since there may be many other concerns that apply to a specific system implementation. Moreover, because technology evolves rapidly, some of the issues discussed here may become moot, while other, new, issues will certainly emerge with new technologies. To minimize the chances that protected health data may be divulged, public health staff and IT system administrators must collaboratively develop and implement a comprehensive data protection plan.

Given the flexibility and popularity of web-based surveillance systems, the data protection information given here assumes that the front end is a web application that the user accesses over a network. System developers can then "piggyback" their protection measures off the same guidelines as those used to safeguard enterprise web applications.

Health data must be protected at all points of the surveillance system's workflow. Unfortunately, there is no "security by obscurity" against would-be hackers and data thieves [45]. Every networked system is a potential target for intruders, who may attempt to hold privileged data for ransom, disrupt the system for "fun," or use the system's computer as a "zombie" machine from which to attack other computers anonymously. Securing data proactively through preventive measures during the development of a surveillance system is far easier and far cheaper than reacting to avoidable security breaches after the system has entered production.

Nevertheless, it is essential to note that there is no way to completely guarantee the security of any IT system. Rather, each preventive measure achieves some limited protection, and the sum total of layering these measures, as shown in Fig. 5.24, may greatly reduce the risk or impact of an intrusion. System owners are *highly* encouraged to become fully aware of their system's security strengths and vulnerabilities.

A successful prevention strategy rests fundamentally on the trustworthiness of every person who has any involvement in the surveillance system. In addition to the expectation that every stakeholder will keep the protected health data confidential, all stakeholders must regard the ongoing security of the data as a *mindset*, not merely a checklist of built-in system features. The various groups of stakeholders and their security responsibilities are listed here in the order in which the groups interface with the system over the system's life cycle:

- *System owners:* have ultimate control of and responsibility for the system. They are responsible for ensuring that all members of every group have received the latest security education needed for their particular roles and have *at least* a high-level understanding of the system's security features and vulnerabilities.

- *System developers:* design the software "blueprints" for a system that will process, store, and transmit data securely; assemble the system; test the system to ensure that it has sufficient technical safeguards; and are responsible for informing system owners about the system's security features and vulnerabilities.

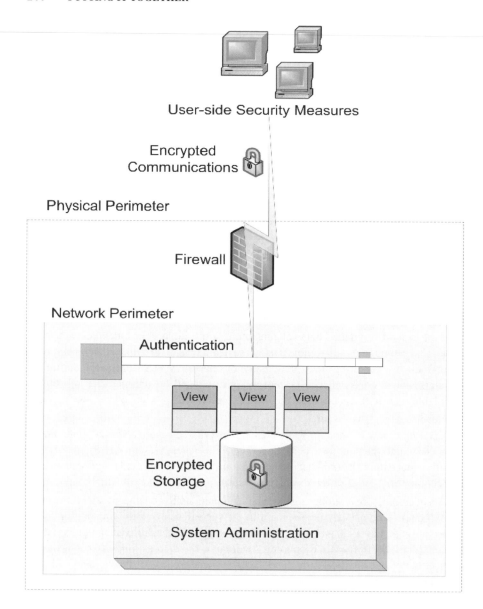

Fig. 5.24 Layered approach to security.

- *System administrators* (SysAdmins): monitor the system's security; perform essential security-related maintenance, such as administering accounts; and have a technical understanding of the system's security features and vulnerabilities.

- *End users:* keep their own account information secret, and as the primary recipients of protected health data, take all steps to ensure that those data are safeguarded and not compromised.

In practice, these roles may be less clearly delineated than they are here.

5.9.1   Design and Implementation of a Secure System

Developing a surveillance system's security entails two steps: design and implementation. The following section discusses security issues to be considered in each step.

5.9.1.1   Design

- **Encryption for Data Storage and Transport.** *Encryption* involves putting data into a representation that can be read only by the intended recipients and will appear unintelligible to all other parties. Designers are responsible for specifying which information in a system must be encrypted, the encryption algorithm, and the level of encryption, which is expressed in terms of bits. Using 128-bit or higher encryption is strongly recommended to assure security. To optimize performance and ensure a greater degree of security, designers should rely on the tried-and-true encryption methods that are already built into programming languages, rather than building their own [46, 47]. The following data should be encrypted:

  - Raw health data files from health care providers
  - Any temporary data created during processing
  - Processed health data and user account information stored in the database
  - All data requests and responses between the front end, or server, and the user's web browser, or client.

  Web communications can be secured through the use of a standard cryptographic protocol, the Secure Sockets Layer (SSL), which establishes a secure channel between the server and the client [48, 49].

- **Access Control.** Access to the system is controlled at two successive levels. Support for these levels must be included in the database structure, and the design must specify code that enforces the policies:

  1. Who may be *authenticated* or is authorized to enter the system. This is a simple binary criterion–a user either may or may not be authorized to enter the system, and any entrance by an unauthorized user is considered a security breach. To increase security, a user's account should be suspended after a set number of repeated unsuccessful login attempts. To

reactivate the account, the user would have to contact the system's administrators and confirm responsibility for the unsuccessful login attempts. This measure would prevent intruders from repeatedly guessing at the user's authentication information until they found the right value.

2. *Privilege separation* or which data an authenticated user is allowed to view. Unlike the question of authentication, there could potentially be many different sets of access privileges, depending on the number of individual viewing privilege criteria (e.g., zip code, county, state). Here, the goal is to guarantee data confidentiality by ensuring that legitimate users view only the data they are allowed to see [50].

- **Reinforce the Network Perimeter.** Firewalls are hardware or software devices that are "gatekeepers" (i.e., they stand between the surveillance system and the outside world). Using firewalls to filter the requests that are allowed to enter the surveillance system is an excellent way of blocking unrecognized networks from seeing the system. Additionally, firewalls help to protect against a common type of attack known as *denial of service* (DoS), in which a hacker sends a massive number of requests at one time to overwhelm a target system. Nonetheless, firewalls cannot protect against every possible network attack [51, 52].

5.9.1.2   Implementation

- **No Encoding of Sensitive Information in Hyperlinks.** It is strongly recommended that surveillance system implementers not encode any sensitive public health or system information in hyperlinks because other users of the same computer may be able to see the links from the web browser's history. This information includes user names, passwords, and details of specific public health data. Following this policy also has the benefit of keeping URLs relatively short—browsers have length limits for hyperlinks, so the user's browser may truncate a long URL. Instead, use the POST method to pass information from the client to the server.

- **Exception Handling.** When a program experiences any sort of error condition, such as a crash or receipt of bad data, it sends out a special message with the error's details, called an *exception*. Although exceptions are a valuable tool for software developers, they present a security risk on the front end because they may divulge implementation details that would be useful to a hacker. Mitigating this risk requires writing exception "handlers" in the code that return only minimal error information to the user, such as the error number and a very general problem description. To help developers debug the problem, detailed exception information could simultaneously be recorded "silently" to an error log on the surveillance system computer. A consistent exception-handling policy should be applied when implementing the system's code [46, 47].

- **Input Validation.** All information that the user enters into the system, from every hyperlink that "hits" the system to search parameters typed in by users, should be checked to ensure that the data are not intended to gain unauthorized system access, to control the system itself, or to harm legitimate users' computers. Users should not be allowed to upload files to the system because they may be contaminated with malicious programs, such as viruses or worms [46, 53, 54, 55].

- **Web Communications Encryption.** Given the sensitivity of public health data, SSL should be used for communications between the system and the user's web browser [46]. As part of securing the channel, the server must have a digital "certificate" that it then shares with the client so that the client may decrypt the server's messages. There are two ways to obtain digital certificates:

    1. Use widely available tools to create digital certificates, such as the "key-tool" in Java.
    2. Purchase a certificate from one of the major certification authorities, such as VeriSign, GeoTrust, or Thawte. Purchasing a digital certificate adds the advantage of allowing the server to prove its identity to a client [48, 49, 56, 57].

- **Build User-Side Security.** Although it is difficult to completely ensure that users will not let their clients be compromised, there are technical safeguards that can be put into place during development to help users keep a system secure:

    – Give the user a means of logging off when a session is finished, such as a logoff button in the upper right corner of each page.
    – Require the user to re-login after a set amount of time has passed since the user last interacted with the system.
    – Implement password security measures.
    – Provide a page on the system that discusses good user security practices, and link to it prominently from all other pages. Users might even be required to read it the first time that they enter the system.

- **Testing the System.** Once these and other safeguards have been implemented, test them thoroughly. Try to break into your own system, and invite trusted others to do so on a system with phony data. In fact, even a "white-hat hacker" or a "good guy" who knows hacking techniques could be consulted on finding and preventing vulnerabilities [58]. Each surveillance system computer should be "locked down" or set to the minimum configuration that will allow it to perform only its intended functions. Locking down systems enhances both their security and their performance. In fact, a public health organization's IT department will probably require that public health computers go through a security process, including lockdown, before the surveillance system may be hosted publicly by the organization's computers. This security process may be lengthy, so it is advisable to start well in advance of the date that the surveillance system is to come online.

Ideally, each computer should be dedicated to just one purpose in the surveillance system to simplify its configuration. To lock down a computer, work with a systems administrator to implement these steps before installing the surveillance system software:

1. *Clean install.* Start building the surveillance system computer by newly installing the operating system and just those applications that are used by the system, such as a database server or web server. Install only the minimum necessary components of the OS and applications to decrease exposure to vendor bugs.

2. *Remove or disable default accounts.* For account-based applications, such as operating systems and database servers, install special accounts with preset passwords and privileges. These "default" accounts, which may have names such as "Administrator" or "Guest," are turned on automatically at startup and represent a security threat because the account names and passwords are publicly known. When possible, these accounts should be removed after the application is installed. If the application does not allow the removal of the accounts, deactivate the accounts.

3. *Create minimum privilege accounts for the surveillance system.* Because the surveillance system is user-supplied software and is not built inherently into the OS or database, the surveillance system itself will need to run as a "user," with dedicated user accounts. OS and database accounts created for the surveillance system should be given only the minimum privileges necessary for the surveillance system to function. As a rule of thumb, surveillance system computers should only have permissions to process, read, and as necessary, transmit data. Then, if someone were to break into the surveillance system computer through the surveillance software, they would not be able to access sensitive information or disrupt the system.

4. *Close all unneeded ports.* There are thousands of channels on each networked computer, known as *ports*, over which Internet applications communicate. For example, a web server computer sends pages over its port 80 to port 80 on the client machine that requested the pages. A few ports must remain open on each surveillance system so that they can transmit data among themselves and to end-user machines, but the surveillance system does not require the use of most ports. Leaving open unneeded ports exposes a computer to risk of attack because hackers typically find unprotected computers by scanning for open ports [59].

- **Initiation of Administration Activities.** More system administration details may be found in Section 5.10.

5.9.2   User Authentication

There are three classes of tools that may be used to authenticate users:

- Passwords

- Smart cards

- Biometrics

Each class has its own advantages and disadvantages. Currently, passwords are by far the most widely used authentication mechanism; password-based solutions may be built into the surveillance system without the need for additional software or hardware and are the easiest to deploy [60].

An approach that is gaining acceptance in enterprises is *two-factor authentication*, where a combination of two authentication mechanisms is used to authenticate a single user. This method makes unauthorized authentications harder because the unauthorized party would need to obtain two pieces of information and have at least one physical object on hand while logging in. One prevalent example of two-factor authentication is RSA Security's SecurID system, which requires both a password value and a "key fob" or separate hardware device that displays a frequently changing authenticator value. Two-factor authentication has disadvantages: it requires both the purchase and integration of a separate authentication system and the deployment of a physical authenticator component to every system user [61, 62].

5.9.2.1 *Passwords*   A password is a sequence of characters used to authenticate a user into the system. In theory, the password is known only to its user. A surveillance system's designers and developers may either build their own custom password authentication component or install a commercial password authentication product.

Passwords suffer from the major disadvantage that they are easily compromised. Intruders may find a password that a user has written down, trick the user into giving away the password, or guess the password. In addition to the database and SSL transmission safeguards for handling sensitive data, both good user management and implementation-level safeguards may reduce the risk of compromising passwords:

- **User Management**

    - *Education.* Remind users frequently and emphatically to memorize passwords instead of writing them down and to keep passwords confidential.

    - *Accounts.* Create a separate login account for each user rather than giving a group of users shared access to the system through one account. Besides keeping account passwords more secure, separate acccounts help create an audit trail of user activity.

- **Implementation Safeguards**

    - *Password complexity.* To prevent would-be intruders from guessing user passwords, require users to create passwords that satisfy certain character and combination guidelines. Although guidelines vary by system, they generally suggest passwords which, at a minimum:

1. Contain six or more characters
2. Contain a mix of at least uppercase, lowercase, and numerical characters
3. Are not similar to any English words or proper nouns [46]

- *Frequent password changes.* Require users to change passwords at regular intervals, such as every 90 days, to passwords that they have not used previously [46].

5.9.2.2 Smart Cards

5.9.2.2 ***Smart Cards***   Unlike passwords, which are known to the user, the user may use a physical item, called a smart card or key fob, for authentication. Smart cards are devices that display a random number that the user must provide at login. This number changes at frequent intervals, typically every minute, on both the smart card and at the server, so if the value were intercepted, chances of intrusion would be minimal because it would be valid for only a brief period of time. RSA Security's SecurID, Aladdin Knowledge System's eToken, and WiKID Systems' Strong Authentication System are examples of authentication products that use smart cards [63, 64].

Challenges with smart cards include:

- Distributing smart cards to users
- Managing who has which smart card
- Synchronizing smart card clocks to the server's clock so that the random number matches at both ends
- Costs—Each smart card costs approximately $50 [65, 66]

5.9.2.3 ***Biometrics***   Biometrics leverages a user's intrinsic, unique biological characteristics, such as fingerprints, voice, or retinal patterns. Most enterprises are only beginning to deploy biometrics authentication, but biometrics will probably become a useful authentication tool for surveillance systems as the hardware and software become cheaper and more standard. Already, fingerprint scanning has become the most commercially available form of biometrics authentication product: high-end laptops are starting to appear with built-in scanners. Although biometrics is an excellent new solution to authenticate users, it is worth noting that like other authentication tools, it can be tricked into providing system access to creative intruders.

5.9.3   Access Privilege Management Overview

Each user should be granted only the minimum privileges necessary for job performance. Health data access should be controlled by the data fields that describe the type and location of health care encounters, such as:

- Zip codes (e.g., the health care encounter's zip code, the patient's residential zip code)

- Health regions, which may be defined by county or by another officially defined geographic grouping

- States

- Data sources, such as ER, OTC, and military; access may be regulated by an individual item within a data source, such as a specific hospital

To prevent user confusion, fields of health care data that the user does not have privileges to view, such as specific zip codes or hospitals, should not even appear on the user's view of the system as menu options or choices.

Access privileges may be administered in one of two ways:

1. *By individual user accounts.* Each user is independently granted privileges to view data on a need-to-know basis. This model has the weakness of making privilege administration a laborious and error-prone process for surveillance systems with large numbers of users, particularly when multiple users should share the same privileges.

2. *By user groups.* Groups of privilege settings are defined for users with different information needs, and every user's privileges are determined by assigning that user to one group [67]. Privilege administration is simplified because privileges can be set just once for a group of users with an equal need to know, and setting up permissions for new users involves less work.

5.9.4   User Responsibilities

System users will need to take several security measures on their own computers that cannot be imposed by the system's software. Note that the users themselves may not have administrative control over their computers, which means that they may not be able to modify system settings. In that case, they must coordinate with their IT organizations.

5.9.4.1   Minimum Computer Configuration   Because browsers that support 128-bit or higher encryption are relatively new and run on newer platforms, a minimum client computer configuration may be required as a prerequisite for using the surveillance system.

5.9.4.2   Location from which Client Accesses the Surveillance System   Technologies that enhance mobility, such as laptops and wireless networks, are popular with many users. Naturally, with greater mobility comes the need for users to exercise more discretion as to the location from which they choose to access the system, as well as the way they go online remotely. Security threats in this area range from a stranger casually looking over a user's shoulder to a hacker scanning the airwaves for unsecured wireless links. Some tools do exist to solve parts of the location problem, such as laptop display screen filters for privacy and virtual private networks (VPNs) for secure wireless networking [68].

5.9.4.3 *Finding and Disabling Malware*
Users should regularly sweep their machines for viruses, worms, and spyware using the latest antivirus and anti-spyware applications. Some malware infections secretly install programs that record the user's keystrokes, such as the web pages visited and login information, or gather data from the user's hard disk and quietly transmit the information back to the malware's authors.

5.9.4.4 *Webpage Caching*
Many web browsers cache (save a copy of) web pages that a user visits so that the browser can load the page more quickly on future visits. Caching surveillance system data is risky because it saves protected health data to a client without the user's knowledge. Confidentiality is jeopardized because the user may be accessing the site from a shared computer. Users are strongly encouraged to disable the "Save" function for encrypted pages if the browser provides that option.

5.9.4.5 *Relaxing Certain Browser Security Measures*
Depending on the surveillance system's features, users may need to disable pop-up blockers on just the surveillance system's website. The user may also need to enable the web browser to run code components, such as scripts or plug-ins for query forms and charts. However, enabling code components in a particular browser for some users may enable code components for all sites. Consult a system administrator before enabling or disabling a web browser's execution of code components.

5.10 SYSTEM ADMINISTRATION

Developing the surveillance system is only the first half of the challenge. To fulfill its purpose of surveillance, the system must be made "available" to receive data and host its intended users. Of course, the question is: What does "available" mean for my system? The quick answer is "it depends"–on the requirements and how the system will be used.

Some questions that will need to be answered are:

- How many users are expected to be on the site at one time?

- When should the system be online?

- How quickly should the system respond to user requests?

- How should the system administrator respond if something catastrophic happens?

All of these concerns related to keeping the system up and running, and many more not mentioned, fall under the area of administration.

System administration is just as crucial as developing the system; without either stage, there will be no surveillance. However, administration is too often an inconvenient afterthought because system development draws most of system owners' attention and therefore most of the budget. Like owning a house or any other large asset, the cost of owning the surveillance system will be greater than just the one-time purchase price. There will be "hidden costs" afterward that were not directly factored into the purchase–costs to secure the asset, insure it, and keep it in good shape. Offsetting at least the known post-purchase costs requires a dedicated funding stream.

Fortunately, system administration tasks are generally far easier than system development and can even be automated to a great degree. Ongoing maintenance pays for itself by giving users a faster response time and keeping the system online with up-to-date protection against computer viruses and other major threats. Additionally, in concert with security, good system upkeep can drastically reduce the chance that confidential data will be compromised, which preserves trust in the system [69].

Although administrative tasks are, by themselves, simpler than development tasks, successfully managing all of the aspects of administration often still requires full-time attention. Given users' expectations that the system will be available when it is supposed to be and the importance of maintaining data confidentiality, it is recommended that system owners work with experienced system administrator personnel rather than attempting to have someone "learn the ropes" while the system is in production. Alternatively, if a web-hosting provider can certifiably protect health data, system owners may choose to have their surveillance system hosted by an experienced third party.

5.10.1   Physical Administration

There are three facets to administering a surveillance system's physical space: location, facility security, and electricity and network access. For mission-critical surveillance systems or larger clusters of computers in a system, greater precautions should be taken, and more resources may be necessary. Ideally, multicomputer surveillance systems should be housed in their own physical room(s), due to the noise and heat that they generate.

Finding a place for a system is the first challenge. When possible, surveillance systems should be located where they have ample access to electricity and the network, are least likely to be tampered with, and are least likely to be damaged physically. If the user population is likely to grow, the system's site should have capacity for additional computers. Systems need to be protected from flood, fire, and exposure to nature, so installing a system near an outside door or below ground level may be risky.

Moreover, the surveillance system's physical site should be secured when not in use. Guidelines for who may enter the facility should be established, and depending on how important the system is, security cameras may be installed. Doors should remain locked when the room is not in use.

Finally, surveillance systems need enough electrical and network outlets to handle their demands. Because of the heat generated by large computer clusters, surveillance systems may require industrial-scale air conditioning. Furthermore, surveillance system computers should have an emergency power system that will keep mission-critical systems running and shut other systems down. Large or mission-critical clusters may need to be placed on separate electrical circuits and/or high-bandwidth network links.

5.10.2   Maintaining Software

Most of a system administrator's time will be spent monitoring, backing up, and updating software subsystems. The administrator's first and primary task is to safeguard each surveillance system computer from attack. Antivirus and anti-spyware software should be installed and maintained on all machines and checked frequently to ensure that these utilities have the latest threat definitions. System administration also means keeping up with the constant stream of bug fixes and security updates or *patches* that are released by vendors for the OS, other necessary applications, and perhaps even the surveillance system software itself. Delays in installing the latest definitions and updates may give hackers time to find and exploit newly identified vulnerabilities that may harm surveillance system operations.

Administrators ae also responsible for setting up and storing backups for surveillance system data. Backups are vital but are not a complete solution on their own. Because any event from a computer failure to a hurricane could knock the system down and render it unavailable when it is most needed, organizations need to prepare additional measures to ensure that they will be able to recover in a catastrophe. Regularly scheduled backups, multiple separate storage locations, and disaster response plans that include the immediate setup of a secondary system are prudent parts of a surveillance system's ongoing maintenance policies.

To monitor system performance and activity, administrators may examine a variety of logs that are maintained by different programs, either by hand or with an automated software tool. They may look at the computer's OS logs to identify any performance lags, error states, or unusual activity. To understand how the surveillance system is being used, they may use the system's logs as an audit trail to discover what page requests were made, how often during the day a request entered the system, and who entered the request. With this information, they can "tune" the system to respond more quickly to requests to find out which features are helpful to users, spot any unusual user activities, and investigate intrusions.

5.10.3   User Management

System administrators and owners need to work together to regulate and ensure authorized access to a system. Depending on how the system is implemented, administrators may or may not need to be actively involved with day-to-day account management. Owners should be responsible for approving new accounts, but new accounts could be registered either manually by the administrator or automatically through the system. When users forget passwords, administrators might reset their accounts manually, or the website could perform the reset automatically.

Account deactivation is a more complex task because there is often no efficient mechanism for determining when users should no longer have access. Depending on the system's implementation, deactivation may entail disabling the account rather than removing it entirely in order to preserve the audit trail of system usage. Although a user may have changed jobs, the owners and administrators may not be aware that the user should not enter the system. Possible solutions are to provide a means for users to deactivate themselves when their status changes and to designate points of contact at each user agency who are responsible for updating system owners when personnel changes occur. Given the circumstances, account deactivation is usually performed manually.

An outbreak of disease may drive up system traffic in the short term, so the system should have additional capacity to handle spikes in the number of users online at any particular time. This capacity may be 20-50%, or more, of the average load [44]. In the long run, as more users or greater levels of usage create more demand for system and network resources, it may become necessary to add more computers and bandwidth to maintain the same level of service. As part of their duties, administrators should monitor system performance and logs on a frequent basis and make the case to system owners to add capacity if usage rises.

5.11   SUMMARY

The information presented in this chapter should be kept in mind when a health juris-diction begins the process of implementing a disease surveillance capability. Many times, the decision to obtain such a system resides with individuals who are keen to address the health threats facing their communities, but who may not be knowledge-able about information technology strategies that make a disease surveillance system a successful endeavor. As will be discussed in Chapter 6, it is important for public health personnel to initiate and continue communication with their IT staff, data providers, and stakeholders throughout the development and implementation of a surveillance system.

5.12   STUDY QUESTIONS

5.1 Consider a hypothetical disease surveillance system that is entirely developed in mathematical analysis software such as SAS or MATLAB. *Q: What sort of drawbacks would such a system have versus a system developed as a web application?*

5.2 Visualizing health indicator data is an important feature of a disease surveillance system. *Q: What are some of the common queries you might perform on your health data? Which data sets would benefit from being overlaid on the same display, such as displaying multiple data sets on the same time-series graph or map?*

5.3 *Q: Given your organization's surveillance activities, would a stand-alone desktop or web client-server application best fit your needs, and why?*

5.4 *Q: Given that data may arrive throughout the day, how might you structure a surveillance workflow to accommodate once-a-day transmissions versus multiple or real-time transmissions?*

5.5 *Q: What are the trade-offs in resources and infrastructure between receiving transmissions once a day, several times a day, and in real time?*

5.6 *Q: What are some of the major hardware and software components required for a health surveillance system? If you were designing a simple health surveillance system on a very tight budget, what sort of hardware and software choices would you make, and why? If you were designing a large-scale full-featured system with high performance and responsiveness requirements, how would your hardware and software choices change?*

5.7 Geographic information systems provide important tools for displaying data in a geographic context. *Q: Identify several types of data that could be useful to display alongside health indicator data, and explain what value the users of a health surveillance system might find in these data sources.*

5.8 *Q: Develop a user-friendly end-user security education and training program for a nationwide group of users. Assume that the users collectively have an average level of computer familiarity. To proceed, first identify all ways in which the users themselves are responsible for safeguarding surveillance data, from not inadvertently disclosing privileged information they may view on the system to memorizing their own login information. Then, develop messages to communicate the importance of keeping data secure and the ways in which users may do so. Given the geographic spread of users as well as their computer literacy, deliver the messages through several different channels, such as posting prominent notices on the website, holding web conferences, and an annually requirement that users reaffirm in writing their responsibility for using the site securely.*

REFERENCES

1. Center for Disease Control and Prevention. CDC Early Aberration Reporting System (EARS). Available at `http://www.bt.cdc.gov/surveillance/ears/`. Accessed August 15, 2006.

2. World Wide Web Consortium. Available at `http://www.w3.org/`. Accessed August 15, 2006.

3. Sun Developer Network, AJAX Developer Resource Center. Available at `http://developers.sun.com/ajax/index.jsp?cid=216424`. Accessed August 15, 2006.

4. Adaptive Path. Ajax: a new approach to web applications. Available at `http://adaptivepath.com/publications/essays/archives/000385.php`. Accessed August 15, 2006.

5. Wikipedia. Three-tier (computing). Available at `http://en.wikipedia.org/wiki/Three-tier_%28computing%29`. Accessed August 16, 2006.

6. Microsoft Corporation. Available at `http://www.microsoft.com/`. Accessed July 31, 2006.

7. Corel. Available at `http://www.corel.com/`. Accessed July 31, 2006.

8. dBASE. Welcome to dBASE. Available at `http://www.dbase.com/`. Accessed July 31, 2006.

9. Oracle. Database 10g. Available at `http://www.oracle.com/database/`. Accessed July 31, 2006.

10. IBM. IBM software: DB2 product family. Available at `http://www.ibm.com/db2`. Accessed July 31, 2006.

11. MySQL. MySQL AB. Available at `http://www.mysql.com/`. Accessed July 31, 2006.

12. PostgreSQL. Available at `http://www.postgresql.org/`. Accessed July 31, 2006.

13. Advanced Micro Devices. Available at `http://www.amd.com/us-en/`. Accessed July 31, 2006.

14. Intel. Available at `http://www.intel.com/`. Accessed July 31, 2006.

15. Wikipedia. RAID. Available at `http://en.wikipedia.org/wiki/RAID`. Accessed July 31, 2006.

16. GNU Project. Free Software Foundation, GNU general public license. Available at `http://www.gnu.org/copyleft/gpl.html`. Accessed September 5, 2006.

17. Open Source Initiative. The BSD license. Available at `http://www.opensource.org/licenses/bsd-license.php`. Accessed September 5, 2006.

18. Apache. The Apache HTTP server project. Available at `http://httpd.apache.org/`. Accessed July 31, 2006.

19. Open Geospatial Consortium, Inc. Available at `http://www.opengeospatial.org/`. Accessed July 31, 2006.

20. Environmental Systems Research Institute. Available at `http://www.esri.com/`. Accessed July 31, 2006.

21. GRASS GIS. Available at `http://grass.itc.it/`. Accessed July 31, 2006.

22. SAS. Business intelligence and analytics software. Available at `http://www.sas.com/`. Accessed September 8, 2006.

23. MapInfo Corporation. Available at `http://www.mapinfo.com/`. Accessed September 8, 2006.

24. Centers for Disease Control and Prevention. PHIN: BioSense. Available at `http://www.cdc.gov/phin/component-initiatives/biosense/index.html`. Accessed August 15, 2006.

25. The ESSENCE II Disease Surveillance Test Bed for the National Capital Area. Available at `http://www.jhuapl.edu/techdigest/td2404/Lombardo.pdf`. Accessed September 8, 2006.

26. RODS Laboratory. Realtime outbreak and disease surveillance. Available at `http://rods.health.pitt.edu/`. Accessed September 8, 2006.

27. New York City Syndromic Surveillance Systems. Available at `http://www.syndromic.org/syndromicconference/2003/mmwr/mm53su01_027_to_029.pdf`. Accessed September 8, 2006.

28. Syndrome definitions for diseases associated with critical bioterrorism-associated agents. Version of October 23, 2003. Available at `http://www.bt.cdc.gov/surveillance/syndromedef/index.asp`.

29. Annotated bibliography for syndromic surveillance: data sources and case definitions. Available at `http://www.cdc.gov/epo/dphsi/syndromic/analytic.htm`.

30. Mitchell TM. Machine learning. Boston, MA: The McGraw-Hill Companies; 1997.

31. Yang YM. An evaluation of statistical approaches to text categorization. J Inf Retriev. 1999;1:67-88.

32. Yang YM, Liu X. A re-examination of text categorization methods. Proc ACM SIGIR. 1999:42-49.

33. Olszewski RT. Bayesian classification of triage diagnoses for the early detection of epidemics. In: Recent Advances in Artificial Intelligence: Proceedings of the 16th International FLAIRS Conference, 2003. Menlo Park, CA: AAAI Press. 2003:412-416.

34. Hripsak G, Friedman C, Alderson PO, DuMouchel W, Johnson SB, Clayton PD. Unlocking clinical data from narrative reports: a study of natural language processing. Ann Intern Med. 1995;122:681-688.

35. Haug PJ, Christensen L, Gundersen M, Clemons B, Koehler S, Bauer K. A natural language parsing system for encoding admitting diagnoses. In: Proceedings of the AMIA Annual Fall Symposium 1997;814-818.

36. Chapman WW, Christensen LM, Wagner MM, Haug PJ, Ivanov O, Dowling JN, Olszewski RT. Classifying free-text triage chief complaints into syndromic categories with natural language processing. Artif Intell Med. 2005;33:1-10.

37. Heffernan R, Mostashari F, Das D, Karpati A, Kulldorff M, Weiss D. Syndromic surveillance in public health practice, New York City. Emerg Infect Dis [serial on the Internet]. May 2004. Available at http://www.cdc.gov/ncidod/EID/vol10no5/03--0646.htm.

38. Sniegoski CA. Automated syndromic classification of chief complaint records. Johns Hopkins APL Tech Dig. 2004;25(1).

39. Shapiro AR. Taming variability in free text: application to health surveillance. In: Syndromic Surveillance: Reports from a National Conference 2003. MMWR. 2004; 53(suppl): 95-100. Available at http://www.cdc.gov/mmwr/PDF/wk/mm53SU01.pdf.

40. Chapman WW, Bridewell W, Hanbury P, Cooper GF, Buchanan BG. A simple algorithm for identifying negated findings and diseases in discharge summaries. J Bio Inf. 2001; 34: 301-310. doi:10.1006/jbin.2001.1029.

41. Mutalik PG, Deshpande A, Nadkarni PM. Use of general-purpose negation detection to augment concept indexing of medical documents: a quantitative study using the UMLS. J Am Med Inf. November – December;8(6):598-609.

42. Chapman WW, Bridewell W, Hanbury P, Cooper GF, Buchanan BG. Evaluation of negation phrases in narrative clinical reports. Proc AMIA Symp. 2001:105-109.

43. US Department of Health and Human Services, Office of the Secretary. 45 CFR Parts 160, 162, and 164 Health Insurance Reform: Security Standards; Final Rule. Available at http://www.cms.hhs.gov/SecurityStandard/Downloads/securityfinalrule.pdf. Accessed June 22, 2006.

44. Jernigan DB, et al. Data standards in public health informatics. In: O'Carroll PW, et al., gen. eds. Public Health Informatics and Information Systems. New York: Springer-Verlag; 2003, Chap 10.

45. Schneier B, Shpantzer G. GAO report says FAA still has cyber security problems to address (September 26, 2005). SANS NewsBites. September 28, 2005;7(39).

46. Meier JD, et al. Design guidelines for secure web applications. In: Improving Web Application Security, Chap 4. Available at http://msdn.microsoft.com/library/default.asp?url=/library/en-us/dnnetsec/html/thcmch04.asp. Accessed April 19, 2006.

47. Meier JD, et al. Architecture and design review for security. In: Improving Web Application Security, Chap 5. Available at http://msdn.microsoft.com/library/default.asp?url=/library/en-us/dnnetsec/html/thcmch05.asp. Accessed April 19, 2006.

48. Wikipedia. Public-key cryptography. Available at http://en.wikipedia.org/wiki/Public_key. Accessed April 19, 2006.

49. Wikipedia. Transport layer security. Available at http://en.wikipedia.org/wiki/Transport_Layer_Security. Accessed April 19, 2006.

50. Wikipedia. Computer security. Available at http://en.wikipedia.org/wiki/Computer_security. Accessed April 19, 2006.

51. Tanase M. Always on, always vulnerable: securing broadband connections. March 26, 2003. Available at http://www.securityfocus.com/infocus/1560. Accessed June 24, 2006.

52. Tanase M. Barbarians at the gate: an introduction to distributed denial of service attacks. December 3, 2002. Available at http://www.securityfocus.com/infocus/1647. Accessed June 24, 2006.

53. Open Web Application Security Project. A1: Unvalidated input. 2005. Available at http://www.owasp.org/documentation/topten/a1.html. Accessed April 19, 2006.

54. Open Web Application Security Project. A4: Cross site scripting. 2005. Available at http://www.owasp.org/documentation/topten/a4.html. Accessed April 19, 2006.

55. Wikipedia. Cross site scripting. Available at http://en.wikipedia.org/wiki/Cross_site_scripting. Accessed April 19, 2006.

56. Acme Internet. How SSL works. Available at http://support.acmeinternet.com/howtofaqs/ecommerce/ssl-howitworks.htm. Accessed April 19, 2006.

57. Pakala S, et al. AppSec FAQ. Available at http://www.owasp.org/documentation/appsec_faq.html. Accessed April 19, 2006.

58. Wikipedia. White-hat hacker. Available at http://en.wikipedia.org/wiki/White-hat_hacker. Accessed June 24, 2006.

59. Wikipedia. Computer port (software). Available at http://en.wikipedia.org/wiki/Computer_port_%29software%30. Accessed June 24, 2006.

60. Skoudis E. Counter Hack. Upper Saddle River, NJ; Prentice-Hall; 2002:289. As quoted in Beverstock D. Passwords are DEAD! (Long live passwords?) [practical paper for SANS GSEC certification]. 2003. Available at http://www.sans.org/reading_room/whitepapers/authentication/1144.php. Accessed June 22, 2006.

61. RSA Security Inc. RSA Security: RSA SecurID authentication. Available at `http://www.rsasecurity.com/node.asp?id=1156`. Accessed April 19, 2006.

62. Wikipedia. Authentication. Available at `http://en.wikipedia.org/wiki/Authentication`. Accessed April 19, 2006.

63. Aladdin Knowledge Systems Ltd. eToken strong authentication and password management. Available at `http://www.aladdin.com/etoken/default.asp`. Accessed April 19, 2006.

64. Timberline Technologies LLC. Alphabetical list of authentication products. Available at `http://www.timberlinetechnologies.com/products/authentication.html`. Accessed April 19, 2006.

65. searchSecurity.com, 2002. Define key fob: a Whatis.com definition. Available at `http://searchsecurity.techtarget.com/sDefinition/0,,sid14_gci795968,00.html`. Accessed April 19, 2006.

66. Wikipedia. SecurID. Available at `http://en.wikipedia.org/wiki/Securid`. Accessed April 19, 2006.

67. CafeSoft LLC. Tomcat security overview and analysis. Available at `http://www.cafesoft.com/products/cams/tomcat-security.html`. Accessed April 19, 2006.

68. Wikipedia. Virtual private network. Available at `http://en.wikipedia.org/wiki/Virtual_private_network`. Accessed June 22, 2006.

69. Radcliff D. After a security breach. Network World. October 24, 2005:42-44.

Part II: Case Studies

6 Modern Disease Surveillance Systems in Public Health Practice

Sheri Happel Lewis, Kathy Hurt-Mullen, Colleen Martin, Haobo Ma, Jerome I. Tokars, Joseph S. Lombardo, Steven Babin

Chapters 1 through 5 of this text addressed the various topics that must be considered in the design and implementation of an automated disease surveillance system. Chapter 5 focused on the individual components needed to process and display data and information as well as the knowledge needed by IT personnel to operate and maintain a web-based disease surveillance system.

The second part of this book addresses the use of disease surveillance systems by health departments. Chapter 6 is directed at the epidemiologist or surveillance analyst/public health monitors who will use the disease surveillance system that has been implemented. This chapter first reviews the health department's requirement to monitor the health of the population it serves, then discusses the systems in operation, and provides examples of public health events that have been identified. The chapter ends with an introduction to a Centers for Disease Control and Prevention (CDC) initiative to conduct surveillance at the national level by capturing data locally across the country.

6.1 PUBLIC HEALTH SURVEILLANCE REQUIREMENTS

Public health officials are tasked with the broad mission of protecting and promoting the health of their communities [1]. This obligation consists of three core functions: *assessment*, *policy development*, and *assurance*, which are outlined by the CDC's *10 Essential Services*:

1. Monitor health status to identify community health problems.

2. Diagnose and investigate health problems and health hazards in the community.

3. Inform, educate, and empower people about health issues.

4. Mobilize community partnerships to identify and solve health problems.

5. Develop policies and plans that support individual and community health efforts.

6. Enforce laws and regulations that protect health and ensure safety.

7. Link people to needed personal health services and assure the provision of health care when otherwise unavailable.

8. Assure a competent public health and personal health care workforce.

9. Evaluate effectiveness, accessibility, and quality of personal and population-based health services.

10. Conduct research for new insights and innovative solutions to health problems [2].

To be effective, public health officials require timely, accurate, and complete data to guide their efforts. This chapter focuses on the first two essential services: monitoring health status and investigating health problems. Public health practitioners can support these objectives more efficiently by utilizing advances in public health informatics.

6.1.1   Disease Reporting Requirements

Until the advent of automated disease surveillance systems, health departments relied on manually intensive reporting. Manual reporting introduces significant time lags in monitoring the status of a community's health. Analyses by public health personnel are reliant on health care providers (such as physicians, infection control practitioners, and diagnostic laboratories), who were required to inform the health department of diseases termed "reportable" by law.

National requirements for public health reporting efforts began as early as 1878 with the collection of information by the U.S. Marine Hospital Services on infectious diseases such as cholera, smallpox, plague, and yellow fever. The reporting of specific infectious disease continues today, in addition to the collection of information on the occurrence of many other diseases. Figure 6.1 represents a typical morbidity report form to be completed by health care providers upon determination of a reportable health event. Reportable conditions are stipulated by state law and include both clinically diagnosed findings and certain laboratory results. Guidance for the designation of reportable conditions is provided by the CDC, but variation exists among individual states.

Most states specify the data elements to be reported by health departments within their jurisdiction. These data are typically limited to information needed for characterization of the case with respect to person, place, and time; evaluation of the potential for spread, which might require public health or clinical intervention; or association with other cases. Information regarding risk factors and specific clinical and laboratory findings are also included to support the diagnosis. The morbidity report shown in Fig. 6.1 provides an example of data elements required by the state of Maryland.

The process of notifiable disease reporting was standardized by the U.S. Surgeon General in 1902. At that time, standards were instituted for the collection, compilation,

MARYLAND CONFIDENTIAL MORBIDITY REPORT (DHMH-1140)
(For use by physicians and other health care providers, but not laboratories. Laboratories use form DHMH-1281)

STATE DATA BASE NUMBER (Completed by Health Department)

SEND TO LOCAL HEALTH DEPARTMENT

NAME OF PATIENT – LAST | FIRST | M | DATE OF BIRTH MONTH DAY YEAR | AGE | SEX M☐ F☐ | ETHNICITY (Select independently of RACE) HISPANIC or LATINO YES☐ NO☐ UNKNOWN☐

(Maryland law prohibits the reporting of a patient's name for HIV infection.)

TELEPHONE NUMBERS Home: Workplace: | RACE (Select one or more. If multiracial, select all that apply.) American Indian/Alaskan Native☐ Asian☐ Black/African American☐ Hawaiian/Pacific Islander☐ White☐ Unknown☐ Other (Specify):

ADDRESS | UNIT# | CITY OR TOWN | STATE | ZIP CODE | COUNTY

OCCUPATION OR CONTACT WITH VULNERABLE PERSONS (Check all that apply - include volunteers) ☐ HEALTH CARE WORKER (Include any PATIENT CARE, ELDER CARE, "AIDES," etc.) ☐ DAYCARE (Attendee or Provider) ☐ PARENT of a child in DAYCARE ☐ FOOD SERVICE WORKER ☐ NOT EMPLOYED ☐ OTHER (SPECIFY): | WORKPLACE, SCHOOL, CHILD CARE FACILITY, ETC. (Include Name, Address, ZIP Code)

DISEASE OR CONDITION | DATE OF ONSET MONTH DAY YEAR | ADMITTED YES☐ NO☐ | DATE ADMITTED MONTH DAY YEAR | HOSPITAL

CONDITION ACQUIRED IN MARYLAND YES☐ NO☐ (IF NO, INTERSTATE ☐, or INTERNATIONAL ☐) | SUSPECTED SOURCE OF INFECTION | DIED YES☐ NO☐ | DATE DIED MONTH DAY YEAR | PREGNANT YES☐ NO☐ UNKNOWN☐ NOT APPLICABLE☐ WEEKS PREGNANT ___ DUE DATE ___

LABORATORY TESTS - VIRAL HEPATITIS (POS NEG DATE) HAV Antibody Total ☐ ☐ ___ HAV Antibody IgM ☐ ☐ ___ HBsurface Antigen ☐ ☐ ___ HB core Antibody Total ☐ ☐ ___ HB core Antibody IgM ☐ ☐ ___ HB surface Antibody ☐ ☐ ___ HCV Antibody ELISA ☐ ☐ ___ HCV Antibody RIBA ☐ ☐ ___ HCV RNA (e.g. by PCR) ☐ ☐ ___ ALT (SGPT) level ___ ALT - Lab Normal Range ___ to ___ NAME of LAB ___ | ADDITIONAL LAB RESULTS + PERTINENT CLINICAL INFORMATION + OTHER COMMENTS (For lab results give SPECIMEN - TEST - RESULT - DATE - NAME of LAB. Please attach copies of lab reports whenever possible.)

ACQUIRED IMMUNODEFICIENCY SYNDROME (AIDS) – ADDITIONAL CASE INFORMATION
ONLY physicians should report AIDS. Physicians reporting AIDS should use this form. ONLY laboratories should report HIV infection. Laboratories reporting HIV infection should use form DHMH-1281 and the patient's Unique Identifier instead of the name. Maryland law prohibits reporting of the patient's name for HIV infection.

CONDITIONS | HIV LAB TESTS | DATE | RESULT
WEIGHT LOSS OR DIARRHEA ☐ | CD4+ T cells < 200 per microliter | |
SECONDARY INFECTIONS (PCP, etc.) ☐ | ELISA | |
OTHER CONDITIONS ATTRIBUTED TO HIV INFECTION ☐ (SPECIFY): | WESTERN BLOT | |
| OTHER (SPECIFY) | |

SEXUALLY TRANSMITTED DISEASE (STD) – ADDITIONAL CASE INFORMATION
SYPHILIS: PRIMARY☐ SECONDARY☐ EARLY LATENT (LESS THAN 1 YR)☐ CONGENITAL☐ OTHER (STAGE)☐ (SPECIFY):
GONORRHEA: UNCOMPLICATED☐ PID☐ RECTAL☐ PHARYNGEAL☐ OPHTHALMIA NEONATORUM☐ OTHER☐ (SPECIFY)
OTHER STD (Specify):

STD LABORATORY CONFIRMATION AND TREATMENT
Specify STD Lab Test (e.g., RPR or VDRL, FTA – ABS, FTA – IgM, Darkfield, Smear, Culture, Other)
DATE | TEST | RESULT | DATE | DRUG | DOSAGE
| | | STD Treatment Given | |

TUBERCULOSIS (Suspect or Confirmed) – ADDITIONAL CASE INFORMATION
MAJOR SITE: PULMONARY☐ EXTRAPULMONARY☐ ATYPICAL☐ (SPECIFY): | ABNORMAL CHEST X-RAY: ☐
COMMENTS:

REPORTED BY | ADDRESS | TELEPHONE NUMBER | DATE OF REPORT MONTH DAY YEAR
☐ Check here if completed by the Health Department

NOTE: Your local health department may contact you following this initial report to request additional disease-specific information.
☐ Check here if you need more confidential morbidity report forms

DHMH-1140 REVISED AUG 2003

Fig. 6.1 Notifiable condition report from the Maryland Department of Health and Mental Hygiene. *Source:* Maryland Department of Health and Mental Hygiene, Office of Epidemiology and Disease Control Programs [3].

and distribution of data at the local, state, and national levels. The CDC took over the duties of this system, known as the National Notifiable Diseases Surveillance System (NNDSS), in 1961 [4] with continuing responsibilities to act as a data repository and to support efforts at the state and local levels. The process begins at the patient encounter with either a qualifying diagnosis made by a clinician or a qualifying laboratory finding. In such instances, the clinician or laboratory director is required to report information to the local health department within a certain time period, depending on the nature of the disease. The staff of the health department compiles reports in weekly cycles for transmission to the state health department. The state, in turn, passes the information to the CDC. The surveillance information is used for purposes that vary at each level of report, but reducing the time between the onset of illness and its report improves the outcome of public health interventions for all purposes. A recent study of reporting lags across states and diseases found that the median number of days to report was 12 for meningococcal disease and 40 for pertussis. This study concluded that because of such lags in reporting, the NNDSS cannot support timely identification of and response to outbreaks at a national level [5].

An established practical application of disease surveillance is the seasonal monitoring and reporting of influenza through a sentinel physician program coordinated by the CDC. Volunteer physicians report influenza activity from their practice on a weekly basis during the months of October through May. Reporting includes data on the total number of patient visits for the week and the number of visits for influenza-like illness by age group. Although valuable, this information suffers in timeliness from the weekly reporting cycles. In addition, only a small proportion of the U.S. population is actually covered by this surveillance activity because participation in the sentinel physician program is strictly voluntary [6]. During the 2004–2005 influenza season, the CDC reported that 2200 physicians were included in the network from 46 states; however, in any given week, approximately 50% of the physicians did not complete reports [7]. Finally, the data from this network are statistically weighed using state population and background influenza rates, so estimates produced by the system cannot be used for understanding influenza activity at the state, regional, or local levels.

These disease reporting processes, namely notifiable disease and sentinel surveillance, remain in place today. The utility of the data from these systems for recognition of important changes in community health status is seriously limited by a reliance on clinical providers to initiate reports to authorities in a timely manner and by the inherent delays in weekly reporting cycles. Additionally, there is a heavy staffing burden inherent in a system that relies on exchanging information on paper with subsequent manual data entry to support reporting and analysis.

The need for improved timeliness and automation in surveillance efforts was understood even before the terrorist events of 2001. The CDC began promoting enhanced surveillance activities through their 1998 plan entitled *Preventing Emerging Infectious Disease: A Strategy for the 21st Century, Overview of the Updated CDC Plan* [8].

Goals and objectives were put forth by health officials in four categories, one of which was surveillance and response. The objectives for improved surveillance included:

1. Strengthening infectious disease surveillance and response

2. Improving methods for gathering and evaluating surveillance data

3. Ensuring the use of surveillance data to improve public health practice and medical treatment

4. Strengthening global capacity to monitor and respond to emerging infectious diseases [9]

The terrorist attacks on the World Trade Center and the Pentagon on September 11, 2001, and the anthrax letters that followed in the autumn of that year accelerated the development of improved disease surveillance systems [8]. Many efforts had already been made to conduct surveillance via "drop-in" systems during large events [10, 11]. Such systems operate by collecting information on emergency department (ED) visits in 24-hour cycles via the ED logs. Although potentially useful in the short-term, these systems are typically difficult to sustain given the amount of labor required to support them and the absence of any historical information to provide context for evaluation of detected anomalies.

The threat of bioterrorism caused many health departments to extend the operations of their manually intensive drop-in surveillance systems. In the National Capital Region (NCR), for example, ED logs containing the chief complaint or discharge diagnosis for each patient from the previous day's visits were faxed to health departments daily. Health department staff then assigned encounters to mutually exclusive syndrome groups [12] and performed aberration detection using CDC-provided algorithms. Such approaches are extremely labor intensive at every point in the process, which makes this form of surveillance prohibitively expensive over time. Automated systems have reduced much of this burden by exploiting advances in clinical information systems and public health informatics. The scope of responsibilities for public health officials has become increasingly broad in recent years; therefore, it is imperative that tools developed to support their work impose as little burden as possible while providing meaningful information for action in a timely, coherent fashion.

Many surveillance activities have been taking place at various government levels in recent years. All types of surveillance come with their own inherent advantages and disadvantages. Each health department or locality must determine what type of system will best meet its needs. Table 6.1 summarizes various types of surveillance systems that have been used and lists the potential advantages and disadvantages of each.

6.1.2 Existing Automated Disease Surveillance Systems

There are a variety of modern disease surveillance systems in use today by health departments. These systems vary greatly between localities, ranging from locally

Table 6.1   Types of Syndromic Surveillance Systems [8].

TABLE. Types of syndromic surveillance — selected characteristics, advantages, and disadvantages

Surveillance type	Selected characteristics	Advantages	Disadvantages
Event-based surveillance Drop-in (20,21)	Active Defined duration Emergency departments (EDs) Large clinics	Develop relationships with ED staff and infection-control professionals Transportable to various sites	Labor-intensive Not sustainable Not scalable
Sustained surveillance Manual (22)	Active and passive Fax-based reporting ED triage staff typically log and tally sheets	Develop relationships with hospital staff Easy to initiate Detailed information obtainable	Labor-intensive Difficult to maintain 24 hours, 7 days/week Not sustainable

Electronic (8,19,23,24)	Passive
	Automated transfer of hospital (usually
	  ED triage or diagnosis) or outpatient data
	Use of data collected for other purposes
	Data mining of large collections or from
	  multiple sources
		Can be scalable
		Requires minimal or no provider input
		Data available continuously
		Data are standardized
			Need programming and
			  informatics expertise
			Confidentiality issues

Novel modes of collection (25)	Passive Hand-held or touch-screen devices	Easy to use; rapid provider feedback; can post alerts and information	Requires provider input Not sustainable

Novel data sources (26)	Active and passive
	Medical examiner data
	Unexplained death or severe illness data
		Clearly defined syndrome
		Can be supplemented with laboratory
		  data
			Not an early warning
			Unclear whether it can be
			  rapidly and broadly
			  expanded

maintained systems to application service provider (ASP) systems that collect and maintain data at a remote site for analysis and access by users. There are also a variety of analytical tools available for users. The differences in systems extend to the types of data they utilize, the frequency of reporting, and the role and capability of the users that review the output. Although not exhaustive, Sections 6.1.2.1 through 6.1.2.5 provide a brief overview of a few systems in use today.

6.1.2.1   ESSENCE

Multiple versions of the Electronic Surveillance System for the Early Notification of Community-Based Epidemics (ESSENCE) are in use today. For example, one version of ESSENCE is used for disease surveillance of all U.S. military personnel and their dependents, and another version exists for the Veterans Health Administration. Several ESSENCE versions, integrating numerous data sources, are also in different civilian localities [13].

ESSENCE is a flexible and scalable application that allows for the import of a variety of data sources, including physician outpatient visit data, OTC pharmaceutical sales, ED chief complaints, nurse advice data, 911 calls, school absentee data, and many other data sources that health departments may want to include in their own version of the application. While ESSENCE employs an alerting capability that identifies and flags statistical anomalies for the end user, it is also customizable, permitting epidemiologists to monitor a variety of health issues of interest within their communities.

ESSENCE allows users to select the algorithms that are used to detect aberrations in their version of the application. For example, if a health department elects to use the CDC Early Aberration Reporting System (EARS) algorithms, these algorithms can be selected and their performance compared to that of other algorithms contained within the application. Analyses within ESSENCE can be performed by data source, region, syndrome group, etc. [14].

ESSENCE utilizes a password-protected encrypted website to allow users to view the information regardless of their location. The user has the ability to drill down into the cause of an alert to see line listings of patients in the case of ED and office visit data or listings of products sold in the case of OTC medication sales. ESSENCE is an information system that is fully queriable to permit users to customize analyses. For instance, new case definitions can be developed and maintained by linking a string of key words or ICD-9 codes. This feature is particularly useful for newly identified health concerns, such as severe acute respiratory syndrome (SARS) or West Nile virus. For example, once a SARS case definition is established, a user can query specifically for those defined strings (key words or ICD-9 codes) to identify patients that may have SARS or SARS-like illness.

Another useful feature of ESSENCE is its ability to generate and save graphs in various image formats, such as .jpegs, with customized titles, axes, and labels for use in presentations, thereby allowing the user to rapidly communicate findings to others. Data can be exported from ESSENCE for use in other software applications. ESSENCE was developed by The Johns Hopkins University Applied Physics Laboratory (JHU/APL) and the Department of Defense Global Emerging Infections System (DoD-GEIS).

6.1.2.2 *RODS*

The Real-Time Outbreak Detection System (RODS) was developed by the University of Pittsburgh and the Auton Lab of Carnegie Mellon University's School of Computer Science to detect a large-scale outbreak due to an outdoor release of anthrax [15]. Like ESSENCE, RODS is used widely by health departments throughout the United States.

RODS uses HL7 admission, discharge, and transfer (ADT) messages from EDs and walk-in clinics to capture chief complaint data for incorporation into the application's seven predetermined syndrome groups. The University of Pittsburgh also operates an OTC pharmacy data-monitoring system known as the National Retail Data Monitor (NRDM).

Like ESSENCE, RODS utilizes a variety of algorithms to identify anomalies in data streams, in particular, the recursive-least-square (RLS) adaptive filter [16], moving average, wavelet [17], and CUSUM with EWMA. The health department can set the alerting algorithms to generate alarms at various sensitivities. If a syndrome reaches a level that exceeds the preset health department limit, RODS automatically sends the health department an e-mail with a link to the RODS site that gives the user the pertinent charts and also the individual-level data that generated the alert [18].

RODS uses a password-protected encrypted website that allows users to log in to view clinical and OTC data. Because this surveillance system is predominantly an ASP model, data are stored at the central RODS laboratory rather than at the local health departments. Users can view summary information, customizable plots, geographical views, and alerts. Drilldown capabilities provide more detailed information to the public health user [17].

6.1.2.3 EARS   The Early Aberration Reporting System (EARS) was originally developed as a "drop in" surveillance system for large-scale events such as national sporting events and political conferences. For example, EARS was used in New York City following the attacks on the World Trade Center on September 11, 2001 [10].

The EARS application is a SAS-based program available via download over the internet and one requires only a web browser to run the program. It uses aberration-detection algorithms to look for changes in frequency or distribution of health events compared with historical data [19]. Data are sent via e-mail or file transfer protocol (FTP) to the user for analysis by EARS.

EARS uses three limited baseline algorithms based on CUSUM calculations: C1-MILD, C2-MEDIUM, and C3-ULTRA, named for their sensitivities [19]. CUSUM detects shifts in a particular syndrome away from its historical mean [20]. EARS is currently being used in many U.S. health departments, as well as internationally.

6.1.2.4 RedBat   RedBat is a commercial software product marketed to health departments for detection of infectious disease outbreaks. In addition to infectious diseases, it may also be used for surveillance of more chronic illnesses, such as asthma, and injuries. RedBat automatically imports ASCII data from existing data streams and uses data mining technology to identify uncommon syndrome clusters. The data can be analyzed either directly within RedBat, or can be exported for analysis in another surveillance system.

Patient demographic data, such as name, ID, age, and address, are collected in an ASCII file at the location of service (e.g., the hospital). This information is read into a natural language processor, which then parses the information into the appropriate syndrome group. Information is then made available to the health department on a daily basis.

RedBat has additional features that assist the health department with the collection of other data that may be useful, including reportable diseases, injuries, classification of clusters, and tracking of victims during disasters. Redbat is currently being used in portions of North Dakota and Texas and other localities [21].

6.1.2.5 SYRIS   The Syndrome Reporting Information System (SYRIS) is a surveillance tool aimed at collecting data entered by physicians, veterinarians, nurses, coroners, emergency management personnel, animal control officers, environmental health practitioners, and microbiologists. The data entered into SYRIS are made available to public health officials. Once the data are entered, the system determines if they meet the criteria for a public health alarm. Only public health officials can set the parameters for public health alarms. Public health officials are also able to do routine statistical analysis and mapping with the SYRIS system. One region currently using SYRIS is the health region around Lubbock, Texas [22].

6.2   IDENTIFICATION OF ABNORMAL HEALTH CONDITIONS

Many modern syndromic surveillance systems use a variety of analytical processes to determine whether the level of disease exceeds the norm for the community. These processes alert the user that a statistically significant increase has occurred and the user must then determine the public health significance of the alert. However, these systems enable important health events to be detected in other ways as well. For example, epidemiologists can use disease surveillance systems to monitor disease trends systematically and to identify suspicious clusters of disease through ad hoc analyses. Epidemiologists also receive information about unusual disease clusters or incidence from local health care providers, which they can then evaluate within their surveillance systems. Both system- and operator-generated alerts may be of equal value. The objective of this section is to examine how existing automated surveillance systems are being used by health departments.

6.2.1   Monitoring Surveillance System Outputs

Anomaly detection presents jurisdictional challenges that should be accommodated in developing response guidelines. Although public health officials have obligations within defined geographic boundaries, neither the movement of persons nor the distribution of illness is limited by these boundaries. To be effective at detecting cross-jurisdictional disease clusters, anomaly detection should be conducted at multiple levels (local, regional, state, and possibly national) to capture anomalies that might remain undetected within or bordering any single jurisdiction.

The common output of most surveillance systems is an alert or flag generated by algorithms applied to data containing indicators of health status. Algorithms typically compare present data with expected data estimated from the background of several previous days. Some algorithms also compare data from surrounding locations to perform a spatiotemporal statistical analysis. The alerts generated reflect statistical anomalies based on some threshold of the expected values (see Chapter 4 for further discussion). Statistical anomalies, however, do not always reflect true epidemiological or clinical anomalies. Because many of these anomalies depend on how the syndromes are defined in the data, the challenge for the user is to determine which, if any, of these statistically significant anomalies are clinically and/or epidemiologically significant. To perform this task, users must have knowledge of possible confounding variables (e.g., air quality, pollen, temperature, holidays, data dropouts), clinical presentations of diseases (e.g., influenza, infectious gastroenteritis, bioterrorism diseases), and epidemiologically significant disease clustering. One method for reviewing the outputs of analytical processes applied to surveillance data is to categorize alerts according to the following criteria:

1. Alerts that appear to be only a result of a statistical process

2. Alerts with a clinical foundation but that are epidemiologically unimportant from a public health perspective

3. Alerts with the potential to be clinically and epidemiologically interesting enough to warrant further monitoring before their public health importance is determined

4. Alerts clinically and epidemiologically important enough that further action, such as detailed epidemiological investigation and alerting of authorities, might be warranted

Figure 6.2 depicts a general process for reviewing information from an electronic disease surveillance system [23].

6.2.2   Characterization of Anomalies

Depending on the background of users and the priorities of the health department, different features may be required in a disease surveillance system, and different users may use the same system differently. General guidelines have been developed to assist in the characterization of anomalies, but they provide only initial guidance for new users until they develop methods that work within their context. Figure 6.2 illustrates the general steps a health department user could consider when evaluating alerts found on an electronic surveillance system. Regardless of the user, anomalies should be characterized fully to determine whether they are likely to represent an important public health event that requires a public health response. From an epidemiological standpoint, the anomaly should be described with respect to person, place, and time using whatever demographic and geographic information are available. Available clinical data (e.g., chief complaint and discharge diagnosis and disposition) should be evaluated and summarized. In certain cases, even more specific information (e.g., laboratory test requests or results, detailed ED admission data) might be available to characterize the anomaly further.

While a physician is specifically trained for and accustomed to working with pre-diagnostic information, the challenge in analyzing syndromic data is that there is no patient to interview or examine. Instead, the analyst must use the brief text listings and other clues in the different fields of data. Although the ease and accuracy of obtaining a "differential diagnosis" for a particular patient are thereby limited, one can still observe patterns and possibly link etiologies among populations of patients. These patterns can raise the index of suspicion that a true clinical anomaly exists among the statistical anomalies provided by the system. It should be noted that, even in traditional epidemiological analyses, statistical clusters of health events occur for which no clinical anomaly is ever found. These are frequently seen in noninfectious health events for which a common exposure is sought (e.g., cancer clusters), and the CDC has developed systematic investigative techniques to evaluate them [24].

Once the user is convinced that an anomaly represents a true cluster of similar health events, whether the anomaly is expected or unusual should be determined. Normal seasonal and temporal syndrome and disease trends should be reviewed. Influenza-like illness is easily spotted by a majority of disease surveillance systems. An increase in disease causes regular statistical alerts in established syndrome groups as illness

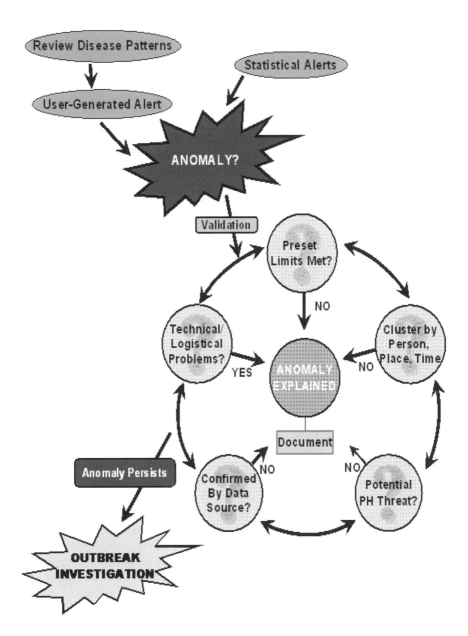

Fig. 6.2 Schematic presentation of daily review of an electronic biosurveillance system (From Coberly et al. [23]).

spreads through the community. Because this increase is expected each winter, the anomaly does not require further evaluation efforts. Similarly, environmental factors should be considered. For example, seasonal increases in pollen generate increases in respiratory illness that might cause statistical alerts in surveillance systems even though these events are expected. If more than one source of data is available within a system, part of the validation effort should be to ascertain whether corroboration is expected from those sources and whether similar patterns do exist in different data sources.

Figure 6.3 provides an overview of the process for the evaluation of potential disease clusters. The process will vary greatly depending on the health department and end user, but the general concept can be applied in any area regardless of the system being used.

Additionally, there may be a condition of particular interest to the epidemiologist. Some systems allow users to query specific text strings or enter a case definition that may be outside the scope of the typical syndrome groups to determine if events of particular interest are occurring. Systems with this functionality run aberration detection for the ad hoc case definition "on the fly" and allow analysts to review the current and historical experience with the particular set of complaints for their communities. Such analyses are common among users of systems with the capacity to create ad hoc case definitions, especially during flu season.

Figure 6.4 demonstrates the time series an epidemiologist can obtain using the ESSENCE system to query the ED chief complaint records for "fever, sore throat, and cough," symptoms commonly associated with influenza. By allowing queries for specific keywords within the patients' chief complaints, ESSENCE enables the user to define new case definitions for a disease of interest.

Epidemiologists may also receive information from other sources throughout the health community. One such source is the Program for Monitoring Emerging Diseases (ProMED). ProMED was started in 1993 and is managed by the International Society for Infectious Diseases. Members of its steering committee include representatives of the CDC, National Institutes of Health (NIH), World Health Organization (WHO), PanAmerican Health Organization (PAHO), and the International Office of Epizootics [25]. ProMED is a global electronic reporting system for outbreaks of emerging infectious diseases and illnesses caused by toxins. With subscribers from over 100 countries, ProMED often provides the earliest public reports of infectious disease outbreaks. Reports of suspicious events are submitted via e-mail or website and are then screened by teams of experts, including physicians, veterinarians, biologists, and epidemiologists. While the screening process results in some delay in dissemination of the information, it minimizes the transmission of erroneous or unclear information and also allows the ProMED editors to comment on the postings and raise pertinent questions for further response and discussion. In addition to providing a service for reporting events, ProMED also provides an online forum for discussion of the reports among subscribers. The amount of relevant information contained in a ProMED report may vary, and the editors make every effort to corroborate information in reports from official sources. Although ProMED exists largely as an educational

Validation of Potential Disease Cluster Seen In An Electronic Biosurveillance System

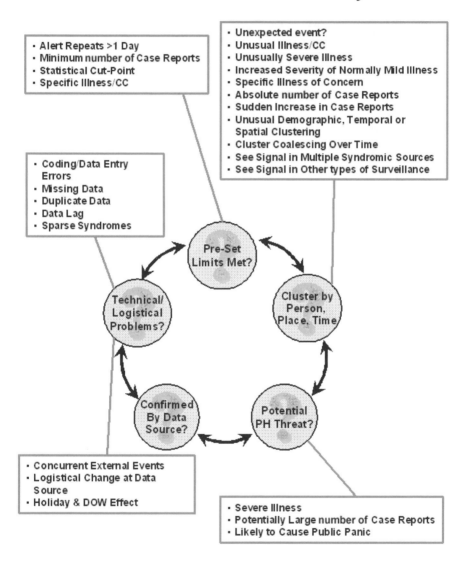

Fig. 6.3   Summation of potential process for evaluating potential disease clusters (DOW is an abbreviation for day-of-week).

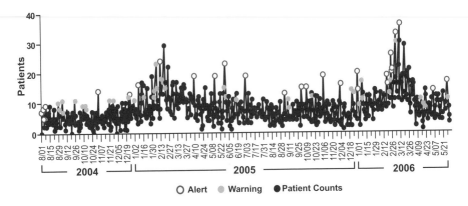

Fig. 6.4 Time series from the Aggregated National Capital Region (ANCR) site showing the daily counts resulting from a query in the chief complaint records for "fever, sore throat, and cough" from August 1, 2005, through June 1, 2006.

resource, it may also provide valuable insight for explaining anomalies observed in electronic surveillance systems.

Different users use different techniques to review and characterize anomalies. Much of this variability can be attributed to the system in place, the education and training of the user, the amount of time a user can devote to reviewing the system, the reliability of data transmission, and the health department's policy on review and follow-up of an electronic disease surveillance system. Some health departments have developed a set of queries (unique syndromes) that are processed and examined in parallel with routine syndromes. Such queries are commonly used where a particular health issue is of ongoing concern, and these issues vary depending on the time of the year. Many users also weigh data sources: that is, they pay more attention to one particular data stream than another because of its clinical significance, completeness, timeliness, or knowledge that it may contain a signal of importance. Some users will continue to follow-up on an alert for a few days after first receiving it, while others will only focus on alerts for a particular day. In addition, while some users will not rely on alerts alone for system review, others will focus primarily on alerts and, if there are none, will cease their review. The amount of attention users devote to pursuing alerts will depend to a large extent on the time available for system review and follow-up. Review and characterization of anomalies will differ greatly among both systems and users.

6.2.3   Case Studies

Several case studies are offered in this section to demonstrate how syndromic systems might be monitored and used. All of these studies are presented using features and findings of the ESSENCE system deployed in Montgomery County, Maryland.

6.2.3.1   Case Study 1: Detection of Influenza-like Illness   The first order of business in the daily review of system findings is to evaluate the overall incidence of each syndrome represented in the region captured. This step is often accomplished by review of the data time series. Figure 6.5 represents the number of ED visits for chief complaints coded into the respiratory syndrome (solid line). Additionally, time-series data are shown for chief complaints containing keywords suggestive of pneumonia and/or influenza (dashed line). From this time series, analysts were able to observe a modest but significant increase in ED visits for respiratory complaints that likely represented the beginning of flu activity in the county. Greater confidence was placed on these findings by the excellent correlation of trends in chief complaints that were strongly suggestive of pneumonia and/or influenza. Based on these data, health officials began discussions with hospital partners about the likelihood of influenza virus circulating in the community. As a result, hospital personnel began reviewing procedures for cough containment, separation of likely influenza cases in treatment rooms, and collection of appropriate specimens for viral isolation. On December 12, 2004, the first suggestion of circulating flu activity was found by querying for specific chief complaint terms. Flu activity was clearly visible in the broad respiratory syndrome group on December 14. The first traditional indicator of flu activity occurred on December 27 in the form of an outbreak of influenza-like illness (ILI) in a nursing home, which was reported to the health department on December 29.

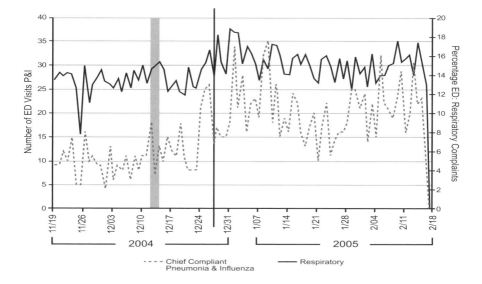

Fig. 6.5   Early detection of ILI in Montgomery County, 2004–2005 (vertical gray bar: range of days over which data began to suggest flu activity; vertical black line: date of onset of first nursing home ILI outbreak).

Figure 6.6 represents a time-series view of multiple data sources available to analysts for determining whether all potential data sources were in agreement regarding

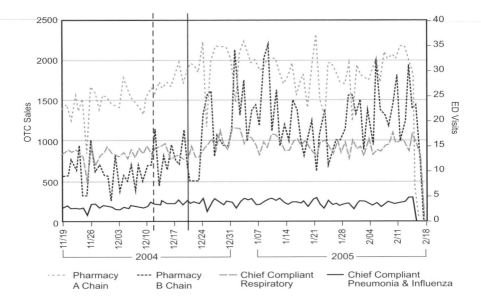

Fig. 6.6 Early detection of ILI in Montgomery County, Maryland, in multiple data sources (dotted black vertical line: earliest data indication of flu activity; solid black vertical line: date of first positive clinical isolate obtained for influenza virus).

the increase in ILI activity in the county. Two OTC pharmaceutical data sources, in addition to the ED respiratory syndrome data and specific ED chief complaints of pneumonia/influenza, exhibit the same general trend with an increase in activity noted and eventually determined to have been sustained in all four sources late in the second week of December. The ability to corroborate findings across data sources is particularly helpful to health officials because most individual data sources lack specificity. A similar finding in multiple streams gives health officials greater confidence in making recommendations based on the findings and can also serve to enhance the data by providing additional information about the geographic areas affected.

6.2.3.2 Case Study 2: Outbreak of Gastroenteritis Routine daily review of the time series of gastrointestinal complaints (shown in Fig. 6.7) revealed an event of concern for the Montgomery County Health Department. Previous statistical alerts had been observed for the past several months without much concern. However, on April 19, 2005, an effort was taken to characterize the alert that occurred. Analysis revealed that the increase in gastrointestinal chief complaints was dominated by patients in the age bracket between 5 and 17 years old.

Figure 6.8 presents the patient-level details that were available for characterizing the cases with respect to person, place, time, and severity of illness. The simple line listing of cases in the 5- to 17-year-old age group demonstrated a clear clustering of gastroenteritis-like complaints among a group of 13- and 14-year-olds who were not

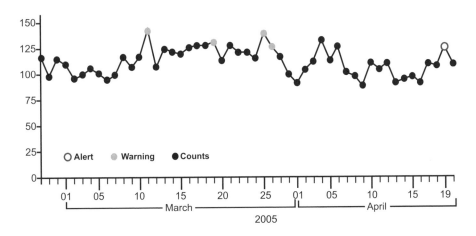

Fig. 6.7 Time series of emergency department visits for gastrointestinal complaints, alert on April 19, 2005.

Date	Time	Hospital	Zipcode	Age	Sex	Chief Complaint Parsed	Discharge Diagnosis	Discharge Disposition	Med Rec No
4/19/05	1:03 Pm	Sgaheroc	20874	5	F	Vomiting	Masked	Disch - Home	Masked
4/19/05	2:59 Am	Waheroc	20783	5	M	Abdominal Pain Vomiting	Masked	Transfer Children's Hosp	Masked
4/19/05	6:29 Am	Holycrosseroc	20853	6	F	Vomiting Abdominal Pain	Masked	Discharge To Home	Masked
4/19/05	4:14 Pm	Holycrosseroc	20906	6	M	Vomiting	Masked	Discharge To Home	Masked
4/19/05	7:17 Pm	Holycrosseroc	20902	7	M	Vomiting	Masked	Discharge To Home	Masked
4/19/05		Sgaheroc	20851	8	F	Abdominal Pain	Masked	Disch - Home	Masked
4/19/05	3:53 Pm	Holycrosseroc	20783	9	F	Abdominal Pain Nausea	Masked	Discharge To Home	Masked
4/19/05	4:15 Pm	Sgaheroc	20874	11	M	Abdominal Pain	Masked	Admit Peds	Masked
4/19/05	4:39 Am	Sgaheroc	Other	13	F	Nausea Vomiting	Masked	Disch - Home	Masked
4/19/05	10:31 Am	Sgaheroc	Other	13	F	Vomiting	Masked	Disch - Home	Masked
4/19/05	12:25 Pm	Sgaheroc	Other	13	F	Vomiting	Masked	Disch - Home	Masked
4/19/05	2:46 Am	Sgaheroc	Other	13	M	Nausea Vomiting	Masked	Disch - Home	Masked
4/19/05	2:58 Am	Sgaheroc	Other	13	F	Vomiting	Masked	Disch - Home	Masked
4/19/05	2:13 Am	Sgaheroc	Other	13	F	Nausea Vomiting	Masked	Disch - Home	Masked
4/19/05	2:15 Am	Sgaheroc	Other	13	F	Nausea	Masked	Disch - Home	Masked
4/19/05	10:32 Am	Sgaheroc	Other	14	M	Vomiting	Masked	Disch - Home	Masked
4/19/05	7:30 Am	Sgaheroc	Other	14	F	Nausea Vomiting	Masked	Disch - Home	Masked
4/19/05	3:04 Am	Sgaheroc	Other	14	M	Vomiting	Masked	Disch - Home	Masked
4/19/05	10:29 Am	Sgaheroc	Other	14	M	Vomiting	Masked	Disch - Home	Masked
4/19/05	2:59 Am	Sgaheroc	Other	14	F	Nausea	Masked	Disch - Home	Masked
4/19/05	3:00 Am	Sgaheroc	Other	14	M	Nausea Vomiting	Masked	Disch - Home	Masked
4/19/05	3:01 Am	Sgaheroc	Other	14	M	Vomiting	Masked	Disch - Home	Masked
4/19/05	2:26 Am	Sgaheroc	Other	14	M	Vomiting	Masked	Disch - Home	Masked
4/19/05	2:13 Am	Sgaheroc	Other	14	F	Vomiting	Masked	Disch - Home	Masked
4/19/05	2:09 Am	Sgaheroc	Other	14	F	Vomiting	Masked	Disch - Home	Masked
4/19/05	2:10 Am	Sgaheroc	Other	14	M	Nausea Vomiting Diarrhea	Masked	Disch - Home	Masked
4/19/05	2:12 Am	Sgaheroc	Other	14	F	Vomiting Nausea	Masked	Disch - Home	Masked
4/19/05	11:24 Pm	Holycrosseroc	20853	15	F	Abdominal Pain	Masked		Masked
4/19/05	11:22 Am	Holycrosseroc	20783	16	F	Abdominal Pain	Masked	Discharge To Home	Masked
4/19/05	6:52 Pm	Sgaheroc	20886	17	F	Lower Abdominal Pain	Masked	Disch - Home	Masked

Fig. 6.8 Line list obtained from system used to characterize patients causing increase in gastrointestinal complaints.

residents of the region, as indicated by "other" in the zip code column. This finding prompted a rapid response of public health officials to contact hospital officials to ascertain the details of these patient presentations. It was learned that these patients were members of a student group visiting the area on a school trip. The name and contact information for the chaperone and the hotel where they were lodging were obtained. Efforts to gather information about the status of illness in the group and to identify potential exposures for investigation were at first unsuccessful because the chaperone declined to cooperate with investigating authorities. When it was revealed that this group of students was scheduled to depart by air later that afternoon, officials had a substantial concern about the public health propriety of allowing this group of children to fly, given an illness that could easily be spread in the close quarters of an airplane during a transcontinental flight.

Eventually, the chaperone agreed to allow the children to be interviewed by health authorities only if the school principal concurred. However, the principal could not be reached because of the 3-hour time difference between the location of the outbreak and the school principal. With the departure of the flight becoming imminent, local health authorities worked to resolve the situation with their partners in the state health department and with authorities at the CDC. Information from the line list in Fig. 6.8 provided sufficient details to enable local health authorities, the state health department, and the CDC to persuade the airline's medical director to prohibit air travel of these students until their condition at the time of departure could be assessed. The chaperone then became much more cooperative and allowed interviews with the children. As a result, the airline allowed all children in the group to fly home with the stipulations that none were actively ill at the time of travel, they were all seated as a group, and a single bathroom was set aside for the children who had been ill or those who might become ill in travel.

The time from identification of this finding to the successful intervention was under 6 hours. Without the information provided by the syndromic surveillance system, it seems unlikely that public health authorities would even have been able to completely identify the patients involved as a single group in the limited time available. It should also be noted that there were 19 patients in this group, all were seen in one ED, and most presented within 1 hour in the very early morning after having been transported by ambulance. However, this event did not prompt hospital personnel to notify the health department.

6.2.3.3 Case Study 3: Detection of a Gastroenteritis Outbreak   Aggregating across an entire region for all age groups, can sometimes mask signals of interest. Only normal variations are present in the total Gastrointestinal syndrome time series provided in Fig. 6.9. It is sometimes necessary to evaluate the syndromic data and algorithm outputs by specific groupings of age, location, or sex. In this particular scenario, an interesting finding was noted in a specific age-group during the same time period as shown in Fig. 6.10.

Figure 6.10 shows on August 8, 2005, there was nearly a threefold increase in the number of 5- to 17-year-old patients reporting to county EDs with Gastrointestinal

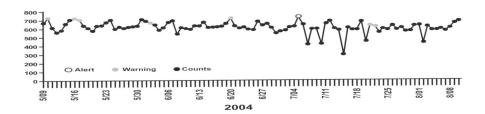

Fig. 6.9   Daily data counts of the total Gastrointestinal syndrome group for all ages in Montgomery County.

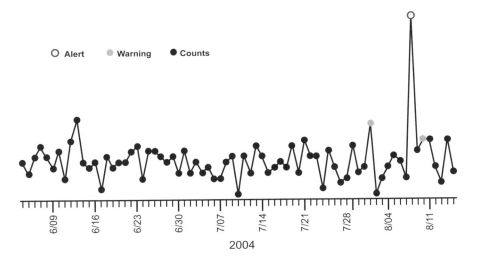

Fig. 6.10   Daily data counts of the Gastrointestinal syndrome group in 5- to 17-year-olds.

syndrome complaints. This increase required further investigation in order to characterize the cases causing the increase. Hyperlinks embedded within the surveillance application provide users the ability to view the underlying details about the cases represented in the daily syndrome counts.

The underlying data for the 5- to 17-year-old gastrointestinal cases on August 8, 2005, is provided in Table 6.2. The listing reveals a group of 17-year-olds presenting in the last 6 hours of the 24-hour reporting period. An investigation by the county

Table 6.2   Data Details from the 5- to 17-Year-Old Time Series for the Gastrointestinal Syndrome Group

Date	Time	Hospital Name	Region	Age	Sex	Chief Complaint
8/8/04	8:17 PM	B	Montgomery	5	F	Diarrhea Rash
8/8/04	8:58 AM	B	Montgomery	6	M	Fever Vomiting
8/8/04	8:07 AM	A	Montgomery	7	F	Fever Vomiting
8/8/04	5:42 PM	B	Montgomery	7	F	Stomach Pain
8/8/04	1:06 AM	C	Prince Georges	10	M	Abdominal Pain
8/8/04	8:19 PM	C	Prince Georges	12	F	Fever, Vomiting, Headache
8/8/04	5:11 PM	B	Montgomery	13	M	Abdominal Pain, Sickle Cell Crisis
8/8/04	8:46 PM	A	Charles	16	F	Nvd
8/8/04	6:12 PM	A	Montgomery	17	F	Abdominal Pain
8/8/04	7:37 PM	B	Montgomery	17	F	Fever, Vomiting, Headache
8/8/04	4:10 AM	B	Montgomery	17	M	Abdominal Pain, Side Pain
8/8/04	12:24 PM	A	Prince Georges	17	F	Abdominal Pain
8/8/04	11:31 PM	C	Prince Georges	17	F	558.9-Noninf Gastroenterit Nec
8/8/04	11:29 PM	C	Prince Georges	17	M	Vomiting, Dizzy
8/8/04	9:46 AM	A	Washington	17	F	RLQ Pain

health department revealed that a number of young adults had become ill at a summer leadership forum in a neighboring county. When the hospitals in the neighboring jurisdiction became full, some of these patients had been transported across county lines. Officials were able to use the unique identifiers provided within the surveillance system to obtain summaries of the medical encounters for these students to facilitate the outbreak investigation.

6.2.4   Summary of Anomaly Characterization

The previous case studies describe how epidemiologists were able to use knowledge of disease processes and relevant community attributes to rapidly review statistical anomalies generated by a syndromic surveillance system. In most cases, the investigation can be done by examination of individual records to identify common etiologies. Patterns suggestive of linked etiologies may be found within or across different syndrome categories and data streams. Each data stream has unique characteristics that must be taken into account. Sometimes, non-clinical data may be useful, such as air quality, aeroallergen levels, weather (temperature and rainfall), and news media reports (e.g., ProMED).

Data completeness must be assessed to determine the significance of each alert. For example, an alert for a county based on ED data from fewer than half the hospitals may not have become an alert if all the hospitals had been reporting. Alternatively, there may be no alerts for that county simply because most hospitals have not yet reported.

Assessments of data completeness for physicians' office visits may not be possible, depending on the data-acquisition strategy in place; because many systems rely on data from insurance claims clearinghouses, the denominator of reporting physicians is never known. It should be possible, however, to determine data completeness automatically for hospital ED and OTC data.

6.2.5   Assessing the Public Health Importance of Findings

Once an anomaly is fully characterized, its public health importance should be considered. First, the magnitude and continuity of the increase generating the anomaly should be evaluated in the context of the particular syndrome group in question. Regardless of statistical significance, a substantial 1-day increase warrants more scrutiny than a smaller increase; similarly, a relatively modest increase over multiple days that deviates from known seasonal and historic patterns should also be evaluated closely. In each of these instances, the size of the actual increase is characterized by the nature of known patterns of the data source and syndrome being evaluated; these considerations require an understanding of the usual frequency distribution for the particular event of concern. Certain signals can be expected and, when detected, are of less concern, especially when the public health response is well established (e.g., the beginning of the influenza season, winter increases in cases of viral gastroenteritis). However, observations of such anomalies at unexpected times of the year, or when frequency is much different than expected, or when presentations are unexpectedly severe, are more likely to represent important public health events [26].

6.3   UTILITY OF DISEASE SURVEILLANCE SYSTEMS AT THE LOCAL LEVEL

Studies were performed by Feighner and Coberly [18] to understand how automated disease surveillance systems were being used by state and local health departments and the utility of the local system. This section presents information gathered from interviews and surveys of users of automated systems.

Many localities describe the purpose of their disease surveillance system as the early detection of any event of public health significance, whether human-made (bioterrorism) or naturally occurring [27]. Many support the notion that optimization of their system for one type of event (e.g., illnesses caused by bioterrorism) should also lead to development of a system optimized for detection of naturally occurring disease. All health departments describe their disease surveillance system as only one of a group of surveillance tools that must be used in concert to understand the public's health. Additionally, health departments use their systems not only for early detection, but also to gauge the extent of known outbreaks or threats. Examples of other uses of enhanced surveillance systems are data mining and public health research. Lastly, a secondary gain for public health departments from the implementation of disease surveillance is improved communication with clinicians, hospitals, and other organizations involved with public health.

Many public health practitioners feel that enhanced disease surveillance represents a promising, yet unproven, initiative [28, 31]. Although rigorous cost-benefit analyses have not been conducted in most jurisdictions, many feel electronic surveillance systems clearly help them to identify seasonal waves of respiratory and gastrointestinal illness earlier than traditional surveillance methods. It is also largely felt that a syndromic surveillance system should be one component of a "system of systems." As the field of early-event disease surveillance progresses, research to evaluate the costs and benefits of disease surveillance will be an important task for public health practitioners [32, 35].

6.3.1 Specific System Features and Utility to Public Health Officials

Modern disease surveillance systems use pre-existing data sources to reduce the cost of the system and to minimize the burden on data providers. If the desire is to characterize anomalies with respect to person, place, and time, data streams must be selected to provide adequate demographic, geographic, and temporal information.

The volume of anomalies detected varies between systems, from only a handful in a year to numerous anomalies in a given week. Factors influencing the number of anomalies are number of syndrome groupings, number of age-group-specific event detections, and groupings by time and place in the aberration detection strategy. Some control over number of anomalies is achieved by decreasing algorithm sensitivity; however, reducing sensitivity should be considered carefully because increased sensitivity over traditional surveillance methods is a major objective for these systems [18].

6.3.2 Local Perspective on Implementation

Planning for and implementation of enhanced surveillance systems can be facilitated by the establishment of a work group. These groups provide all parties involved with opportunities to arrive at mutually agreeable and beneficial specifications and procedures. The membership of such groups should include practitioners from the health department and data partners, as well as information technology professionals from those organizations. Depending on the circumstances of funding and implementation, many such work groups include academic informatics groups or clinical information system vendors [27]. In addition to their technological expertise, these designers of disease surveillance packages may also contribute expertise in the administrative and legal issues of disease surveillance implementation.

6.3.2.1 System Facilitation   As a locality implements a local disease surveillance capability, communication between all interested parties is imperative. Ingestion of pre-existing data streams should drastically decrease the reporting effort required for data providers such as hospital EDs. Drafting data-sharing agreements (DSAs) between hospitals and health departments can be the rate-limiting step in the process of establishing an early-event surveillance system because corporate officers and legal staff will consider the many implications of such agreements. Data partners may wish to share data electronically with the health department only when assurances can be provided that this data sharing will not impose an additional burden resulting from health officials' investigations of system findings.

6.3.2.2 Need for Effective Communication with Stakeholders

While an established protocol might exist for communicating concerns in widening circles as the certainty and/or severity of findings warrant, such graduated communication processes should also contain provisions to avoid alarming the general public. Formal meetings between stakeholders in the surveillance system allow for ongoing, consensus-driven refinements to the system and help to maintain engagement of all parties.

Informal communication is equally important, particularly between the health department and those entities associated with data sources such as hospital infection control practitioners, ED health care providers, and laboratory personnel. Users report that an informal phone call to a data source will often quickly clarify the circumstances surrounding an anomaly [18]. This kind of communication allows for the efficient clarification of data findings and supports collegial relationships that are essential to all public health efforts. Communication is essential for sustaining any surveillance system. Users recognize the need for both formal and informal communication frameworks when maintaining a disease surveillance system. Formal communication frameworks are useful for a stepwise or phased approach to anomaly evaluation.

6.3.2.3 Understanding Data at the Local Level

Each type of data and each source within a given data type have idiosyncrasies. Data peculiarities must be appreciated and anomalies evaluated with this knowledge in mind to optimize the public health response. Because this knowledge is acquired by working with data and providers at the local level, such peculiarities may prove challenging when surveillance systems are being monitored at the state and national levels. This point is most appreciated in localities where systems allow analysts to manipulate the data to fit their needs; such a capacity must be supported by solid understanding of community attributes.

6.3.2.4 Training of Staff Is Essential

All staff and system users must be provided with both structured training and opportunities for hands-on experience as they learn. New users to early-event disease surveillance systems are faced with substantial learning challenges given the complexity of most systems. Owners of such systems report that it takes 6 weeks to 3 months to become completely familiar with a robust, multidata-source system [18] — new users of a disease system must learn the peculiarities not only of their data but also of the system itself. Users eventually do become comfortable with their systems, even those with the numerous methods for anomaly detection discussed previously. In addition to expertise in system use and data attributes, users must recognize recurrent patterns in the data over time.

6.3.2.5   Costs of Implementing and Maintaining a System   Much of the cost associated with surveillance systems are incurred during implementation. Initial costs include purchasing hardware and software and addressing the administrative, legal, and technical issues concerning data acquisition, as well as the substantial staffing costs at system start-up. The costs associated with monitoring and following up on system findings vary depending on the number of personnel a health department commits to this task, as well as their pre-existing capacity to support other surveillance efforts. An epidemiologist or other analyst must be assigned to evaluate daily findings. Most surveillance system monitors report spending 1 to 2 hours per day reviewing data.

Implementation costs generally do not include research and development of new technologies. The most economical way to establish a disease surveillance system is to use a prepackaged system (e.g., ESSENCE or RODS) via an ASP deployment. The ASP model, however, generally does not provide easy access to individual-level data due to confidentiality concerns. Furthermore, ASP deployment represents an investment risk in terms of funding sustainability at both the host and user ends.

6.3.3   Regional Perspective

There are a number of reasons that a health department or group of health departments may choose to undertake surveillance at the regional level. Among them are the attributes of the region itself. For example, in sparsely populated rural areas where logistical or fiscal concerns might preclude individual local systems, the pooling of resources and staffing may offer opportunities for a regional surveillance effort. In situations where there are large, multi-jurisdictional, densely populated, interconnected metropolitan areas, regional capacity is required to understand the health experience of a population living, working, and recreating across jurisdictional boundaries. Implementation of regional systems requires careful consideration and planning to ensure that the regional data captured and analyzed are appropriately shared, maintained, and funded.

A regional system is currently in place in the area surrounding Washington, DC, also known as the National Capital Region (NCR). The NCR comprises the District of Columbia; the counties of Montgomery and Prince George's in Maryland; and the counties of Loudoun, Fairfax, Arlington, Alexandria, and Prince William in Virginia. This region, which serves as the home of the U.S. federal government, is culturally, economically, and socially diverse, with residents often living in one location and traveling inter-jurisdictionally for work or recreation. Additionally, tourists and business travelers frequently visit the region, thus increasing the potential for the introduction and rapid spread of infectious disease. Given the cross-jurisdictional nature of this region and its status as a tier 1 city for bioterrorism threats, as per the U.S. Department of Homeland Security (DHS) [36], a regional surveillance view is considered necessary to completely evaluate important changes in community health status. The NCR uses the ESSENCE system. Figure 6.11 illustrates the connectivity of the NCR network. Maryland (MD), Virginia (VA), and the District of Columbia (DC) each operates a stand-alone surveillance application.

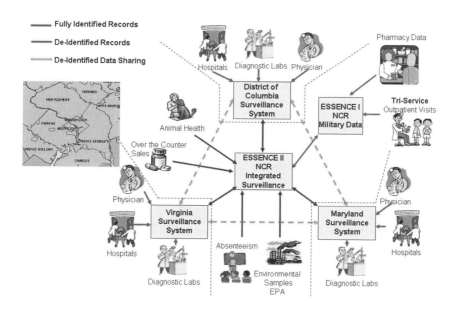

Fig. 6.11   Schematic illustrating the system placement and data flow within the NCR disease surveillance network.

The NCR network permits each health department to collect fully identifiable data regarding their residents, which improves the efficiency of additional investigations and follow-up activities. For sharing across the region, these data are de-identified, aggregated, and sent to the regional node, known as the Aggregated National Capital Region (ANCR) system. The ANCR site provides the regional view, and personnel from the MD, VA, and DC health departments have access to this site. The aggregation and sharing of data between the jurisdictions is supported by a single Data Sharing Agreement (DSA) among MD, VA, and DC and the ANCR host. This DSA sets parameters for the use, sharing, and release of aggregate data.

6.3.3.1   Need for Effective Regional Communication with Stakeholders   Regional systems require another level of communication for both implementation and sustainability. In addition to local communication within each jurisdiction, there must be a forum to communicate effectively among jurisdictions and as a whole group. In the case of the NCR, the Enhanced Surveillance Operating Group (ESOG) was created to facilitate discussions on topics such as system features and functionality, response protocols, and review and approval of all research and functionality developed to address problems unique to regional systems. This group comprises personnel from each participating health jurisdiction as well as members of the surveillance system development team and ANCR host.

6.3.3.2   Understanding Data at the Regional Level   In addition to understanding local data anomalies, users of a regional system are also tasked with monitoring anomalies that may arise at the regional level. In regional systems, spatial and temporal analytics are run both locally and regionally to capture both locally occurring problems and to identify potential regional issues. For example, although there may be a low level of illness in two neighboring jurisdictions such that neither jurisdiction generates an anomaly independently, these illnesses may in fact signal an alert when the jurisdictions are combined. As with other statistical anomalies generated by a system, these may be explained away by using a different level of knowledge than that required in assessing local anomalies alone.

An event/communication feature was designed and developed by a team of epidemiologists and software developers for the ANCR system. This feature allows people conducting daily data reviews to communicate their concerns to one another about specific events, situations, and statistical detection algorithm outputs. This prototype tool is embedded within the regional surveillance system and provides a forum in which users can write free-text comments, rate events based on level of concern, and attach hyperlinks to user screens that relay pertinent information to others. These capabilities aid in resolving specific health alerts at both the local and regional levels.

In addition to meeting the immediate needs of users for better awareness of the community's current health situation, this inter-regional component also enables the information recorded to be used for future enhancements of the overall disease surveillance system. For example, algorithm developers can view the communications logs to better understand and compare which detection alarms were met with concern versus those that were dismissed. This knowledge can aid in the future refinement of alerting algorithms.

6.3.3.3   Costs of Implementing and Maintaining a Regional System   Regional systems are more complex than local systems because each jurisdiction must maintain its own disease surveillance capacity and then transmit data to a regional hub. From a cost standpoint, implementation within each jurisdiction requires funding for hardware and system support. At the regional level, organizations have successfully obtained federal funds to link local systems and create regional nodes. Potential cost savings may be realized in implementations where data are collected and processed centrally in the regional node and then passed to local systems. Similarly, if a system is being set up in a rural area, only one central hub, rather than multiple nodes, may be needed to give users from all localities access. This approach reduces costs to approximately those of a locally maintained system that is shared among the supported jurisdictions. It also eliminates any duplication of effort that might occur if each jurisdiction were to seek data sources individually, and it ensures that all users use the same data set.

System maintenance is more complex in a regional system because any existing local systems must be maintained in addition to the regional node. At a minimum, each system needs to be maintained and updated with the latest version of the software, and, for the purposes of communication, the regional node should have the same software version. This degree of maintenance can be challenging because individual jurisdictions vary in their IT capabilities and financial ability to maintain the hardware.

6.4   ELECTRONIC BIOSURVEILLANCE AT THE NATIONAL LEVEL

BioSense, a national program developed by the CDC, is intended to improve the nation's capabilities for conducting near real-time biosurveillance and health situational awareness through access to existing data from health care organizations. BioSense is envisioned to provide local, state, and national public health and clinical partners with situational awareness capabilities for suspect illness and disease cases before, during, and after a health event, to assist public health officials with confirming or refuting the existence of an event, and to monitor an event in terms of size, location, and rate of spread. BioSense provides simultaneous access to health data by all levels of public health and supports cross-jurisdictional biosurveillance during a public health event.

6.4.1   BioSense System Description

BioSense was initially developed in 2003 as the early-event detection component of the CDC Public Health Information Network (PHIN) to support enhanced early detection, quantification, and localization of possible bioterrorism and other events of public health concern on a national level. At that time, BioSense began receiving national data feeds from the Department of Veterans Affairs (VA) and Department of Defense (DoD) and a web-based application was developed to enable visualization of these data. BioSense was made available to state and local public health officials in April 2004. In November 2004, a major national clinical laboratory, Laboratory Corporation of America (LabCorp), began sending data to BioSense. Therefore, the initial BioSense data included International Classification of Diseases, Ninth Revision, Clinical Modification (ICD-9-CM) codes and Current Procedural Terminology (CPT) codes from VA outpatient medical centers and clinics ($n = 849$) and DoD medical treatment facilities ($n = 355$), as well as laboratory test orders (local and LOINC codes) from LabCorp.

In mid-2005, the CDC embarked on a major initiative to enhance BioSense by including clinically rich data in real time from hospitals across the United States. In December 2005, BioSense began receiving foundational data (patient chief complaints, diagnoses, and demographics) from hospitals in key public health jurisdictions in real time. To protect privacy, BioSense does not receive patient identifiers. Patient populations include outpatients, ED patients, and inpatients. In early 2006, daily hospital census data (including occupancy rate, admission count, discharge count, and death count at the hospital level, and occupied and available beds at the unit level) began to be transmitted. Additional data, including ED clinical (e.g., vital signs and triage notes), microbiology laboratory orders and results, radiology orders and results, and pharmacy orders, are now being transmitted from some hospitals. In a public health event situation, these data are envisioned to provide a real-time window on community health status that has not been previously available to public health. Rigorous technical and scientific evaluations are needed to determine best practices and utility for BioSense data.

Real-time data are sent to CDC in batches every 15 minutes. Once data are received, they must be pre-processed, categorized, and stored in a data warehouse prior to being visualized in the application. Coded (ICD-9 and CPT) and free-text (chief complaints and working diagnoses) data are assigned as appropriate to 11 syndromes (botulism-like, fever, gastrointestinal, hemorrhagic illness, localized cutaneous lesion, lymphadenitis, neurological, rash, respiratory, severe illness/death, specific infection). A multiagency working group defined these syndromes in 2003 to capture pre-diagnostic data relevant to infectious bioterrorism agents [37]. BioSense medical staff also defined 78 sub-syndromes to allow for surveillance for more specific events and for a wider range of disease indicators. For example, the botulism-like syndrome includes several sub-syndromes, such as paralysis, speech disturbance, and dysphagia. Certain sub-syndromes do not map to a syndrome category; examples include allergy, burns, and excessive heat. For a single patient visit, more than one syndrome or sub-syndrome can be assigned; there is no hierarchical mapping.

ICD-9-CM codes are mapped to sub-syndromes based on definitions created by BioSense medical staff. Free-text data are mapped to sub-syndromes based on a text search for keywords and their associated misspellings, word fragments, and abbreviations. Keywords were derived from terms that appear in the ICD-9-CM descriptions or in the Unified Medical Language System [38]. Free-text search methods include exact match, partial match, and regular expression. A method to account for negation is implemented with keywords within a configurable window. Negations are not mapped to a syndrome or sub-syndrome. Keywords were modified during the initial implementation period based on experience with sample data; continual improvement of free-text data mapping is informed by comparing actual text to final syndrome or sub-syndrome results. BioSense plans to compare this method with natural language processing methods.

As of August 2006, some hospitals were also sending laboratory, radiology, and pharmacy data. BioSense is defining appropriate pre-processing and classification methods for these data. Microbiology laboratory data will be processed to recognize potential bioterrorism agents, notifiable diseases, and certain other organisms of interest (e.g., influenza, respiratory syncytial virus). Radiology data will be processed to recognize features such as pneumonia and widened mediastinum (from chest x-rays), and fracture and dislocation (from extremity films). Both laboratory and radiology data will require text parsing. Pharmacy orders will be classified according to drug classes, such as antibacterials and antivirals; antibacterials will be further broken down into agent classes (penicillins, aminoglycosides, etc.).

Once data are pre-processed and classified into disease indicator categories, statistical algorithms are applied to the data to determine if health activity is higher than expected. BioSense analyzes both counts and rates per 1000 visits. The rate is a proportion of the number of patient visits that map to a syndrome or sub-syndrome out of all visits for that day multiplied by 1000. For example, the rate per 1000 visits for the chief complaint-based respiratory syndrome is the number of patient visits with a chief complaint that maps to the respiratory syndrome divided by the total number of patient visits with a chief complaint times 1000. Initially, BioSense implemented a modified CUSUM [39] approach to identify statistically significant data anomalies. This approach compares the current day to a seven-day moving average with a two day lag, and with the seven-day moving average separated into weekdays and week-ends/holidays. For example, if today is a weekday, today's count is compared with the mean of the previous seven weekdays (with a two day lag). If today is a weekend day, today's count is compared with the mean of the previous seven weekend days (with a two day lag). Analyses are done at the individual hospital facility level, as well as by combining data across hospitals for a state or metropolitan area jurisdiction. A recurrence interval is calculated to indicate the expected days of surveillance needed for one such event of at least the observed magnitude to occur and can be used to characterize the severity of data anomalies.

In early 2006, new application modules were developed to visualize real-time hospital data and were made available in a beta test version to state and local public health officials in jurisdictions with hospitals transmitting data, as well as clinical partners from those hospitals. They include core functionalities found to be useful from experience with the initial BioSense interface and with other well-accepted electronic biosurveillance systems. Once the pre-processing and classification for laboratory, radiology, and pharmacy data have been determined, additional summary tables and customizable reports will be developed to display those data. Continued BioSense development will be guided by data analysis and end-user input.

BioSense modules include:

- *Chief complaint/diagnosis*

    - *Purpose:* Quick overview of syndrome activity by day for chief complaint and diagnosis data stratified by patient class, indicating statistically significant syndrome counts.

    - *Display:* Table of syndrome counts for the reason for visit, chief complaint, reason for admit, working diagnosis, and final diagnosis data (stratified by patient class) for a single day.

- *Statistical anomalies*

    - *Purpose:* Identifies anomalies found by automated statistical testing.

    - *Display:* Line list of statistical anomalies for syndrome count and rate; analyses are performed for individual facilities as well as for all facilities in a metropolitan reporting area (MRA) or state.

  – *Navigation:* To go to the time series for the data type and syndrome, click on an anomaly.

● *Time series*

  – *Purpose:* Displays trends and statistical anomalies over time for a disease indicator (Fig. 6.12).
  – *Display:* Graph of count and/or rate per 1000 visits by day.
  – *Navigation:* To go to the patient list, click on the desired graph point or the patient list link in the table beneath the graph. To go to the patient map, click on the map link in the table beneath the graph.

● *Patient list*

  – *Purpose:* Examine clinical and demographic data for a group of patient visits.
  – *Navigation*: To go to the patient detail for an individual patient, click on the patient of interest in the patient list.

● *Patient detail*

  – *Purpose*: Provides all detailed data for an individual patient.

● *Patient map*

  – *Purpose*: Displays number of visits with a specified disease indicator by zip code of patient residence (Fig 6.13).

● *Describe*

  – *Purpose:* Provides basic descriptive statistics for a group of patient visits (Fig 6.14).

● *Hospital census*

  – *Purpose:* Provides daily inpatient hospital census data.
  – *Display:* Table of hospital-level census data (occupancy rate, admission count, discharge count, and death count) and unit-level census data (occupied beds and available beds).

Future development plans include increasing application customizability for local needs and enhancing statistical analyses. Feedback from BioSense users has indicated that flexibility is extremely important. BioSense plans to incorporate the capability for the user to modify current definitions and create syndromes and sub-syndromes, as well as customize time-series graphs and tables, and set statistical thresholds for defining anomalies. Additional statistical analyses, such as regression methods that include a longer baseline period and spatiotemporal methods to detect clusters in both space and time, are planned. With so many data sources and statistical results for users to evaluate, a signal fusion and dashboard concept will allow users to better combine results to make informed decisions about the data.

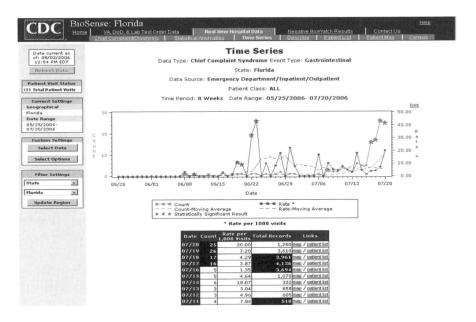

Fig. 6.12   Time-series module (demonstration data).

6.4.2   Monitoring of BioSense Application for National Surveillance

BioSense is intended for local, state, and federal public health officials, and hospital partners use. Users include epidemiologists, bioterrorism response coordinators, and hospital infection control personnel. BioSense Administrators for each state and metropolitan area jurisdiction, for each hospital facility, and for the VA and the DoD must approve BioSense access for personnel in their jurisdiction. Users access BioSense through the CDC Secure Data Network website with user names and passwords that permit viewing of hospital or jurisdictional-specific data. Data from a given hospital are viewable by personnel at that facility. State or metropolitan area public health officials may view data from all facilities in their jurisdiction.

In 2004, CDC initiated the BioIntelligence Center (BIC) to support state and local use of BioSense. The BIC includes data analysts at the CDC responsible for monitoring, analyzing, and interpreting BioSense data. The BIC staff are available to answer questions and assist users as requested. Examples of such aid have included surveillance support for large-scale events (including political conventions, presidential debates, and major sports events), help with interpreting data anomalies, and providing further information for public health follow-up. BIC staff review data for a set of jurisdictions daily; they are familiar with general data trends and can be a valuable resource for users [40].

BioSense does not receive patient identifiers, but during a public health investigation, there is a need for local public health officials to be able to link data in BioSense with the individual seen at the hospital. To facilitate response, each hospital patient is assigned a longitudinal BioSense patient identifier (ID). This ID is used to uniquely distinguish a patient across all visits to a single facility, or in some cases, across all visits to a health care system, over time. This ID may be used only by the health care facility to associate the BioSense patient ID to a patient's identity and medical record. This linking to patient identifiers only occurs at the local level.

BioSense is in the process of developing monitoring protocols with the understanding that state and local jurisdictions may have their own monitoring and response protocols. A current priority activity is determining how, in a systematic and automated way, to characterize anomalies as being of potential public health importance. Various criteria are being explored for an anomaly ranking analysis, including the recurrence interval and a comparison of the current count to the expected count (risk ratio and risk difference) and to previous maximums for that day of the week. Experience with this type of characterization will help the CDC determine the criteria that are useful in daily public health monitoring of BioSense data, and could be incorporated in the application for all users.

Statistical analyses can assist with, but cannot replace, the human element for evaluating anomalies. BIC daily activities involve looking at time series to determine if current patterns vary substantially from historical and seasonal trends, observing geographic patterns, and assessing data quality, as data duplication and errors in categorizing free-text data to syndromes can cause data anomalies. BIC analysts may not be overly concerned with anomalies that occur only for a single day. Epidemiological characteristics are examined to explore patterns with regard to age, sex, location, and disease characteristics. More severe disease, or similar patterns of illness among a

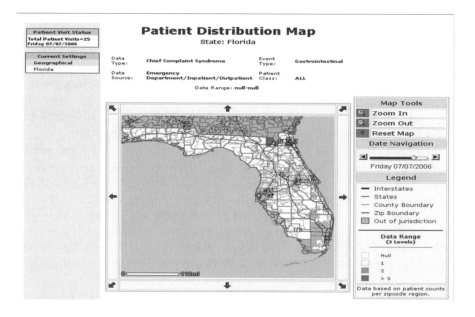

Fig. 6.13   Map module (demonstration data).

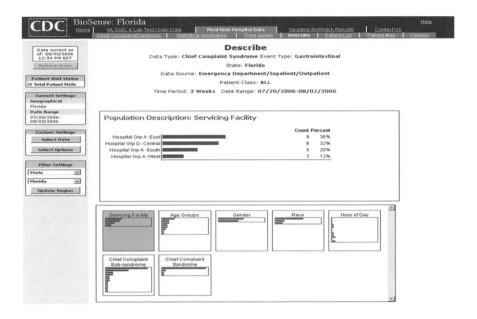

Fig. 6.14   Describe module (demonstration data).

group of patients, may indicate an anomaly of potential public health importance. In a cross-jurisdictional public health event situation, BIC staff can use BioSense data to determine the event location, size, spread, and characteristics to inform public health response activities.

The BioSense vision is to provide local, state, and federal public health and clinical partners simultaneous access to existing health data for biosurveillance related to naturally occurring and bioterrorism-related events, both locally and across jurisdictions. A major goal of BioSense is to add substantial national and local data sources to improve coverage and system utility. Because experience with BioSense data has indicated that statistical data anomalies happen often and syndromic data can be difficult to interpret, including adequate information to support a public health response is essential. BioSense can provide public health officials with access to national data sources and rich clinical data that may not otherwise be available at the state and local levels. To meet the needs of its users, BioSense will continually be expanded, improved, and evaluated.

6.4.3   Movement Toward Surveillance System Standardization

Section 6.4.2 included a discussion of the dual use of BioSense data for surveillance at the national and local levels. Sharing of data is only one aspect of standardization that must be considered in the development of systems that serve a common region. Other surveillance system components must be somewhat similar, or confusion will arise during collaboration between users of the national BioSense and local health department surveillance systems. Commonality needs to exist not only at the data communications level, but also at the receiving, processing, and monitoring levels. The alerts and flags produced by system A will be quite different than those produced by system B if the data are not aggregated similarly into the same syndrome groupings or if different analytics are applied to finding anomalies in similar data streams. An alert in system A may not be an alert in system B, causing confusion among users of different applications viewing the same data streams. Likewise, different visualization techniques applied to similar data streams could represent the data differently, so that an event shown in one format could seem highly significant while going unnoticed in another surveillance system. Thus, there must be a movement toward commonality among systems components that acquire, process, and analyze the same data. As a result of the potential differences among systems, BioSense and ESSENCE developers have agreed to migrate toward the use of common solutions for both applications.

6.5   SUMMARY

This chapter discussed the history of surveillance methods and how electronic surveillance systems have enhanced the capabilities of public health jurisdictions. While community-wide surveillance and epidemiological investigations have long been roles of public health, large amounts of timely data have not been readily available to aid in active day-to-day surveillance. There are many considerations that must be factored into the decision of whether to implement such a system at the various levels of public health, including the cost to set up and maintain a system, availability of staff to monitor, and availability of resources to respond. The case studies included in this chapter illustrate instances when an electronic surveillance system allowed epidemiologists to identify and respond to a health event expeditiously. Similarly, the role of the CDC in national surveillance was discussed.

Public health officials serve a very important but often unrecognized role in a community. Until recently, they have not had access to IT tools to enhance their ability to perform their jobs more efficiently. With the mounting threats of both bioterrorism and emerging infectious diseases, such as pandemic influenza, electronic surveillance systems provide public health officials with an additional tool to assist in early detection and effective response.

6.6   STUDY QUESTIONS

6.1 Through the years, public health has undertaken numerous surveillance responsibilities. The threat of bioterrorism has imposed additional responsibilities on already resource-strapped departments. *Q: How can electronic disease surveillance systems enhance public health's ability to perform surveillance activities?*

6.2 Individual health departments and/or systems users may have unique methodologies for reviewing and responding to an anomaly identified in an electronic disease surveillance system. These methodologies will be based on, among other factors, the resources of the health department and the skill level of the end user. *Q: Describe a generalized method of evaluating system alerts.*

6.3 Requirements and attributes for implementation of electronic surveillance systems vary by locality. *Q: What are some of these requirements and attributes at the local and regional levels? Based on these considerations, what kinds of systems would be more desirable?*

6.4 Information requiring action may vary depending on the particular situation, such as the time of year and the perceived severity of the illnesses. This chapter provided case studies to explain a variety of situations where action by public health officials was required. *Q: Explain what constituted actionable information in each case scenario.*

6.5 Electronic surveillance systems are being implemented at every level of public health, from the local city/county/state level to the national level. The issues public health officials face at each one of these levels are very different. *Q: Describe the challenges faced at the city/county/state, and national levels in establishing an electronic disease surveillance system.*

REFERENCES

1. Committee for the Study of the Future of Public Health, Division of Health Care Services Institute of Medicine. The Future of Public Health. Washington, DC: National Academy Press; 1988.

2. Members of the Essential Services Work Group: members of the Association of State and Territorial Health Officials, National Association of County and City Health Officials, Institute of Medicine (National Academy of Sciences), Association of Schools of Public Health, Public Health Foundation, National Association of State Alcohol and Drug Abuse Directors, National Association of State Mental Health Program Directors, and Public Health Service.

3. Maryland Department of Health and Mental Hygiene, Office of Epidemiology and Disease Control Programs. Reportable diseases and conditions. Provider reporting form. Available at http://www.edcp.org/html/reprtabl.html. Accessed September 28, 2006.

4. Centers for Disease Control and Prevention. National notifiable diseases surveillance system. Available at http://www.cdc.gov/epo/dphsi/nndsshis.htm. Accessed August 29, 2006.

5. Jajosky RA, Groseclose SL. Evaluation of reporting timeliness of public health surveillance systems for infectious diseases. BMC Public Health 2004;4:29.

6. New York State Department of Health. Influenza sentinel provider surveillance. Available at `http://www.nyhealth.gov/diseases/communicable/influenza/recruit.htm`. Accessed August 28, 2006.

7. Centers for Disease Control and Prevention. CDC fact sheet: overview of influenza surveillance in the United States. June 26, 2006. Available at `http://www.cdc.gov/flu/weekly/fluactivity.htm`. Accessed September 28, 2006.

8. Henning KJ. Overview of syndromic surveillance: what is syndromic surveillance? MMWR. 2004; 53(suppl): 5-11.

9. CDC. Preventing emerging infectious diseases: a strategy for the 21st century. MMWR. 1998;47(RR-15):1-19.

10. CDC. Syndromic surveillance for bioterrorism following the attacks on the World Trade Center. MMWR. September 11, 2002;51(special issue):13-15. Available at `http://www.cdc.gov/mmwr/preview/mmwrhtml/mm51SPa5.htm`. Accessed August 29, 2006.

11. Vaz V. Syndromic disease surveillance in the wake of anthrax threats and high profile public events. Prevention (publication of the Bureau of Epidemiology and Disease Control Services). January – February 2002;16(1):1-2. Available at `http://www.azdhs.gov/diro/pio/preventionbulletin/janfeb02.pdf`. Accessed August 29, 2006.

12. Begier EM, Sockwell D, Branch LM, et al. The National Capitol Region's emergency department syndromic surveillance system: do chief complaint and discharge diagnosis yield different results? Emerg Infect Dis. 2003;9(3):393-396.

13. Lombardo JS. The ESSENCE II disease surveillance test bed for the national capital area. JHU/APL Tech Dig. 2003;24(4):327-334.

14. Burkom HS. Development, adaptation, and assessment of alerting algorithms for biosurveillance. JHU/APL Technical Dig. 2003;24(4):335-342

15. Tsui F, Espino JU, Dato VM, et al. Technical description of RODS: a real-time public health surveillance system. J Am Med Inf Assoc. 2003;10(5):399-408.

16. Orfanidis SJ. Optimum Signal Processing. 2nd ed. New York: McGraw-Hill; 1988.

17. RODS version 4.2 user manual. University of Pittsburgh, Pittsburgh, PA; 2006.

18. Feighner B, Coberly J. Four cities, four systems. Report for BioWatch Program, Department of Homeland Security; 2005.

19. Lawson BM, Fitzhugh EC, Hall SP, et al. Multifaceted syndromic surveillance in a public health department using the early aberration reporting system. J Public Health Manage Pract. 2005;11(4):274-281.

20. Hutwagner LC, Thompson WW, Seeman GM, Treadwell, T. A simulation model for assessing aberration detection methods used in public health surveillance for systems with limited baselines. Stat Med 2005;24:543-550.

21. ICPA, Inc. RedBat features and benefits. Available at http://www.icpa.net/redbat-features.html. Accessed September 28, 2006.

22. Ares Corporation, SYRIS. Available at http://syris.arescorporation.com/demo. Accessed September 28, 2006.

23. Coberly J, Feighner B, Holtry R, Lombardo J. Automated surveillance systems: evaluation of anomalous data clusters. Report for Centers for Disease Control and Prevention; 2006.

24. CDC. Guidelines for investigating clusters of health events. MMWR. 1990;39(RR-11):1-16.

25. Kay BA, Timperi RJ, Morse SS, Forslund D, McGowan JJ, O'Brien T. Innovative information-sharing strategies. Emerg Infect Dis. 1998;4(3):465-466.

26. Hurt-Mullen K, Coberly J. Syndromic surveillance on the epidemiologist's desktop: making sense of much data. MMWR. 2005;54(suppl):141-146.

27. Mandl KD, Overhage JM, Wagner MM, et al. Implementing syndromic surveillance: a practical guide informed by the early experience. J Am Med Inf Assoc. March 1, 2004;11(2):141-150.

28. Weber SG, Pitrak D. Accuracy of a local surveillance system for early detection of emerging infectious disease. JAMA. 2003;5:596-598.

29. Stoto MA, Schonlau M, Mariano LT. Syndromic surveillance: is it worth the effort? Chance. 2004;17(1):19-24.

30. Sosin DM. Syndromic surveillance: the case for skillful investment. Biosecurity Bioterrorism. 2003;1(4):247-253.

31. Reingold A. If syndromic surveillance is the answer, what is the question? Biosecurity Bioterrorism. 2003;1(2):77-81.

32. Buehler JW, Hopkins RS, Overhage JM, Sosin DM, Tong V, Group CDCW. Framework for evaluating public health surveillance systems for early detection of outbreaks: recommendations from the CDC Working Group. MMWR. 2004;53(RR-5):1-11.

33. Karras BT, Lober WB, Smith GT. Evaluating the new electronic disease surveillance systems. University of Washington School of Public Health and Community Medicine. Fall–Winter 2002: 22-23.

34. Sosin DM. Draft framework for evaluating syndromic surveillance systems. J Urban Health. 2003;80(2 suppl 1):i8-i13.

35. Bravata DM, McDonald KM, Smith WM, et al. Systematic review: surveillance systems for early detection of bioterrorism-related diseases. Annals Int Med. 2004;140(11):910-922.

36. US Government Accounting Office. GAO-06-663R. Report released May 23, 2006. Available at http://www.gao.gov/htext/d06663r.html. Accessed August 29, 2006.

37. Centers for Disease Prevention and Control, Syndrome definitions for diseases associated with critical Bioterrorism-associated agents. October 23, 2003. Available at http://www.bt.cdc.gov/surveillance/syndromedef/index.asp. Accessed September 15, 2006.

38. National Library of Medicine, Unified medical language system. Available at http://www.nlm.nih.gov/research/umls/. Accessed September 15, 2006.

39. Hutwagner L., et al. The bioterrorism preparedness and response early aberration reporting system (EARS). J Urban Health. 2003;80:89i-96i.

40. Bradley CA, Rolka H, Walker D, Loonsk J. BioSense: implementation of a national early event detection and situational awareness system. MMWR. 2005;54 (suppl):11-19.

7 Canadian Applications of Modern Surveillance Informatics

Jeff Aramini, Shamir Nizar Mukhi

Chapter 6 examined the operational aspects of disease surveillance systems in settings that ranged from local public health practice perspective to national disease surveillance. The intent of Chapter 6 was to learn from the experience of leaders in implementing automated disease surveillance systems in the United States.

The remaining chapters in Part II of the book explore advanced disease surveillance applications outside the United States. Chapter 7 describes an initiative within the Public Health Agency of Canada (PHAC) to establish automated disease surveillance. The chapter begins by outlining the processes used within PHAC to develop surveillance applications. The architecture and functionality of the Canadian Early Warning System (CEWS) are then presented. The Federated Area-Based Result Management System (FARMS), an application used to manage large data sources and various analytics in CEWS, is also described. Finally, the chapter presents insights and recommendations based on experiences of the PHAC in implementating these automated surveillance applications.

7.1 INTRODUCTION: DISEASE SURVEILLANCE IN CANADA

7.1.1 Understanding the True Public Health Needs

Over the past several years, a number of widely publicized health events have sparked much reflection, debate, and subsequent action relating to the state of public health surveillance in Canada. Two large waterborne outbreaks (an *E. coli* outbreak in Walkerton, Ontario, in 2000 and a cryptosporidiosis outbreak in North Battleford, Saskatchewan, in 2001), the 2003 limited SARS episode in Toronto, Ontario, and fears of bioterrorism since September 2001 have all prompted local, provincial/territorial, and federal health authorities to critically assess their surveillance capacities, particularly with respect to infectious diseases.

New technologies and informatics methods are central to the current activities to improve public health surveillance capacities at all levels of government. Web-based and wireless technologies, data extraction and exchange tools, and sophisticated modeling and forecasting methods all have roles in enabling surveillance. However, along with potentially facilitating public health surveillance in Canada, information technology also has the potential to further complicate an already complex public health activity. Over the past several years, there has been an explosion in technologies that are potentially applicable to public health surveillance. The challenge from an applied perspective is not whether processes are technically possible, but which technologies to harness and for what purposes, and how to implement and integrate them with existing systems and business processes. The growing divide in technical knowledge between the ultimate users of surveillance systems (i.e., public health stakeholders) and information technology professionals has the capacity to result in surveillance systems and tools that do not fully meet —or do not efficiently meet— their intended goals. Given the rapid expansion of new technologies, it is critical that in the development and implementation of new surveillance systems, the ultimate purpose for harnessing new technologies is defined clearly and understood.

An assessment of the Canadian public health surveillance environment indicates that improvements are needed along the entire surveillance life cycle — from data to information, to the sharing of analysis results. Sharing the results of analyses is important because public health surveillance includes not only data exchange and analysis, but also the dissemination and sharing of information. Communication among and between stakeholders is often overlooked as a piece of the surveillance puzzle. To the contrary, communications may be the most critical component of an effective public health surveillance system. This understanding of health surveillance is in line with Naylor's definition in his 2003 report, in which he reflects upon the 2003 SARS episode in Canada:

Health surveillance is "the tracking and forecasting of any health event or health determinant through the continuous collection of high-quality data, the integration, analysis and interpretation of those data into surveillance products (for example reports, advisories, alerts, and warnings), and the dissemination of those surveillance products to those who need to know" [1].

7.1.2 Developing and Harnessing the Right Technology

The Public Health Agency of Canada, working with public health stakeholders, has undertaken several efforts to improve public health surveillance through the application of new technologies. As noted, with so many technical options available, matching the right technology with the right problem can be a challenge. A number of guiding principles were developed to assist in choosing the right technologies:

- Where possible, make use of existing legacy systems/applications by creating interfacing adapters and single-sign-on (SSO) methods to provide a seamless user experience.

- Develop systems that are flexible and scalable to meet changing public health needs over time.

- Adhere to international standards when they exist; attempt to create new standards where they do not.

- Implement user interfaces that are intuitive and appropriate for the intended users.

- Choose technologies that align with current fiscal realities.

- Implement hosting infrastructures that allow for expansion, using clustered setups for inherent redundancy and load balancing to manage increasing traffic loads during critical periods (e.g., during a disease outbreak) and provide scalability.

Clearly, there are many technologies that could (if applied correctly) contribute to an effective public health surveillance system. But when a deliverable can be achieved with two servers rather than 12, or a function can be accomplished with a few lines of code rather than thousands, the most cost effective choice should be made.

These principles were applied to the development and implementation of a new information management/information technology/knowledge management (IM/IT/KM) architecture and framework, the enhanced Federated Architecture for Collaborating Technologies (eFACT). As an overall architectural strategy, eFACT provides a mechanism for standardizing how applications and users communicate and data are captured, stored, and analyzed. Based on core J2EE (Java 2 Platform, Enterprise Edition) technology, eFACT is a scalable and flexible architecture that enables many useful features (Fig. 7.1):

- *Data center server* (DCS). DCS enables data extraction and collation and supports multiple communication methods. One of the key components of DCS is newly developed middleware referred to as *smart engine technology* (SET). SET facilitates data extraction, interrogation, analysis, and communication between disparate databases within a federated environment, independent of data format and database type. SET allows full control by the user of field-level data sharing. The DCS is being designed and developed to continuously enhance capabilities to support various technology and nomenclature standards, including XML (extensible markup language), HL7 (health level seven), SOAP (simple object access protocol), WSDL (web services description language), ICD (international classification of disease), LOINC (logical observation identifiers, names, and codes), and SNOMED (systematized nomenclature of medicine). This capacity allows interfacing with existing legacy systems, such as emergency room triage systems, case management systems, tele-health systems, and pharmacy databases.

- *Data exchange server* (DES). DES is a central processing device that enables seamless communication between applications — for example, between two eFACT instances, between an eFACT instance and an external web services compliant application, or between an eFACT instance and an external application with an arbitrary communication protocol.

- *Intelligent alert notification* (IAN). IAN is an automated escalation-based communication management device for the delivery of notifications via multiple communication channels, including e-mail, phone, fax, pager, and text messaging.

- *Registration system* (RS). The RS performs user registration, authentication, and access control (role-based and target-based) for each of the data sets and applications within the eFACT framework. It allows communication and synchronization between different registration systems. The RS ensures data confidentiality while allowing controlled access to multiple databases and applications.

- *Single-sign-on server* (SSOS). The SSOS is responsible for interfacing with external application authentication systems to enable seamless access and navigation. In addition to supporting standard protocols such as LDAP (lightweight directory access protocol), SSOS supports proprietary application adapters and custom solutions ranging from token-based access control systems to proxy-based access.

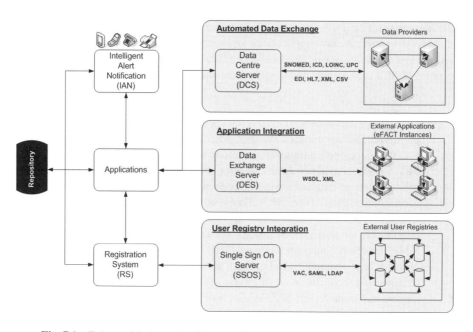

Fig. 7.1 Enhanced federated architecture for collaborating technologies (eFACT).

All technologies developed and described in the remainder of this chapter have been implemented using the eFACT framework.

7.2 DISEASE-SPECIFIC SURVEILLANCE ENABLED THROUGH TECHNOLOGY

7.2.1 Introduction

With the exception of some very recent advances in syndromic surveillance and other close-to-real-time surveillance approaches, the methods used for public health surveillance have not changed over the past century. Data on deaths and specific diseases are gathered, aggregated at a central location, analyzed, and summarized. For the most part, public health surveillance is still very much disease or program specific. The mechanism by which data are gathered, aggregated, analyzed, and summarized may be quite different for influenza than for enteric illnesses, and different again for sexually transmitted diseases. Many disease-specific surveillance systems still rely on the manual collection of data from the providers, mail and fax (and now e-mail) to deliver data to a centralized location, manual execution of basic statistical procedures to summarize the data, and mail and fax (and e-mail) to distribute analytic results.

Over the past few years, there has been much discussion among public health stakeholders of the need for an integrated approach to surveillance. An integrated approach would ultimately involve different program areas working together to standardize and streamline data and information management. Ideally, all programs would use the same basic IM/IT/KM framework to share and analyze surveillance data and to distribute surveillance products. Although a laudable final goal, experience from working with many program groups leads to the conclusion that a stepwise transitional approach is needed. It is unrealistic to expect program areas to abandon surveillance systems they have used for a decade or more and migrate to an entirely new system in one step. To begin with, a "standard system" that meets the current exact needs of each and every program area simply does not exist. Furthermore, the standardization of definitions (e.g., alert levels, influenza activity levels) and processes (e.g., information distribution preferences, communication channels) is not an IM/IT/KM challenge–it is a program and business challenge.

In many respects, new technologies can be used as facilitators to change how public health surveillance is done. As described in Section 7.2.2, the implementation of new technologies has helped create real advances in the efficacy and efficiency of public health surveillance in Canada. A prominent public health stakeholder in Canada recently commented that if implemented strategically in public health, technology could be "the tail that wags the dog" [2].

7.2.2 Working with Stakeholders to Improve Disease-Specific Surveillance Through the Implementation of Technology

Work with Canadian stakeholders to map the processes of a given disease-specific surveillance system showed that technology has a significant role to play in improving both the efficiency of existing surveillance systems and the quality of the outputs. The National Enteric Surveillance Program (NESP) is one program-specific surveillance system that has been augmented through the application of technology. Established in 1997, NESP is a system for monitoring short-term fluctuations in the numbers of human enteric pathogen isolates in Canada to enable the timely identification of disease outbreaks. Provincial laboratories fax/e-mail weekly summary sheets to the Public Health Agency of Canada (PHAC), National Microbiology Laboratory (NML), where the data are entered manually into a database. ML microbiologists work with PHAC epidemiologists (from a separate office) to analyze and interpret the data, and a weekly report is generated that is faxed to stakeholders. The report includes tables with isolate numbers, together with comments and interpretation. The audience includes federal and provincial/territorial stakeholders involved directly in the identification, prevention, and control of enteric disease in Canada. Figure 7.2 outlines the basic NESP business prior to technology enhancement.

Under the underlying IM/IT/KM framework described in Section 7.1.2, the Public Health Agency of Canada was engaged to work with NESP stakeholders to technically augment NESP to improve its timeliness and usability. The existing system was labor intensive and prone to delays. Working with NESP stakeholders, a web-enabled application (wNESP) was designed, developed, and implemented. The basic approach taken throughout the development of wNESP was to augment, not necessarily change, the system. Although a radically new approach to real-time enteric disease surveillance could have been developed, where all data were exchanged automatically and sophisticated algorithms and GIS (geographic information system) techniques were used, experience has shown that stakeholders respond best to a stepwise approach to technology implementation. No matter how technically advanced a system, without stakeholder buy-in and adoption, it will not serve its intended purpose. To ensure success, stakeholders were engaged in all stages of the project, from design to implementation.

wNESP was developed as a secure web-based application with the following goals:

- *More efficient data collection and analysis and information dissemination.* Data can be entered either online or extracted automatically from existing laboratory databases. Data (including historical data) and information are accessible to appropriate users 24 hours a day, 7 days a week, via a secure web interface. Statistical procedures are automated, and custom queries and statistical procedures can be conducted.

- *Increased data security.* Data collection, transfer, and storage are enabled through a secure web infrastructure. The infrastructure includes server redundancy and strict user registration policies.

- *Flexible user interface.* Users can define what information is displayed: for example, time period, organism, and view options.

- *Online tools to empower users.* wNESP links to a suite of resources to facilitate decision making, including discussion boards, news boards, and keyword searches.

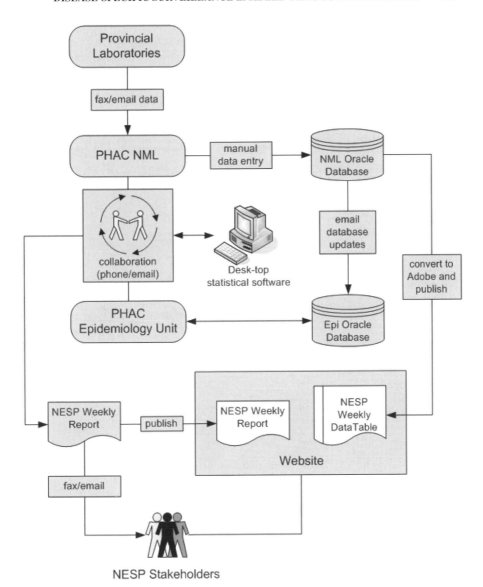

Fig. 7.2   NESP business before technology enhancement.

- *Developing and implementing wNESP transformed the business of NESP.* The new business framework is shown in Fig. 7.3.

For the most part, wNESP is a straightforward web application. It includes role-based access control, data input screens, charting and graphing resources, etc. Two aspects of NESP, however, presented challenges that required the development of

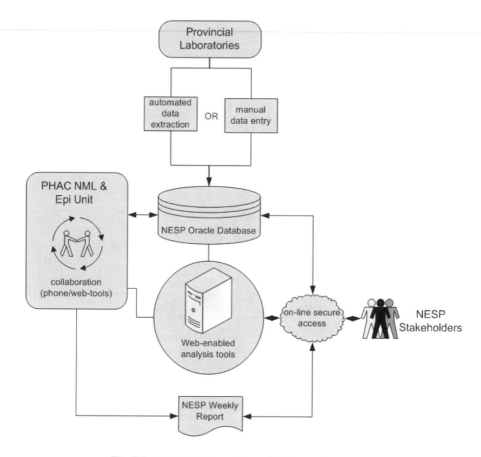

Fig. 7.3   NESP business after technology enhancement.

unique technical solutions: an automated aberration-detection algorithm and a mechanism to extract data from legacy systems automatically.

7.2.2.1 *Anomaly Flagging Algorithm for Enteric Surveillance*   A proprietary algorithm (called a *progressive scan*) was developed to flag anomalies based on a comparison of a week's current organism count for each classification (genus, species, serovar, etc.) and jurisdiction (provincial/territorial, and national) of interest with previous years' values around the same calendar time. The progressive scan algorithm depends on the following generic parameters (Fig. 7.4): granularity (g), which defines the unit time of primary interest (e.g., day, week, month); step size (s), which defines the time unit size to consider in each calendar direction from the time of interest; walking distance (w), which is the number of steps (and thus number of values) to consider; period (p), which indicates the time blocks for historical comparison with the current value; and reference block (r), which denotes the overall time to consider in the comparison. In general, the total number of comparative values to be used is

$N = r/p * w$. For NESP, $g = 1$ week, $s = 1$ week, $w = 5$ weeks, $p = 1$ year, $r = 5$ years. The value of interest (the current week's count) is compared to a reference value, which, for this case of NESP, is the mean (μ) of the previous 25 values.

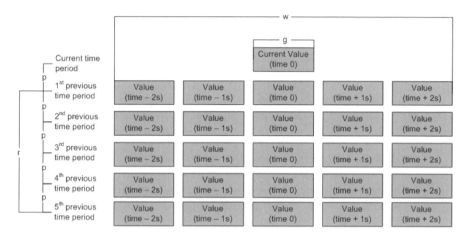

Fig. 7.4 Progressive scan parameters.

A standard colored alert/threshold framework was also implemented for wNESP. The alert/threshold takes into account both statistical and biologically relevant parameters: Ψ is the current week's value for a given organism classification for a given jurisdiction, μ is the comparative mean based on up to 25 values, σ is the standard deviation of the 25 values, and β is a minimum critical value.

- If $\beta > 1$:
  Alert level = orange (warning) if $\Psi > \mu + \sigma$ and $\Psi \geq \beta$
  Alert level = red (urgent) if $\Psi > \mu + 2\sigma$ and $V \geq \beta$
  Alert level = black (no problems) if not orange or red

- If $\beta = 1$:
  Alert level = red (urgent) if $\Psi \geq 1$
  Alert level = black (no problems) if $\Psi < 1$

The minimum critical value (β) was introduced (1) to help prevent excessive alerting for very common organisms, and (2) to enable alerting for very rare organisms of interest.

7.2.2.2 Smart Engine Technology   wNESP, together with other program-specific surveillance systems (including a web-enabled FluWatch application), presented significant challenges with respect to data extraction and exchange. Although potential public health data providers were willing to share relevant data for the purposes of surveillance, their existing legacy data management systems did not offer simple solutions for data sharing. Furthermore, the same data providers had limited resources available to help implement costly new technologies. To meet this challenge, the new SET middleware was developed. SET facilitates data extraction, interrogation, analysis, and communication among disparate databases, independent of data format and database type, via extract, transform, and load (ETL) processes.

A vocabulary of common SET functions was defined to facilitate the development of a generic data exchange engine for disparate data source formats and structures:

- *Data receiver*: allows importing of multiformat data from flat files and/or databases using ODBC (open database connectivity) and JDBC (Java database connectivity). Provides support for various communication protocols and standards, including HL7, XML, and EDI (ASCX12: electronic data interchange).

- *Data mask*: allows for field-level control by data providers. For example, if the database being accessed has 100 fields, the data provider might be willing to share only 10 fields. Data providers need the ability to control/modify field-level access easily because data exchange needs may differ depending on the situation: for example, during an outbreak period.

- *Data validation*: applies predefined logical rules to incoming data sets to filter any records that are missing key data elements.

- *Data fixer*: applies logical rules to specified data using XML configuration files and fixes raw data (if possible) that failed validation rules. For example, if city = WINNIPEG and province = MANITOBA, then country = CANADA.

- *Data duplicate detector*: detects duplicates in the data based on both simple and complex statistical matching algorithms. An example of a simple algorithm could be to match first name, last name, and address.

- *Data translator*: maps (or transforms) incoming data fields into a common format to facilitate data collation. This process is responsible for implementing lookup tables and format scripts to convert incoming data to match the predefined common data format.

- *Data coder*: converts data values into standard codes: for example, LOINC, SNOMED. A key requirement for surveillance in a federated environment is the standardization of fields, especially test results.

- *Data aggregation*: provides the capability to aggregate data at specified classifications (e.g., geography, disease classification). This key process is required for disease surveillance and offloads processing from central servers.

- *Data logger*: provides the ability to log various events during the data transformation process: for example, dropping a record because of missing data.

- *Data export*: facilitates exporting of data in various formats, including text and database tables. Once data are transformed, they must be stored in a format that can be transmitted.

- *Data transmitter*: provides the capability to transmit data based on standard protocols.

- *Workflow manager*: manages the workflow of tasks based on the specific needs of the data provider. As shown in Fig. 7.5, an XML-based state machine controls the sequence of operations necessary to manage the processes. A bit map is used to control the enabling of each process in the state machine, where a value of 0 disables a specific process.

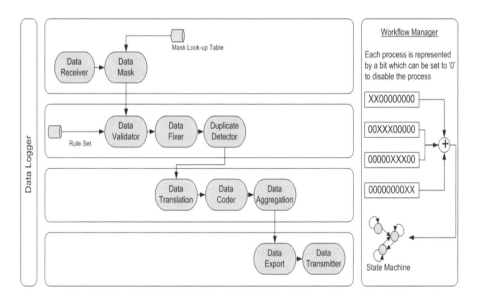

Fig. 7.5   Smart engine technology state machine and associated workflow manager.

SET has been used successfully to connect and exchange data with a number of data providers. Although expensive and hardware-intensive proprietary solutions can be purchased, effective data exchange can be achieved through implementation of SET with standard equipment and software.

7.2.2.3   wNESP Is Helping to Improve Enteric Disease Surveillance in Canada

Although implemented only recently, wNESP has already been successful in achieving its ultimate goal of improving enteric disease surveillance in Canada. Data are entering the database in a timelier manner. Aberration detection is now standardized to allow for meaningful comparisons across jurisdictions. Data and analysis results are available online, 24 hours a day, 7 days a week. Users have tools to facilitate data exploration, result sharing, and collaboration. The Public Health Agency will continue to work with NESP stakeholders to implement additional decision support resources and technologies, including real-time GIS and more sophisticated aberration-detection algorithms.

7.2.3 Lessons Learned Through Disease-Specific Surveillance Application Development

The cooperative efforts between the Public Health Agency and the many program stakeholders to develop and implement disease-specific surveillance applications highlighted the need for a new approach to public health IM/IT/KM resource development and implementation. Most stakeholders have had negative IM/IT project experiences in the past. For the most part, public health program stakeholders expressed dissatisfaction with the traditional IT approach to application development. They felt that the traditional approach of endless requirements collection and documentation was tedious and unproductive. Furthermore, they felt that the end result rarely met their expectations.

In an attempt to break this unproductive cycle, a *program-centric approach* was developed. The current strategy brings program users (e.g., epidemiologists, microbiologists, administrators) into the core project team. People with experience and training in the program areas were recruited to work with their regional/provincial/territorial/national colleagues and with a team of engineers and computer scientists to guide end users through the entire business cycle from needs assessment to product implementation.

For each of the business cycle stages, new approaches were developed and tested. Most important, it became apparent that rarely are user needs well defined from the outset. Hence, the business cycle used is based on an iterative and visual approach to needs assessment. The primary objective is to provide an environment in which users can explore options and, together with the application development team, create innovative solutions. The users are buffered from the traditional tedious IM/IT process of formal change requests and endless documentation during development stages. Applications evolve quickly, and versions are released rapidly. This, user-friendly approach to application development has necessitated changes in how applications are coded. For example, very little is hard-coded, providing architects and developers with a malleable framework. The end result of this approach has been overwhelming buy-in and user ownership. It has resulted in an environment of trust, respect, and mutual appreciation.

Another key element of the strategy used is the *building block approach* to IM/IT/KM resource development. Although infectious disease surveillance and response programs have developed in a "siloed" environment (particularly at the federal level), there are many similarities in business processes (data flow, analysis needs, communication needs, etc.) among the many disease-specific areas. The traditional siloed approach has resulted in fragmented IM/IT systems and, as a by-product, has encouraged fragmented business approaches. Fragmented public health business approaches are a barrier to establishing the much sought-after "integrated" surveillance approach alluded to earlier (Section 7.2.1).

The approach used leverages similarities in business processes among program areas to achieve considerable efficiencies in IM/IT/KM resource delivery. The surveillance framework allows for the rapid configuration and implementation of solutions.

Common business needs include real-time data extraction, analysis, and decision support; structured alerting/notification; team communication and collaboration; syndromic surveillance; laboratory-based surveillance; and quality assurance processes. The interaction among many program areas has resulted in a rich and diverse suite of "infostructure" building blocks that has provided the opportunity to leverage tools developed for one specific program across all program areas. Not only has this approach been well received by programs, it is also contributing to standardization and integration in business functions across public health programs.

The adoption of a program-centric, stepwise approach to IM/IT/KM implementation is intended to help program areas achieve an integrated approach to public health surveillance. As mentioned previously, in many respects, new technology can be a facilitator for change in how public health surveillance is conducted.

7.3   REAL-TIME SYNDROMIC SURVEILLANCE

As is emphasized throughout this book, recent advances in technology have made it possible to gather, integrate, and analyze large amounts of data in real time or near-real time. For the most part, the traditional purposes of health surveillance have been to monitor long-term trends in disease ecology and to guide policy decisions. With the introduction of real-time capabilities, surveillance now holds the promise of facilitating early event detection and assisting in day-to-day disease management.

Once detected, disease events must be monitored and assessed accurately and in real time. Ongoing information on the prevalence, incidence, characterization, severity, and location of cases will provide health professionals with the information necessary to mobilize and allocate resources, monitor progression, and plan subsequent steps. Mass numbers of persons presenting to one emergency room will require a different type of response than modest numbers presenting to several emergency rooms in the same city. People phoning into a tele-health service with similar symptoms from throughout an entire region would probably indicate the need for greater resource mobilization than the case where calls originate from only one neighborhood.

Taken together, the need for early detection and for the real-time monitoring of disease dynamics suggest that existing traditional surveillance capabilities are not optimal. The potential benefits of early disease event detection have been demonstrated by a number of Canadian experiences:

- Retrospective analyses of a large waterborne outbreak of cryptosporidiosis in North Battleford, Saskatchewan, in 2001 demonstrated that sales of OTC antidiarrheal medication increased approximately 2 weeks prior to the recognition of a widespread outbreak by public health officials [3].

- Retrospective analyses of a waterborne outbreak of *E. coli* O157:H7 in Walkerton, Ontario, in 2000 showed that sales of OTC antidiarrheal medication increased 3 days prior to the first reported laboratory-confirmed case. Early detection and implementation of a drinking water advisory would have prevented several hundred cases of diarrhea and might have minimized loss of life in Walkerton [4].

- Many foodborne outbreaks (particularly those involving distributed food products) are not identified until increases in laboratory-confirmed gastroenteritis cases are reported to public health authorities. The time between symptom onset and laboratory diagnosis is typically between 7 and 14 days. The opportunity to identify foodborne-related clusters of disease before laboratory confirmation clearly exists.

It is well recognized that a comprehensive early warning system must identify as many people as possible early in the disease process when they have nonspecific symptoms, such as cough or diarrhea, and then use statistical algorithms to find any interesting patterns among the sick that suggest that an unusual event is occurring. Such a system needs to receive data directly and within an acceptable time frame. Candidate sources of early warning data are many and include emergency departments, laboratories, pharmacies, and tele-triage systems.

Despite their promise for facilitating early-event detection and real-time disease monitoring, the evolution of real-time surveillance systems, particularly syndromic surveillance systems, have not been a main priority in the health care community.

Canada (among other countries with some sort of universal publicly operated health care program) has a role to play in helping to test and evaluate syndromic surveillance methods. The goal of the Canadian "public" health care system is to give everyone equal access to basic health care services, including primary care physicians, hospitalization, dental surgery, tele-health, and so on. For example, Canadians may visit any emergency room in Canada without a direct charge. Canadians are also not charged directly when visiting a physician's office. For the most part, the data associated with publicly funded health care services are centrally managed, stored, and accessible. Depending on the data management systems used, much of these data can be accessed in real time.

Concerns about the timeliness of traditional surveillance systems have led to the creation of the Canadian early warning system (CEWS), a syndromic surveillance system being developed and piloted in Canada. The development of CEWS has highlighted some of the unique challenges of syndromic surveillance.

7.3.1 Canadian Early Warning System

Prompted by fears of bioterrorism-related disease events, resources have been made available in Canada to develop, pilot, and evaluate real-time syndromic surveillance technologies. The Public Health Agency of Canada has partnered with the local health authority in Winnipeg, Manitoba [the Winnipeg Regional Health Authority (WRHA)], to develop and test a syndromic surveillance system. Winnipeg is the largest city in Manitoba, with a population of approximately 650,000. The WRHA oversees all health care services for the city of Winnipeg and is, in essence, the "owner" of all relevant data sources, except for OTC data, which are owned by individual pharmacy chains. OTC data access has been facilitated through a related national project to investigate the utility of OTC data for gastroenteritis surveillance. By negotiation with WRHA, the Public Health Agency secured access to real-time data from all seven emergency rooms and the regionwide tele-health system. All seven emergency rooms use the same electronic triage system. The tele-health system is a free telephone health service for all Manitobans, manned by nurses 24 hours a day, 7 days a week. The basic goal of the pilot project is to work with front-line public health care providers to develop and pilot a real-time syndromic surveillance system. Ultimately, it is the utility of the system as viewed from the perspective of front-line users that will determine the likelihood of system sustainability.

7.3.1.1 *CEWS — Application*

In designing and developing CEWS, the Public Health Agency worked hand-in-hand with potential users. The first challenge was determining who the users might be. It quickly became clear that potential users of a syndromic surveillance system were very diverse and varied in a number of dimensions, including jurisdictional role (local, provincial/territorial, federal), discipline/expertise (e.g., microbiology, epidemiology, statistics, occupational health), education (e.g., MD, DVM, MSc, BSc), and responsibility (e.g., medical officer of health, senior epidemiologist, communicable disease nurse, data analyst, clerk). Not surprisingly, the diversity of users led to diversity in required functionality. End users requested that the system be able to accommodate many different types of potential data inputs, including emergency room visits, OTC sales, tele-health calls, laboratory data (submissions and results), weather data, and air quality data. Some users wanted a very simple user interface with standard default settings; others required the ability to manipulate most parameters.

The initial business requirements, which evolved through the development cycle, were used as the basis for a syndromic surveillance system concept design. Central to the overall design is the ability to control user access to all aspects of the system. For example, access to data could be restricted by type (e.g., OTC data only) and by granularity (e.g., provincial aggregate only). Similarly, it would be possible to restrict which algorithms and what results were available to each user. The CEWS application was then designed from the basic syndromic surveillance system concept design. The application design is based on four primary modules: *handler*, *processor*, *analyzer*, and *presenter* (Fig. 7.6).

- The *handler's* primary function is to receive incoming data in various formats [e.g., HL7, EDI, comma-separated value (CSV)] and efficiently store the data to optimize analytical computations and database access. The *handler* is responsible for parsing the data, organizing them in an optimal object structure to facilitate manipulation, and storing the raw data in the system repository. Data can be presented to the handler by a number of different mechanisms, including via SET (Section 7.2.3).

- The *processor's* primary function is to perform all necessary data processing, preparing it for analysis and presentation. The *processor* is responsible for

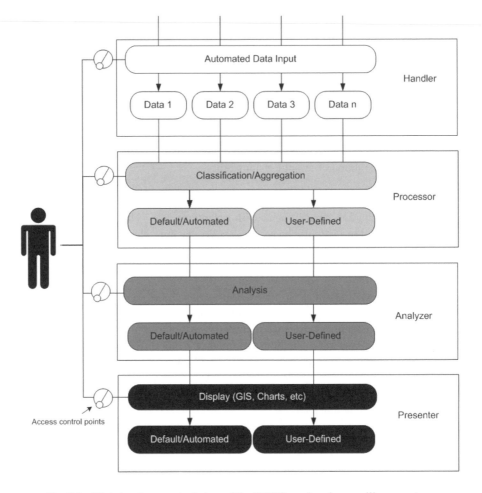

Fig. 7.6 High-level conceptual view of the CEWS syndromic surveillance system.

classifying the data based on standard codes — for example, SNOMED, UPC (universal product code) — and aggregating data at various classifications (e.g., syndrome, province, health unit, city).

- The *analyzer's* primary function is to execute analytical anomaly detection algorithms on the aggregate data and to flag anomalies. The *analyzer* supports both automated and manual algorithm execution.

- The *presenter's* primary function is to manage the user interface of the system, how results are presented, and how anomaly alerts are distributed. The *presenter* is responsible for controlling user access to data and information based on profile parameters, including data type (e.g., emergency room visits, tele-health,

OTC), geo level, organization, and function (e.g., mapping, charting, algorithm execution, data management).

Based on this high-level modular design, the system's technical framework was developed. The technical framework consists of a number of independent functional blocks that provide flexibility and scalability to accommodate an increasing number of data feeds and analysis tools. The technical framework was designed to promote functional clarity and manageability. As illustrated in Fig. 7.7, the technical framework is composed of six main functional blocks, each addressing specific logical requirements.

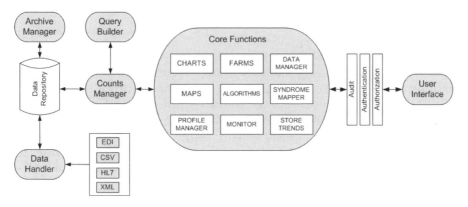

Fig. 7.7   CEWS technical framework.

- *Data handler.* The system is required to support multiple data feeds with a number of different data standards. For example, some data feeds are in a simple comma-delimited format, while others consist of HL7-encoded data that require HL7 listeners.

- *Archive manager.* As the system receives large amounts of data, a facility is needed for managing raw data such that older data that no longer contribute to the automated anomaly detection process are archived for historical purposes. The system manages two sets of tables that store raw data: *active* and *archived*. Active tables hold all current data up to a total of 5 years. Data are transferred to archived tables at the beginning of each new year.

- *Counts manager.* Once the data are received, they are stored in raw format for potential reverse linkage if needed. For example, someone with the proper authority may wish to review an emergency room chart associated with a particular CEWS record. Once stored, data are aggregated based on system and user-defined parameters to facilitate anomaly detection and trend analysis at various geo levels and classifications groupings.

- *Query builder.* To simplify code manageability and repeated access to data for analysis and presentation, a query builder was developed that manages queries in structured query language (SQLs) for data access. The approach utilized focuses all database access logic into one area of the code base, thus making it simple to manage.

- *Core functions.* There are a number of core system functional requirements from the user's perspective, ranging from simple charting to the execution of complex algorithms and mapping. A set of core resources was developed which, combined with the user interface module, provides users with access to data and results in various ways.

- *User interface.* The system provides a browser-based interface enabling Internet access for users.

7.3.1.2   CEWS — Initial Experiences   CEWS has been operational in Winnipeg since the fall of 2005. The application continues to evolve with the addition of new data streams and user feedback. Challenges to date have included interruptions in data flow resulting from technical complexities experienced by the data providers; user interface design and development to enable the required level of configurability; and manipulation while maintaining intuitive navigation, algorithm implementation, and results management. Solutions developed and implemented to address challenges related to algorithm implementation and results management are described in Section 7.3.2.

A major goal of the pilot study has been to help answer many of the questions relating to the utility of syndromic surveillance. For example, which data sources are best suited for which syndromes? With respect to emergency room data, are some chief complaints better than others? Which algorithms should be used and for what purposes? Which disease events are more likely detected sooner using syndromic surveillance? As part of the Winnipeg CEWS pilot, a comprehensive evaluation study was designed. Included in this study is a descriptive and comparative analysis of the data sources, a retrospective analysis of traditional outbreak information compared to algorithm results, a simulation study to compare the sensitivity and specificity of different algorithms, and a prospective study to examine how CEWS can best be integrated into WRHA surveillance practices. The results of these studies will be presented as they become available in the future.

7.3.2   Unique Solution for a Unique Problem: FARMS

With increasing access to data from a wide range of data providers (e.g., hospitals, tele-health systems, laboratories), vast amounts of surveillance data can potentially be collected, processed with a large array of aberration-detection algorithms, and analyzed over many variables (e.g., age, sex, syndromes, geography). Because data can be accumulated in real time (or near-real time), continual reanalysis is possible, leading to many results sets and the need for results management. This huge quantity of data not only leads to technical and computational challenges, it presents significant usability issues. The ultimate purpose of a real-time surveillance system should be to help the end user make informed decisions regarding early event detection, not further complicate the decision-making process.

There are many technical approaches to dealing with potential data and analysis overload. For instance, a surveillance system could allow only for the manual execution of algorithms, eliminating the need for automated result management in its entirety. Another solution is to allow for the automated execution of algorithms on a limited number of data strata (e.g., syndrome, geo level) to reduce the amount of results to be stored and managed. Clearly, neither approach is optimal. To advance the efficiency, effectiveness, and usability of real-time surveillance, a collection of processes, definitions, and algorithms is being developed, called the Federated Area-Based Result Management System (FARMS). The main elements of FARMS are discussed in Sections 7.3.2.1 through 7.3.2.5.

7.3.2.1 Source–Classification–Spatial (SCS) Hierarchy

The complex nature of disease syndrome and geo-level hierarchies adds significant complexity to syndromic surveillance analysis and results management. Some data sources have clear definitions of syndromes: for example, emergency room data from which syndromes are defined using chief complaints. Some data sources have a rather complicated syndrome definition: for example, pharmaceutical OTC sales data from which a syndrome is defined as a collection of drugs. Further complication arises because not all data sources provide data in a standard format, nor do they provide data at the same granular level (such as product UPC). Without some way to standardize and classify incoming data to enable "apple-to-apple" comparisons, aggregation prior to analysis becomes problematic.

Syndrome specification/classification aside, geography also presents a significant challenge. In Canada, health surveillance data have been analyzed at numerous geo levels, including postal code point locations (based on a six-digit postal code), forward sortation areas (based on the first three digits of the postal code), city, county, province/territory, health unit, and health region. Given the epidemiology of some illnesses and the needs of different users, analysis is required over several different geographic levels. Complexity arises because different data types are often more amenable to classification at one geographic level than another, and different levels of geography are not necessarily hierarchical.

The SCS hierarchy (Fig. 7.8) provides a means of defining a data organization structure to enable aggregation and analysis at various levels based on source, classification, and space.

- A data *source* is the type of data, such as emergency room visits, laboratory results, and pharmaceutical OTC sales. Each data source has unique characteristics. For example, emergency room visits typically provide such data elements as arrival time, presenting complaint, patient demographics (potentially), and hospital location. Tele-health data provide patient call time, symptoms, initial diagnosis, and demographics (potentially). On the other hand, OTC data provide time and place of drug sale, UPC, drug name, or drug category.

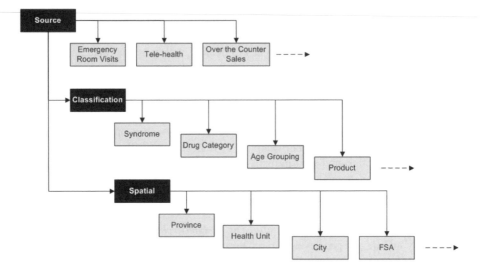

Fig. 7.8   SCS hierarchy example.

- *Classification* is the outcome of interest. In the case of emergency room data, it is probably the chief complaint. The setup of a specific classification hierarchy is dictated primarily by the granularity of the data elements provided. For example, if one OTC supplier provides products by drug category (e.g., anti-nauseants), but another provides drug UPCs, the lowest possible classification level must be category.

- The *spatial* element is the actual geographical decomposition of the area under consideration. Syndromic surveillance within Canada typically considers the following geographic levels: province or territory, health unit, city or town, and forward sortation area (FSA). Because geographic levels are not always perfectly hierarchal, systematic interpretation is often required. For example, whereas most FSAs are contained within a city or town, some can span more than one. The selection of geo level for analysis is again dictated primarily by the granularity of the data elements provided.

Careful design and implementation of the SCS hierarchy is critical when setting up a syndromic surveillance system.

7.3.2.2 Algorithm Execution Management   Depending on the SCS hierarchy, frequency of analysis, and suite of algorithms chosen, significant computational power may be required to perform the necessary analyses. Accordingly, a dynamic Algorithm Execution Management (AEM) framework was created to facilitate algorithm execution and results management in a multiserver environment. AEM enables algorithm scheduling and results collation. The basic concept of execution management is to execute the algorithms in a systematic manner so that results can be written to a database in a format that enables intuitive access for results presentation. Figure 7.9 illustrates an execution management workflow algorithm for a three-level SCS hierarchy. As shown, the process requires three steps to address the corresponding three levels in the SCS hierarchy. The first level addresses the data sources by providing a loop for all available data sources; the second level addresses each classification; the third level addresses the spatial hierarchy.

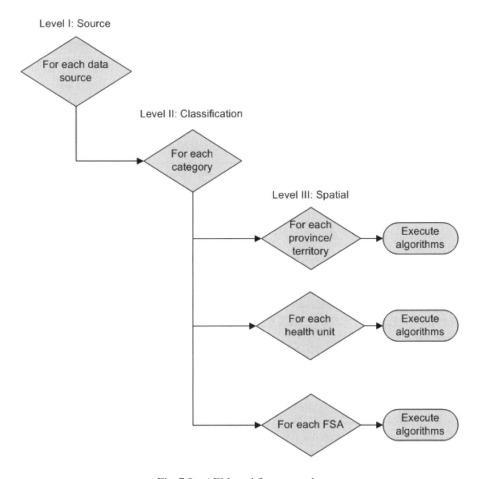

Fig. 7.9   AEM workflow example.

Central to AEM is the task coordination manager table (CMT). The CMT resides in a database and houses information necessary for the coordination of all algorithm executions (herein referred to as *tasks*). Figure 7.10 illustrates a typical multiserver environment setup. The application server hosts the front-end application, including the web server and user interface with which a user may manually request tasks to be executed. Tasks may also be predefined to enable routine automated executions. The algorithm execution server is responsible for monitoring the CMT and performing pending tasks. The CMT comprises seven key data elements: ID, a unique identifier for each task; TASK, a categorical variable describing instructions for the execution server (request, abort, and resume); TIME SUBMITTED, a timestamp when the task was submitted by the application server; SERVER, which identifies the physical algorithm execution server that is processing the task; STATUS, a categorical variable describing task state (pending, active, and completed); START TIME, a timestamp indicating when an execution server started working on a task; and END TIME, a timestamp indicating when an execution server ended working on a task.

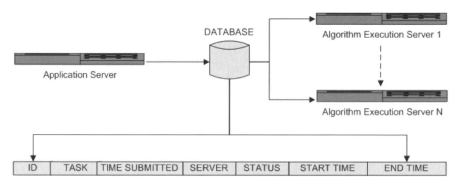

ID	TASK	TIME SUBMITTED	SERVER	STATUS	START TIME	END TIME

Fig. 7.10   Typical multiserver environment.

Each algorithm execution server manages the execution of algorithms using a state machine. Figure 7.11 depicts a high-level state machine to manage three possible states. To date, the algorithm set includes 3-day moving average, 5-day moving average, 7-day moving average, weighted moving average, exponentially weighted moving average, CUSUM, EARS C1, EARS C2, EARS C3, and progressive scan (Section 7.2.2) [5, 6, 7].

7.3.2.3   Results Storage Management   As might be expected, the execution of several algorithms over a complex SCS hierarchy can lead to many large results sets. The number of results sets is further amplified if algorithms are executed automatically on a specified schedule (e.g., daily). A structured system is needed to manage results so that they can be accessible for presentation in an effective manner. Furthermore, storage of results over a specific time frame is critical to save computation power as well as for quick access to retrospective results.

A result storage management (RSM) system framework was created to address the needs. Central to RSM is the result storage table (RST), also housed in a database. The RST holds information necessary for the coordination of algorithm results. The RST consists of the following variables: DAY, the date of analysis; SCS triplet (i.e., source, classification, spatial region); VALUE SET, the actual results of the algorithm executed for a specific time period (also known as an epidemiologically significant window); and RESULT SET, the results from the heuristic approach to alert-based result mapping (haARM) analysis (activity rate, activity direction, and alert level) for each algorithm. (haARM is discussed in Section 7.3.2.4.)

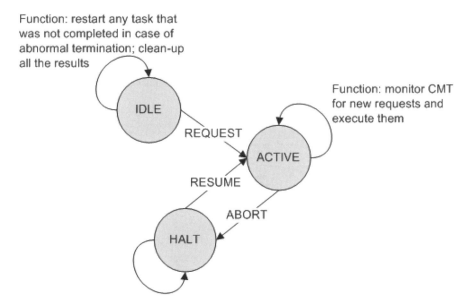

Function: restart any task that was not completed in case of abnormal termination; clean-up all the results

Function: monitor CMT for new requests and execute them

Fig. 7.11   High-level AEM state machine example.

7.3.2.4   *Visual Impact Analysis*

The ultimate purpose of a syndromic surveillance system is to facilitate decision making by the end user. The huge amount of data produced by daily results from multiple algorithms over multiple classifications from multiple data sources and with multiple presentation methods (charts, graphs, maps) can potentially complicate rather than facilitate the decision-making process. Whereas most surveillance systems provide information to the end user through the analysis of data, one of the goals of FARMS is to help the end user to create intelligence. To facilitate system usability and decision-making utility, therefore, methods are being developed to enable the presentation of results, both spatially (geographic) and temporally (time-based) in an intuitive, seamlessly accessible and navigation friendly view. This overall approach is called visual impact analysis (VIA).

haARM is a recently developed and implemented VIA method that is based on heuristic approaches as well as mathematical methods for collating results from multiple algorithms. Currently, the haARM approach is based on two main parameters: activity rate (β) and activity direction (δ) computed for a specific geographical level. Other parameters, including "area under the curve," are being considered. Activity rate (β) is defined as the rate of change in parametric values (e.g., moving average, CUSUM) over a specific epidemiologically significant window (Δ), which is typically defined in number of days. For the purpose of this discussion, this window is assumed to be a 7-day period. Consider a scenario of algorithm result values represented as h_n, where n is the day within Δ, as illustrated in Fig. 7.12. The y-axis represents the parametric value and the x-axis represents the epidemiologically significant window starting with the oldest possible day and ending with the current day under investigation. The activity rate is computed using linear regression to fit the best straight line among the h values. The average rate of change over Δ, normalized to variation for a specific algorithm, is defined by $\beta = m/\sigma$, where m is the slope and σ is the parametric standard deviation computed over Δ. Normalization of slope to obtain activity rate is crucial for ultimately facilitating cross-algorithm comparison and metaalgorithm analysis.

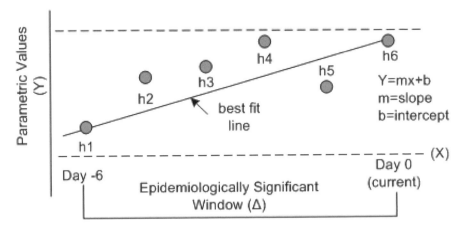

Fig. 7.12   Typical algorithm daily results.

Activity direction δ is used to describe the direction of the activity rate based on Δ. It is computed based on the sign of the slope value (m). Once δ and β have been computed, the results can be visually represented with some simple angle-based shading via the minima concept from elementary calculus, as shown in Fig. 7.13.

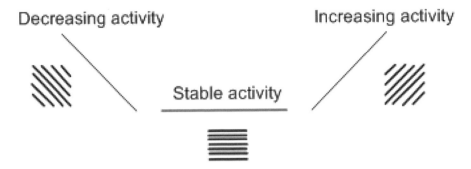

Fig. 7.13   Representation of activity rate direction.

Over time, haARM has been further refined to account for epidemiologically significant nuances encountered in the interpretation of surveillance data. For example, during a very dramatic and quickly developing outbreak, the average slope over Δ days may not capture a sudden and significant change in activity rate direction. To capture these types of scenarios, a new slope parameter was defined: the average-based activity rate (see Fig. 7.14).

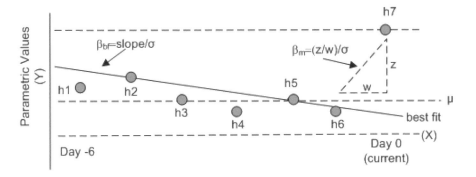

Fig. 7.14 Example of a rapidly developing outbreak.

Here β_{bf} is the activity rate using linear regression best-fit approach, and β_m is the activity rate computed using the mean value (μ) such that $\beta_m = (h_7 - \mu)/\sigma$. The final activity rate β is then computed as the average of β_{bf} and β_m. Once generated, δ and β values can be displayed using GIS layers on an area- or geo-level-specific basis, yielding a temporal-spatial visualization of the results (Fig. 7.15).

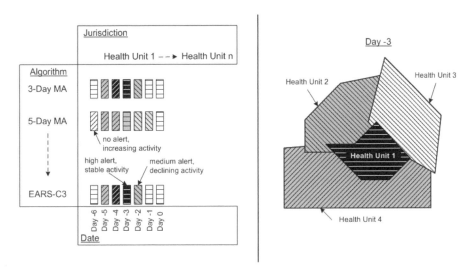

Fig. 7.15 Temporal-spatial visualization of algorithm results.

To facilitate visualization, δ has been categorized as *positive*, *negative*, and *no change* based on preset cutoff values. Colors represent predefined *alert* levels. For example, a green alert is generated when the parametric value is less than a specified mean (e.g., a seasonal rolling average), a yellow alert is generated when the parametric value is between the mean and 1 standard deviation; an orange alert is generated when the parametric value falls between the mean plus 1 standard deviation and 2 standard deviations; and a red alert is generated when the parametric value is more than the mean plus 2 standard deviations.

7.3.2.5 Ongoing FARMS Research   In further work on haARM, methods are currently being developed to provide decision-making intelligence based on the results of several different algorithms executed on the same data set. With the availability of dozens of different algorithms, it is possible, if not probable, to get different results from different algorithms executed in parallel on the same dataset. A new approach, called confidence-based aberration interpretation, may help to address this current gap in syndromic surveillance utility.

7.4   CONCLUSIONS: PUBLIC HEALTH SURVEILLANCE

7.4.1   Importance of Communication and Collaboration

Communication, collaboration, and information sharing are often afterthoughts when the necessary elements for an effective and efficient public health surveillance system are being considered. Historically, communication among public health stakeholders was the cornerstone of surveillance. Even today, many, if not most, disease events are still identified by astute health care professionals (physicians, nurses, epidemiologists, microbiologists, etc.) recognizing abnormal patterns in disease or illness parameters. The importance of epidemiologists and microbiologists comparing notes on disease counts or risk factors across jurisdictions cannot be overstated.

Together with generating public health information and intelligence, public health surveillance systems should facilitate the sharing and distribution of this information and intelligence among the appropriate people. Furthermore, an effective public health surveillance system should provide tools and resources to facilitate stakeholder interaction and seamless collaboration. This collaboration will become even more important as the World Wide Web continues to evolve, and web-based surveillance technologies potentially replace direct person-to-person interactions.

The assessment of the needs of public health surveillance in Canada identified the need for a mechanism for both structured alert-based communication and informal communications and collaboration. Resources were needed not to *replace* phone, fax, and e-mail, but to *augment* them. To fill these gaps, the Public Health Agency developed a national alerting system that now connects more than 2000 public health stakeholders countrywide. Furthermore, a suite of Web-based communication and collaboration tools was developed and implemented. A unique approach was developed to package and provide access to communication and collaboration tools to reflect the business needs of public health professionals. The response to such tools has been overwhelmingly positive. Current plans are to integrate communication and collaboration resources with all of the agency's surveillance and response management applications.

7.4.2   Integrating Surveillance into a Comprehensive Public Health Information Management Framework

Public health surveillance applications and resources should not be developed in isolation from other public health information management resources. Efforts should be made to achieve a comprehensive IM/IT/KM framework that integrates all public health functions (alerting, surveillance, response, data and information management, case management, etc.), thus providing a seamless environment of resources to meet the continuum of needs, including disease detection, investigation, response, and evaluation. Although it is not necessary for specific applications to be on the same technical platform or from the same software provider, it is essential that public health applications be able to communicate and integrate.

The syndromic surveillance resources and activities discussed in this chapter were developed within a national IM/IT/KM framework [the Canadian Network for Public Health Intelligence (CNPHI)]. Figure 7.16 shows how disease-specific surveillance applications (including wNESP) and CEWS fit into this much larger framework. Key elements of CNPHI are:

- *Data Exchange:* includes SET (Section 7.2.2), which facilitates data extraction, interrogation, analysis, and communication among disparate databases, independent of format and database type. SET allows for full user control of field-level data sharing. This component of middleware is required to allow data sharing within a federated system of databases. Epi Assist is a generic online record management tool based on proprietary formbuilder technology that enables nontechnical users to collect and manage data.

- *Decision support:* designed to provide users with easy access to a number of resources (e.g., GIS, modeling tools). Users can create custom dynamic queries to interrogate data to which they have access. The data can also be presented on a GIS map depending on business rules. Decision-support resources are available to all application users, and data access is controlled through tiered and targeted access control.

- *Collaboration tools:* comprise a number of management and collaboration tools. These resources are constantly evolving to accommodate newly emerging tools that facilitate peer-to-peer collaboration.

- *Knowledge management:* provides a secure environment for the sharing of documents, publications, online texts, protocols, training materials, etc.

- *Public health alerting/notification:* a role-based resource that allows for jurisdictional flexibility and is targeted to tailored audiences. It is secure and integrated into all other CNPHI resources. It has multiple levels to facilitate the flow of information among jurisdictional levels. This module currently connects 100% of federal, provincial/territorial, and local public health authorities in Canada.

- *Disease-specific surveillance:* utilizing a common architecture and set of functional resources, the applications that make up this module facilitate program-specific surveillance needs. They accommodate program-specific data, analysis, distribution, and communication requirements. wNESP (Section 7.2.2) is one example of a disease-specific surveillance application.

- *Real-time surveillance:* with advances in technology, the real-time exchange of data has created the potential for more timely surveillance of health events. CEWS (Section 7.3.1) was developed to investigate and evaluate the utility of real-time surveillance.

- *Registration system:* performs user registration, authentication, and access control (role-based and target-based) for each of the data sets and applications within the entire framework. It is implemented to allow communication and synchronization among different registration systems. This module ensures data confidentiality while allowing access to multiple databases and applications.

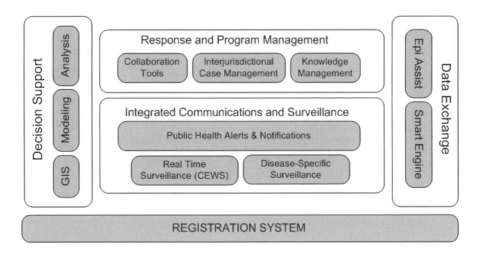

Fig. 7.16 High-level modular overview of a comprehensive public health IM/IT/KM framework: the Canadian Network for Public Health Intelligence.

7.4.3   Future Opportunities in Public Health Surveillance

Opportunities to further advance public health surveillance through the adoption of technologies are limited only by the imagination. Consider the following examples:

- In Canada, it is expected that most, if not all, health records will be in electronic format and available online to appropriate persons within the next decade or so. Electronic health records (EHRs) provide the opportunity to improve both clinical care and public health through advances in evidence-based medicine and evidenced-based public health. Envision a system that automatically recommends to a physician a differential diagnosis list, based not only on a patient's presenting symptoms, but also on current population disease dynamics in his or her community. Similarly, envision the same system aggregating EHR data, providing surveillance information to local public health officials in real time and allowing the public health official to push requests for additional required data elements (history, tests, etc.) down to the physician to test an hypothesis.

- Consider air quality and drinking water advisories based not only on air and water sampling results but also on real-time health parameters reported from a given community (e.g., emergency room visits, physician visits, sales of OTC medications, tele-health activity). Current air and water quality guidelines assume the offending chemical/microbe can be detected in the air or water in a timely manner. However, some tests are performed only daily or not at all. What about pollutants and chemicals that cannot yet be measured?

- Occasionally, grocery store receipts are used to help identify a common food item during a presumed foodborne outbreak. Could electronically monitored transactions (which most are these days) and health records be monitored automatically to identify a suspect food item or restaurant?

- Could wireless devices be used to monitor individual health parameters in real time, such as heart rate and respiratory rate? In the event of a heat advisory, real-time surveillance of the elderly and shut-ins would probably prevent loss of life.

- Many infectious diseases in Canada can be traced back to travel to a foreign country. Could air and sea travel data be monitored and integrated with health information to help identify risk areas outside Canada's borders?

These examples are just a few of many surveillance possibilities, all of which are technically feasible today or in the near future. The real challenge will be in working with stakeholders to evaluate both the need and the potential benefits of new surveillance methods. The future of surveillance will inevitably provide many exciting challenges and opportunities.

7.5   STUDY QUESTIONS

7.1 One of the greatest challenges facing public health surveillance today is achieving some degree of standardization and integration among jurisdictions (local, state/provincial, national, etc.). Because of this, it is difficult to compare findings among jurisdictions and achieve a "surveillance picture" over a large geographical area. This challenge exists for a number of reasons, including the large number of different applicable technologies, and because (for the most part) each jurisdiction controls and funds its own surveillance systems. *Q: Given the current situation, please discuss what approaches could be used to help achieve a truly national public health surveillance system.*

7.2 Currently in Canada we have implemented a national alerting system to facilitate rapid communication of disease events to appropriate persons. *Q: Describe how public health surveillance and communication tools such as alerting and syndromic surveillance can play a significant role in disease outbreak identification and management within and among jurisdictions (including across national borders).*

7.3 Although stakeholders and contributors to public health surveillance primarily include those working directly in the public health sector (e.g., physicians, epidemiologists, microbiologists, nurses), many disciplines, public-sector agencies, and industries have a role to play in public health surveillance. *Q: Make a list of potential "nontraditional" public health stakeholders and describe what role each could and should play in a comprehensive public health surveillance system.*

7.4 For the most part, public health surveillance systems discussed in this chapter assume that stakeholders have reliable and high-speed Internet access. In Canada (as in most parts of the world), health care providers in rural and remote communities often do not have such facilities. *Q: Describe how processes and technologies could be used to address these technology gaps.*

7.5 Over the next decade, electronic health records will likely become a standard tool in the health care sector. Just like Internet banking, detailed personal health information will be accessible online. *Q: Discuss what potential challenges and opportunities electronic health records provide to public health surveillance.*

Acknowledgments

The authors of this chapter would like to thank the many persons who have contributed to the work presented here. It would be impossible to name all members of the respective teams, but we would like to mention a few Public Health Agency of Canada scientists in particular. Many thanks to Dr. Victoria Edge for leading the charge on OTC sales surveillance. Thanks also to Laura McDonald for her involvement in the Winnipeg CEWS pilot, and to Walter Demczuk and Nadia Ciampa for their efforts in the development of wNESP.

REFERENCES

1. Naylor D, ed. Learning from SARS: Renewal of Public Health in Canada. Ottawa, Ontario: Health Canada; 2003. Available at `http://www.phac-aspc.gc.ca/publicat/sars-sras/naylor/`. Accessed July 2006.

2. Kettner J. Chief Medical Officer of Health, Winnipeg, Manitoba. Personal communication; 2005.

3. Stirling R, Aramini J, Ellis A, Lim G, Meyers R, Fleury M. Waterborne *Cryptosporidiosis* outbreak, North Battleford, Saskatchewan, Spring 2001. Ottawa, Ontario: Health Canada; 2000. Available at `http://www.health.gov.sk.ca/ mc_dp_health_can_epi_report_NB_part1.pdf`. Accessed July 2006.

4. BGOSHU (Bruce Grey Owen Sound Health Unit). The investigative report on the Walkerton outbreak of waterborne gastroenteritis, May – June 2000. Owen Sound, Ontario: Bruce Grey Owen Sound Health Unit; 2000. Available at `http://www.publichealthgreybruce.on.ca/_private/Walkerton/ SPWalkerton.htm`. Accessed July 2006.

5. Morton A, Whitby M, Mclaws M, Dobson A, Stackleroth J, Sartor A. The application of statistical process control charts to the detection and monitoring of hospital-acquired infections. J Qual Clin Prac. 2001;21:112-117.

6. Hutwagner L, Thompson W, Seeman G, Treadwell T. The bioterrorism preparedness and response early aberration reporting system (EARS). J Urban Health. 2003;80:i89-i96.

7. NIST/SEMATECH. e-Handbook of statistical methods. Available at `http://www.itl.nist.gov/div898/handbook/`. Accessed July 2006.

8 Case Study: Use of Tele-health Data for Syndromic Surveillance in England and Wales

Duncan Cooper

Chapter 7 discussed initiatives within the Public Health Agency of Canada to implement and manage an automated disease surveillance system and provided a good example of issues arising during the development and implementation of the Canadian Early Warning System. This chapter looks at the experiences of the UK Health Protection Agency in using data from a national health service phone triage system (NHS Direct). NHS Direct supplies call data that are grouped into syndromes and analyzed on a daily basis to detect abnormal trends in disease. Examples of health events detected through this system are presented and recommendations are provided to those interested in using similar data sources for surveillance.

8.1 INTRODUCTION

In recent years, there has been a growth in the number of tele-health systems, which provide the public with health advice and information via the telephone. This chapter describes the experience of using telephone call data from a national UK National Health Service telephone triage system (NHS Direct) for syndromic surveillance. The aim of the Health Protection Agency (HPA) NHS Direct syndromic surveillance system is to identify, as early as possible, an increase in syndromes indicative of early stages of illness due to common infections or the deliberate release of a biological or chemical agent. This chapter outlines the design of the surveillance system and the methods used by a multidisciplinary public health team to investigate increases in syndromes reported to NHS Direct call centres. Results are presented that demonstrate the system's usefulness for providing early warning of rises in infectious disease and disease caused by environmental factors, as well as reassurance when there is a perceived threat to public health. Two methods of enhancing NHS Direct syndromic data are described: (1) a self-sampling study that links syndromic data with traditional surveillance data (laboratory testing) and (2) a straightforward statistical modeling technique to provide added confidence in the interpretation of syndromic surveillance data. Also included are recommendations for the design, operation, and evaluation of syndromic surveillance systems based on telephone triage data.

8.1.1   What Is Tele-health?

Tele-health enables a clinical process to be conducted remotely, thus combining the power of health telecommunication and information technology to improve the efficiency and quality of health care. The innovative use of technology to deliver tele-health services, such as by video or audio-conferencing, means that health care services can be provided to those who are some distance from the provider, thus reducing geographic barriers to accessing care. Tele-health applications now cover a diverse range of health care services, including consulting, psychiatry, cardiology, gastroenterology, rehabilitation, ultrasound, remote diagnostics, dialysis, and robotic surgery. The current value of the annual U.S. tele-health market alone is in excess of $300 million [1]. Tele-health is also becoming increasingly vital to developing nations by providing health care to rural or underserved areas. In 1997, the World Health Organization (WHO) announced that it would make tele-health a global strategy area for the twenty-first century, advocating its use for disease prevention, education and training, and, interestingly, disease surveillance [2].

Telenursing or telephone triage is a subset of tele-health in which the focus is on nursing practice via telecommunications (usually the telephone). Such systems have gained in prominence as governments and major health care providers have sought to control rising health care costs, reduce inappropriate visits to emergency care, and meet patient demand for round-the-clock health care advice and information. In recent years in countries with largely public health care delivery, telephone triage systems have been operating on a regional (e.g., Tele-health Ontario in Canada [3], HealthDirect in Western Australia [4]) and on a national level (e.g., NHS Direct in England and Wales [5], NHS 24 in Scotland [6], Healthline in New Zealand [7]). Privately run telephone triage systems have also become commonplace, with at least 100 million Americans able to access some form of telephone triage.

8.1.2   The UK Experience: NHS Direct

NHS Direct is a nurse-led health helpline that provides the population of England and Wales with rapid access to professional advice and information about health, illness, and the NHS. The service operates 365 days per year from a network of 21 sites in England and a single site covering all of Wales (22 in total). It is the world's largest online provider of health care advice and answers nearly 7 million calls per year. Other ways of accessing health care information and advice from NHS Direct include a digital television channel and, most important, its website (NHS Direct Online), which receives over 1 million visits per month.

NHS Direct nurses use clinical decision-support software [the NHS Clinical Assessment System (NHS CAS)] to triage, rather than diagnose, NHS Direct callers. NHS CAS is structured around approximately 230 computerized clinical algorithms, each consisting of a "treelike" structure of questions relating to the symptoms of the person calling NHS Direct. Nurses use clinical judgment and the most appropriate clinical algorithm to triage the call. The nature and severity of the reported symptoms (e.g., diarrhea, fever, back pain) dictate the algorithm selected and, ultimately, the recommendation provided by NHS CAS (e.g., self-care, family doctor referral, paramedic dispatch).

8.1.2.1 *Comparison with Other Health Services*

NHS Direct total call rates are still a fraction of total consultation rates for primary care doctors. NHS Direct handles approximately 7 million calls per year compared with approximately 14 million visits a year to accident and emergency departments in England [8] and 190 million consultations with family doctors [9]. So although NHS Direct has national coverage, the majority of primary care visits in the UK are through face-to-face clinician-based services.

8.1.2.2 *Age and Sex of NHS Direct Callers*

The highest symptomatic call rates to NHS Direct are for young children (<1 year: 358 calls per 1000 per year; 1–4 years: 173 per 1000 during 2005; and younger adults: 76 per 1000). Call rates fall with increasing age, and the lowest call rates are for the elderly. This pattern is consistent with telephone triage data from Australia [10]. Women are more likely than men to use the service: the ratio of female to male calls (all ages) is 1.3:1. The distribution of calls by age and sex is largely comparable to that for family doctor services, except for the low NHS Direct call rate from those over 65 years — possibly reflecting the older generation's reluctance to use telephone services for information and services rather than traditional local medical centres.

8.1.2.3 *Social Factors*

Approximately 25% of the population uses NHS Direct [11]. Although questionnaire studies have indicated low awareness [12] and low usage [11, 13] of the service among lower socioeconomic groups, research using call records indicate high call rates from areas where socioeconomic status is low. Studies at three NHS Direct sites have shown that local call rates (all ages combined) rise with increasing social deprivation before falling in the most deprived areas. Call rates were in fact lowest in the least deprived [14, 15] and rural areas [16]. With respect to ethnicity, internal NHS Direct figures indicate that the proportion of callers from different ethnic groups mirrors the census population data in most areas. To limit barriers to accessing the service, NHS Direct has a well-publicized interpreting service, will translate written health information on request, and has a dedicated text phone for the deaf and hearing impaired.

8.1.2.4 *Call Outcomes*

Seventy percent of NHS Direct callers request assessment of symptoms. Of these, 19% receive self-care advice or a pharmacy referral, 51% are referred to their family doctor, 8% are advised to go to an accident and emergency department, and 5% need a paramedic callout. The remaining 17% are directed to a variety of other services (e.g., poison centre, family planning clinic).

8.1.2.5   Main Reasons for Calling NHS Direct   The 10 most used NHS CAS clinical algorithms during March 2005 accounted for 29% of total symptomatic calls (Table 8.1). Gastrointestinal and respiratory illness algorithms, and algorithms designed specifically for triage of young children are used most frequently.

Table 8.1   Ten Most Used CAS Clinical Algorithms (March 2006) by the 21 NHS Direct Sites in England

10 Most Used Clinical Algorithms	% Total Clinical Algorithms Used
Abdominal pain	5.8
Vomiting	3.0
Toothache	2.9
Vomiting, toddler (Age 1-4 years)	2.7
Fever, toddler (Age 1-4 years)	2.6
Chest pain	2.5
Diarrhea	2.5
Headache	2.5
Diarrhea, infants and toddlers (age 0-4 years)	2.4
Sore throat	2.4

8.1.3   Using Telephone Triage Data for Syndromic Surveillance

8.1.3.1   North American Experience   There are few published examples of the use of data from telephone triage or help lines for real-time disease surveillance. In 1998, a time-series analysis showed a 17-fold increase in nurse hotline calls about diarrhea during a citywide outbreak of cryptosporidiosis in Milwaukee [17]. Two retrospective analyses of nurse hotline data from the Baltimore–Washington metropolitan area demonstrated that individual calls can be used to predict respiratory and gastrointestinal final diagnoses [18], and that trends in telephone triage data accurately predict trends in doctor diagnoses [19]. A study correlating after-hours telephone triage data (from physicians' offices) with CDC influenza surveillance data showed no clear early warning advantage to using telephone triage data for surveillance [20]. There are plans to use real-time tele-health data from Ontario's Tele-health helpline prospectively within the province's syndromic surveillance strategy [21].

8.1.3.2   Disease Surveillance in the UK

At present, reports of notifiable disease, data collected by National Health Service and Health Protection Agency (HPA) laboratories, and doctor consultations recorded by the Royal College of General Practitioners (RCGP) sentinel surveillance system [22] are the main modes of communicable disease surveillance in England and Wales. Other sources of data include hospital admissions, death certifications and registrations, and outbreak reports. The HPA also monitors chemical incidents reported from a range of sources, including local health protection units, the fire service, and the National Poisons Information Service [23]. Data from the laboratory and clinical surveillance systems are subject to some reporting delay and generally produce weekly summaries for the public health community, media, and general public.

8.1.3.3   Why Use NHS Direct Data for Surveillance?

NHS Direct sites use clinical software (NHS CAS) and reporting tools to record and report caller details on a daily basis. This timeliness, coupled with the broad national population coverage of NHS Direct and the wide range of recorded syndromes, makes the data suitable for population health surveillance. If a deliberate release of a harmful agent were to cause illnesses with a mild prodromal phase, some proportion of the population would be likely to contact NHS Direct before visiting other health services. This proportion is currently unknown, although in general, 25% of the population use NHS Direct. Consequently, an increase in illness may be identified through surveillance of NHS Direct before it is reported to other primary care or secondary care services.

The aim of the HPA NHS Direct syndromic surveillance system is to identify an increase in syndromes indicative of common infections and diseases or the early stages of illness caused by the deliberate release of a biological or chemical agent. Additionally, information on the age, geographical location, and syndromes of affected callers to NHS Direct could help track a rise in illness over time. The national HPA NHS Direct syndromic surveillance system uses telephone triage data for daily surveillance of 11 syndromes and has been operational since 2001. The surveillance team that oversees all aspects of the surveillance system is drawn from HPA and NHS Direct and consists of data analysts, scientists, epidemiologists, and NHS Direct managerial and medical staff. Section 8.2 outlines the design of this system and the way in which this multidisciplinary team investigates increases in cases detected through surveillance.

8.2   SYSTEM DESIGN AND EPIDEMIOLOGICAL CONSIDERATIONS

8.2.1   Data Availability

The call reporting system linked to NHS CAS was designed for performance manage-ment purposes rather than as an epidemiological or surveillance tool. However, NHS Direct-derived data do provide a valuable snapshot of symptoms in the community, and a number of "off the shelf" NHS CAS reports provide breakdowns of call data (e.g., calls grouped by algorithm or outcome). Daily national data that are routinely available from NHS Direct are used for surveillance. Problems have been encountered with the consistency of syndromic data due to regular software upgrades of NHS CAS, which, at times, have resulted in clinical algorithms being merged, changed, or deleted from the system.

8.2.2   System Design

Total calls and call data relating to 11 algorithm groupings (syndromes) (Table 8.2) are received electronically by the HPA from all 22 NHS Direct sites every weekday (Fig. 8.1). This list of syndromes is intended to be indicative of the early stages of a range of illnesses caused by biological or chemical agents or common infections. Data are broken down by NHS Direct site, syndrome, age group, and call outcome.

Consistent daily data returns were achieved within the first year of the project. Factors that helped in this process were:

1. Using only routinely collected NHS Direct data for surveillance

2. Causing minimal disruption to the work patterns of the data providers (NHS Direct nurses and analysts) and working within existing reporting frameworks

3. Ensuring continual feedback (both verbal and through routine and ad hoc surveil-lance reports) to staff within NHS Direct

Upper confidence limits (99.5% level) of calls for each syndrome, as a proportion of daily total calls, were developed for each NHS Direct site. These confidence limits were derived from the standard formula for proportions [24], with the baseline numbers of total answered syndromic calls adjusted for seasonal effects (monthly adjustment). An *exceedance* was defined as an observed daily proportion of calls above the 99.5% upper confidence limit. A proportional model was used rather than an absolute count or population incidence model to account for the gradual year-on-year increase in calls and sudden and local increases in call rates due to local publicity. Sensitivity/specificity analysis of the NHS Direct syndromic surveillance system's ability to detect a cryptosporidiosis outbreak also confirmed that a proportional model outperformed an absolute count model for NHS Direct data [25].

In addition to the confidence interval analyses, control charts were constructed for 6 of the 10 syndromes (cold/flu, cough, fever, difficulty breathing, diarrhea, and

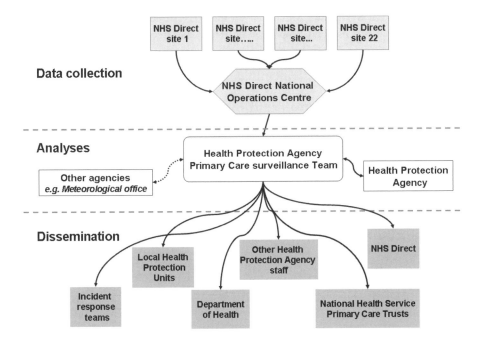

Fig. 8.1   National HPA NHS Direct syndromic surveillance system flow chart.

vomiting) at the 10 NHS Direct sites covering major conurbations in England (London, Manchester, Leeds, Birmingham, Sheffield, and Newcastle). Baselines for the control charts were calculated based on the assumption that the number of syndromic calls followed a Poisson distribution. Total calls were used as an offset. A model was fitted to each site and syndrome separately using data from December 2001 onwards. These models always included a public holiday and seasonal term, a day of the week if necessary (weekday, Saturday, or Sunday), and a linear long-term trend factor. Scaling was performed to account for overdispersion when present.

A normal approximation was not used to calculate the 99.5% upper control chart limit of calls for each symptom because it yielded more exceedances than would be expected (i.e., approximately 2% as opposed to the expected 0.5%). Instead, a transformation to approximate normality with zero mean was performed and then a back-transformation to the original scale. The resulting expression for the 99.5% upper limit of syndromic calls, used for the control charts, was:

$$\left(\sinh \frac{z_\alpha/2 + \sqrt{N - 0.5}\,\sinh^{-1}\sqrt{p}}{\sqrt{N - 0.5}}\right)^2 (N - 0.75) - 3/8 \qquad (8.1)$$

where N is the expected value divided by one less than the scale parameter, p is equal to the scale parameter minus 1, and z_α is the $100 * (1 - \alpha)$th centile of the normal

Table 8.2   Eleven Syndromes Monitored by the NHS Direct Syndromic Surveillance System; Number of Calls and Proportion of Total Calls Recorded by the Surveillance System, 2005

Syndrome	Number of Calls	% Total Calls
Cold/flu	32,462	0.80
Cough	105,740	2.50
Diarrhea	119,399	2.80
Difficulty breathing	49,205	1.20
Double vision	371	0.01
Eye problems	42,613	1.00
Fever	133,761	3.20
Heat/sun stroke (monitored only June–September)	947	0.03
Lumps	31,754	0.80
Rash	170,202	4.10
Vomiting	164,742	3.90
Total from 11 syndromes	*851,196*	*20.30*
Total symptomatic calls to NHS Direct	4,191,779	100.00

distribution. Ad hoc choices of z were used to achieve the desired proportion of purely random exceedances (0.5%). The upper 99.5% control chart limit of syndromic calls as a proportion of total calls is calculated on a daily basis. Statistically significant excesses (i.e., exceedances) in calls for any of the 11 syndromes are automatically highlighted (for the confidence interval and control chart method) and assessed by the surveillance team. These are termed *stage 1 exceedances*. The project analyst and scientist assess the public health significance of exceedances daily with input from a medically trained consultant epidemiologist.

8.2.3   Investigating Exceedances

8.2.3.1   Stage 1   By monitoring 11 syndromes at 22 NHS Direct sites using a 99.5% upper prediction limit, one would expect at least 1 exceedance per day throughout the year. In reality, even after accounting for daily, monthly, holiday, and long-term factors, the temporal distribution of exceedances is far from uniform, with more exceedances occurring during the winter months. The surveillance team must decide which exceedances represent a potential threat to public health and require further investigation. Because the resources are not available to investigate every exceedance fully, the surveillance team takes the following factors into account when deciding whether to progress from a stage 1 exceedance (statistical alert) to a stage 2 investigation:

- Obvious data errors.

- Single-day or multiple-day exceedances. Single-day exceedances may, in the absence of other factors, be left until the next day's data become available.

- The clinical severity of calls. Calls where NHS Direct nurses have recommended an emergency care outcome (e.g., paramedic dispatch or emergency department referral) are used as a proxy for severity.

- The age distribution and time of year of the calls. For example, statistical exceedances during winter are more likely due to self-limiting viral illness and are less likely to be investigated than exceedances of calls about adults in the summer months.

- Levels of call activity and exceedances at neighbouring NHS Direct sites.

- Previous exceedance history at the site.

- Current community levels of disease reported by other surveillance systems.

- Media reports/advertising campaign. Increases in calls have been observed during NHS Direct advertising campaigns and during health problems of global concern (e.g., the SARS epidemic in 2003).

- Upgrades to the clinical decision-support software. Exceedances may occur due merely to a change in the way calls are classified by NHS Direct nurses (CAS upgrades may cause clinical algorithms to be removed, merged, or added to the system). Upgrades will also eventually affect baseline data.

8.2.3.2 Stage 2   If no reasonable explanation can be found for the exceedance, a stage 2 investigation is undertaken in which additional "line listings" of call details (including the call IDs and callers' home postcodes) are requested for the day of the exceedance and the current day. The call ID, which is a unique number, is used to identify duplicate call records, and the current day's data, if available, are used to determine whether the high level of calls has persisted for a particular syndrome. A geographical information system (GIS) may then be used to map calls for obvious clustering. Mapping is not a routine procedure for all exceedances.

Privacy issues have been carefully considered because individual line listings of call details (containing postcodes) are analyzed when there is felt to be a potential threat to public health. In the UK, the use of patient identifiable data is governed by the principles of the Caldicott report (1997) [26] and the UK Data Protection Act

(1998). These principles (Fig. 8.2) provide a sensible guide for the use of potentially sensitive data for surveillance.

1. Justify the purpose of using the data.
   JUSTIFIED

2. Only use when absolutely necessary.
   USEFUL

3. Use the minimum data required.
   MINIMAL

4. Access to data should be on a need to know basis.
   SECURE

5. Everyone must understand their Responsibilities.
   RESPONSIBLE

6. Understand and comply with the law.
   LEGAL

Fig. 8.2 Caldicott's key principles with regard to patient identifiable data. (From U.S. Department of Health [26])

8.2.3.3 Stage 3   When the surveillance team believes that the information provided by the call line listings (stage 2) necessitates further action, the call information is passed to the on-call surveillance team consultant epidemiologist, the NHS Direct medical advisor, and other relevant national or local public health staff. This situation is termed a stage 3 alert and may result in the dissemination of reports to public health teams or, on rare occasions, direct contact of callers by the NHS Direct on-call medical adviser to obtain further clinical information. When this type of action is taken, local or national agencies are normally informed within 24–48 hours of the NHS Direct calls. To obtain a definitive clinical diagnosis for a caller, it may be necessary to collect a sample. Although a mechanism to collect self-testing kits from NHS Direct callers has been developed (Section 8.4.1), this procedure is not currently routine.

8.3   RESULTS FROM THE NHS DIRECT SYNDROMIC SURVEILLANCE SYSTEM

8.3.1   Stages 1 to 3

Table 8.3 lists the number of stage 1 exceedances, stage 2 investigations, and stage 3 alerts during a single year. Of 158 stage 1 exceedances generated by the control chart methodology, 23 were investigated, and a further 3 progressed to stage 3 alerts with local public health officials informed. These figures do not include other relevant syndromic trends issued through the national weekly syndromic surveillance bulletin. Syndromes with fewer exceedances (e.g., fever and cough) were more likely to trigger stage 2 investigations. Figure 8.3 provides an example of a control chart showing the increase in proportion of fever calls to Manchester NHS Direct (shown as dots) rising above the 99.5% upper prediction limit during January 2002 and October 2003. These rises in fever calls provided a timely indication of a substantial increase in community morbidity. Subsequent laboratory data indicated concurrent rises in reports of a new subtype of influenza A (H1N2) during winter 2001–2002 [27] and the emergence of a new antigenic drift variant influenza A (H3N2) Fujian-like strain during winter 2003–2004 [28]. In both these instances, the stage 3 alerts gave national surveillance coordinators and local health protection teams early warning of a substantial and potentially serious rise in influenza-like illness.

Table 8.3   Number of Exceedances (Stage 1), Exceedances Investigated (Stage 2), and Alerts (Stage 3), March 2004–February 2005

	Stage 1: No. of Exceedances	Stage 2: Exceedances Investigated	Stage 3: Alerts
Cold/flu	45	3	1
Cough	8	3	0
Diarrhea	37	6	0
Difficulty breathing	6	2	2
Fever	6	3	0
Vomiting	56	6	0
Total	158	23	3
Percent of total exceedances	100	14.6	1.9

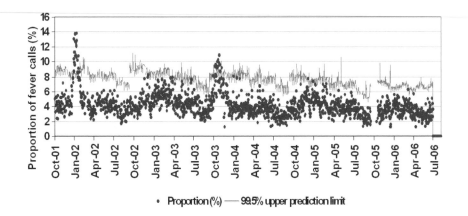

Fig. 8.3   Control chart showing Manchester NHS Direct fever calls as a proportion of total calls, against a 99.5% upper prediction limit.

8.3.2   What Have the Data Detected?

Sections 8.3.2.1 through 8.3.2.3 describe stage 3 alerts where the surveillance system provided early detection and characterization of increases in illness related to infectious diseases, environmental health effects, and, potentially, a major incident.

8.3.2.1   Case Study 1 (Infectious Diseases): Influenza B During the Winter of 2005–2006   The winter of 2005–2006 was characterized by low rates of clinical influenza-like illness reported by the Royal College of General Practitioners Weekly Returns Service and low numbers of influenza laboratory reports prior to Christmas 2005. Sporadic school outbreaks of influenza B were reported in northwest England during December 2005 just before a sudden national increase in reports during January 2006 (689 school outbreaks of influenza-like illness, some also with norovirus, reported during January–February 2006) [29]. At the time, there was media concern that influenza B was hitting schools particularly hard in the West Midlands region of England. The reporting of school outbreaks, however, is not consistent across the country, so it was necessary to examine carefully the various sources of available surveillance data.

On January 25, 2006, the weekly NHS Direct syndromic surveillance bulletin reported a significant rise in the proportion of NHS Direct fever calls for the 5- to 14-year-old age group, reaching its highest level since November 2003. At the same time, clinical and laboratory indicators of influenza remained relatively low. After examination of regional trends in NHS Direct fever calls (5–14 years) (Fig. 8.4), the surveillance team reported that although the West Midlands had one of highest levels in terms of fever calls (peaking at 14.3%), the level was not unusually high. In fact, during this period, the London region had the highest proportion of fever calls for the 5- to 14-year-old age group, peaking at 21% on February 8.

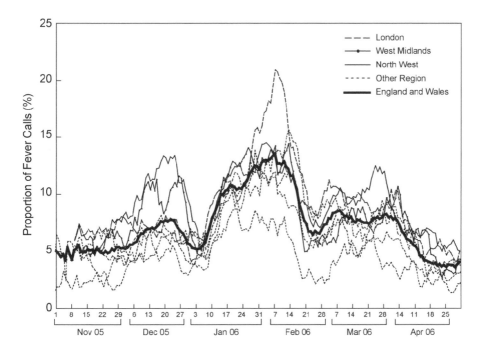

Fig. 8.4   NHS Direct fever calls as a proportion of total calls by English region and Wales (5- to 14-year-olds); November 2005–April 2006.

In this instance, NHS Direct syndromic surveillance data were able to provide an early indication of a community rise of influenza-like illness in school-aged children (late January 2006). At the time, influenza-like illness reported to sentinel general practitioners was still within baseline levels. This case demonstrates how health advice-seeking behaviors (calls to a tele-health system) can provide the first indication of a widespread community rise in illness (before patients present to family doctors). Syndromic data also confirmed that the level of fever calls was not particularly high in the West Midlands (quelling media fears) and provided ongoing regional-specific monitoring (along with other primary care surveillance systems) for the remainder of the national outbreak.

8.3.2.2 Case Study 2 (Environmental Health Effects): Annual Rise in Grass Pollen Counts and NHS Direct Eye Problems Calls   The concentration of pollen grains in the air is monitored at 33 sites throughout the UK. The data collected are used to detect the start and end of the various pollen seasons and the geotemporal variation in pollen counts as the season progresses. Publicly available forecasts are used by doctors to guide diagnosis and treatment and by hay fever sufferers to manage their condition. In the UK, tree pollen affects a small proportion of hay fever sufferers during the spring months. By June, grass pollen is the most important pollen type in terms of allergic reactions. As much as 90% of hay fever sufferers are allergic to grass pollen [30].

The exact timing of the start, peak, and end of the grass pollen season can vary from year to year. The time of day and concentration of pollen spores also influence the incidence levels and severity of hay fever symptom. Within this complex mix of factors, daily NHS Direct syndromic data have provided a way of measuring whether the pollen levels are having a significant public health impact. Figure 8.5 presents daily "eye problems" calls (coded as "eye discharge," "red or painful eye," or "visual disturbance or loss" by NHS Direct nurses) as a proportion of total NHS Direct calls from April 2003 to June 2006. The trend for the 15- to 44-year-old age group shows a series of minor peaks during spring, which might have been caused by a combination of the tree and grass pollen season and other factors. However, there was a sudden peak in eye problems calls for school-aged children (5–14 years) on June 14, 2003 (5.2%), June 13, 2004 (4%), and June 18, 2005 (6.5%) (Fig. 8.5). The high likelihood of a similar sudden peak during June 2006 was highlighted in the national weekly bulletin on June 7. The peak, which actually occurred on June 10 in most parts of England and Wales (6% nationally), was described in a surveillance alert on June 11 and was fully characterized in the weekly bulletin on June 14. The notice forewarned local health protection teams of a likely rise in community morbidity in their areas and alerted NHS Direct sites to expect a change in types of calls received.

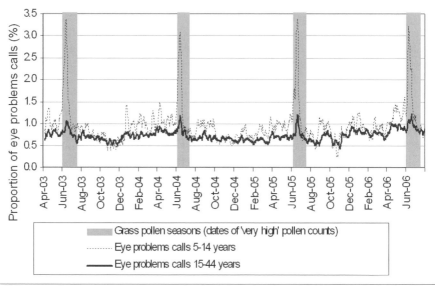

Grass pollen seasons cover approximate dates when 'very high' levels of grass pollen were recorded in parts of the United Kingdom. The pollen season generally starts in the South of England and gradually moves north. Pollen season data provided by the UK National Pollen & Aerobiology Research Unit.

Fig. 8.5   NHS Direct "eye problems" calls as a proportion of total calls (7-day moving averages) for 5- to 14-year olds and 15- to 44-year olds, England and Wales, April 2003–June 2006.

8.3.2.3   Case Study 3 (Major Incident Surveillance): Buncefield Fuel Depot Fire
Early on the morning of Sunday, December 11, 2005, there was a huge explosion
at the Buncefield fuel depot in southern England (Fig. 8.6) [31]. Twenty oil tanks
were destroyed in one of the largest blasts in peacetime Europe. The blast injured
43 people, took 3 days to control, and caused the closure of local schools. A plume
of smoke, largely made up of carbon dioxide, carbon monoxide, and hydrocarbons,
drifted in a southerly direction over London and the surrounding area. As in all major
incidents, a high-level "gold" command team was established, combining emergency
services and other agencies, including the UK HPA.

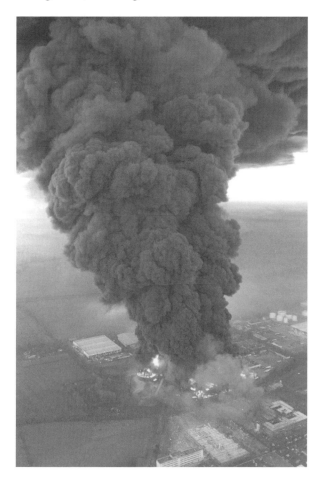

Fig. 8.6   Buncefield fuel depot fire (Photo courtesy of AP Photo/Hertfordshire Police).

The NHS Direct syndromic surveillance system, along with GP surveillance systems, was well placed to monitor the potential short- to midterm health effects of the
blast on the local population. In the immediate aftermath of the blast, and for the next
6 weeks, calls to the eight NHS Direct sites serving the area within the path of the

plume received increased scrutiny with respect to (1) total NHS Direct calls, (2) NHS Direct calls about "breathing problems" and "cough," and (3) the outcomes of NHS Direct respiratory calls. Daily surveillance bulletins were issued to key personnel on the incident response team.

No significant rises in calls to potentially affected NHS Direct sites were observed in the days following the blast. However, an exceedance occurred in "difficulty breathing" calls to Bedfordshire and Hertfordshire NHS Direct on 3 consecutive days between December 31, 2005, and January 2, 2006 (Fig. 8.7). The blast was located in the catchment area of this NHS Direct site. The outcomes of these "difficulty breathing" calls were considered normal: accident and emergency department referral and paramedic dispatch call outcomes of 32% (baseline 37%) and GP outcomes of 63% (baseline 54%). As a precautionary measure, "difficulty breathing" calls were mapped, but no evidence was found of geographical clustering around the blast location or pollution footprint (Fig. 8.8). The surveillance and incident teams concluded that the rise in calls was probably due to the general rise in seasonal respiratory disease (exceedances had also occurred in November and earlier in December 2005) and unusual call patterns possibly associated with the New Year period. The proportion of "difficulty breathing" calls at this NHS Direct site was short-lived and dropped below the exceedance threshold on January 4, 2006. The incident team was informed of these trends via the usual surveillance bulletins.

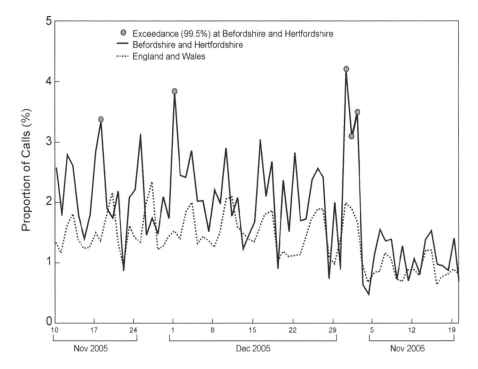

Fig. 8.7 "Breathing difficulty" calls as a proportion of calls to Bedfordshire and Hertfordshire NHS Direct, November 2005–January 2006.

Home postcodes of difficulty breathing callers to Bedfordshire and Hertfordshire
NHS Direct 31st Dec 2005 to 2nd Jan 2006

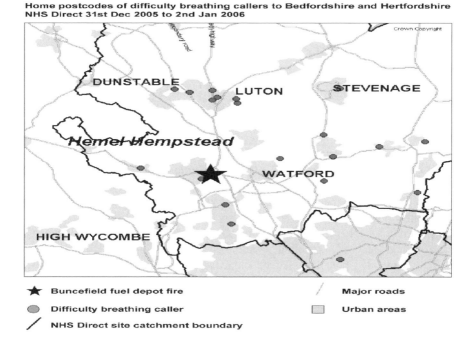

★ Buncefield fuel depot fire   /   Major roads

● Difficulty breathing caller   ▢   Urban areas

/ NHS Direct site catchment boundary

Fig. 8.8 Postcode locations of "breathing difficulty" calls, December 31, 2005–January 2, 2006 (3-day exceedance).

Data from the HPA NHS Direct syndromic surveillance system and other primary care surveillance systems were used to monitor potential health effects immediately after the explosion and in the following weeks (further chemical release was suspected). No increases in NHS Direct respiratory calls (preprimary care) or doctor consultations (primary care) were observed that were attributed to the blast. This conclusion was supported by hospital admissions data (indicating no unusual rise in illness) and environmental sampling results (indicating a lack of ground-level pollution). The syndromic surveillance data with accompanying interpretation provided reassurance to both the incident team and the public that there was no unusual increase in clinical illness.

8.3.3 Weekly Reporting

Weekly bulletins summarizing NHS Direct call activity for all 11 syndromes are e-mailed to local and national health protection teams, surveillance leads, NHS Direct sites, and the NHS every Wednesday. These bulletins and additional surveillance data are also published on the primary care surveillance pages of the HPA website [32].

8.4   ADDING VALUE TO THE SURVEILLANCE DATA

8.4.1   Linking Syndromic Data with Traditional Laboratory Sources

One limitation of syndromic surveillance is the lack of specific medical or laboratory confirmation of diagnosis. The collection and testing of samples from syndromic surveillance systems is not routine. Microbiological sampling of patients captured by syndromic surveillance systems has been attempted in certain settings. For example, samples were collected and tested in a follow-up to a rise in diarrhea and vomiting syndromes in New York City and were found to be positive for norovirus [33]. During the winter of 2004–2005, the NHS Direct syndromic surveillance team explored whether a mechanism could be developed that would enable NHS Direct callers to self-test for influenza, thereby providing early warning of an increase in influenza and complementing syndromic data. Between November 2004 and February 2005, nurses at three NHS Direct sites used predefined scripts to recruit NHS Direct callers over the age of 15 years who reported "cold/flu" symptoms. Subjects accepted into the study were mailed a specimen kit that included an information sheet, two nasal swabs, viral transport medium, instructions, appropriate packaging, and a short questionnaire. Subjects were asked to take a swab from each nostril and mail the swabs to the national influenza reference laboratory of HPA. The swabs were tested by multiplex polymerase chain reaction (PCR) for influenza virus, and positive material was cultured for viable virus isolation.

Several important results arose from this study:

1. *Self-testing by NHS Direct callers can provide early warning of influenza circulating in the community.* During the study period, there were 1,817 NHS Direct cold/flu callers, and 610 agreed to participate in the study. Of these, 294 were identified as eligible, were recruited to the study (Fig. 8.9), and received self-testing kits. Ultimately,142 samples (48%) were returned, 23 of which (16.2%) were positive on PCR for influenza, comparing favorably to a positivity rate of 26% for the existing HPA virological surveillance based on samples supplied through family doctors' surgeries. Eight of the self-testing samples were positive for RSV (respiratory syncytial virus), highlighting the potential of the scheme to detect other viruses, such as those that cause common gastrointestinal infections (e.g., norovirus, rotavirus).

2. *Multiple strains of the virus could be detected through self-testing.* Following culture, three Wellington/1/2204-like influenza A (H3N2) and one Shanghai/361/2002-like influenza B viruses were recovered. The NHS Direct samples included the second community sample of influenza A (H1N1), the fourth sample of influenza A (H3), and the first influenza B sample received by the national reference laboratory during the 2004–2005 influenza season.

3. *Virological samples from callers complemented syndromic call data by providing a syndromic and virological picture of influenza circulating in community.* The early positive NHS Direct samples were obtained between weeks 45 to

50 of 2004 and preceded a general community syndromic rise in cold/flu calls during weeks 51 and 52 of 2005 (Fig. 8.10).

4. *Samples could be collected in a timely way.* The mean time between the date of the NHS Direct call and the date the swabs were received by the laboratory was 7.4 days, with a range of 3–27 days. Despite a week in transit, samples maintained good viability for antigenic characterization and molecular detection.

5. *The self-testing was acceptable to callers and only marginally disruptive to NHS Direct call centres.* Only 7 out of 141 callers reported problems taking the swabs (e.g., "spilt the transport diluent"; "dropped swabs on floor"). What is important is that these samples were collected without the intervention of a health care worker. Also, when questioned, NHS Direct nurses did not feel that the study had markedly increased call length or caused significant disruption during the busy winter period.

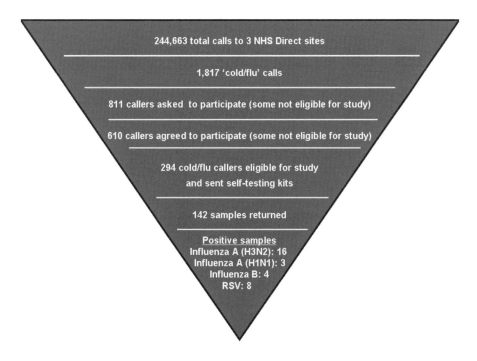

Fig. 8.9 Recruitment of NHS Direct callers for the study (November 1, 2004 through November 2, 2005) and results of positive tests for influenza and RSV viruses (eligible participants were over 15 years and reporting "colds and flu" symptoms).

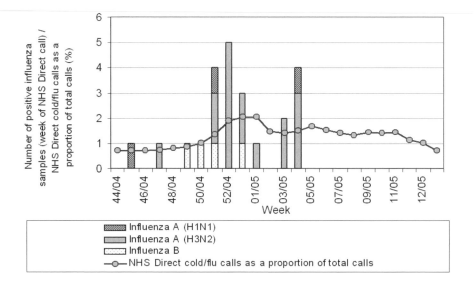

Fig. 8.10 Number of positive NHS Direct samples by week and virus type; weekly NHS Direct cold/flu calls as a proportion of total calls in weeks 46 of 2004 through week 13 of 2005.

8.4.2   A Statistical Model: Types of Infections That Cause People to Phone Telephone Triage Systems

Section 8.4.1 described a mechanism for collecting and testing influenza samples taken by NHS Direct callers. If resource limitations or privacy issues prohibit this type of investigation, other means are available to assess the range of diseases prompting people to phone tele-health systems. Multiple linear regression modeling offers a way of estimating the relative contribution of a range of pathogens to NHS Direct calls without involving the callers directly. This technique has been used previously to estimate the contribution of respiratory pathogens (both viral and bacterial) to hospital admissions [34] and to family doctor consultations [35]. Modeling NHS Direct calls against laboratory reports has helped elucidate the likely cause of a large proportion of NHS Direct respiratory and gastrointestinal calls, which in turn has helped in the interpretation of trends in surveillance data.

For this work, data were collected on the weekly numbers of NHS Direct calls about specific syndromes (respiratory and gastrointestinal) for the period October 2002–October 2004 (outcome variables) and the weekly numbers of laboratory reports of the main respiratory and gastrointestinal pathogens (explanatory variables). Public holidays were added as a dummy variable to account for holiday effects. Multiple linear regression models were constructed for each syndrome, with variables (pathogens) that contributed little to the model removed by backward stepwise regression. The formula used for estimating the number of NHS Direct calls in week j due to pathogen i was

$$Y_j = C + \sum \alpha_i L_j \tag{8.2}$$

where L_j is the number of lab reports in group i (e.g., influenza) in week j, α_i is the number of NHS Direct calls associated with each lab report, and C is the constant number of calls due to other causes.

Figure 8.11 shows the estimated weekly contribution of norovirus and rotavirus to NHS Direct diarrhea calls (age 0-4 years). These pathogens were the only two, from a range of possible causes, that were significantly associated with NHS Direct diarrhea calls within the final model. Table 8.4 provides estimates of the yearly contribution and maximum weekly contribution of individual pathogens to NHS Direct calls. It must be stressed that, as with any model, the quality of the results is determined largely by the quality of the model data. For example, the laboratory data used here are subject to case ascertainment bias because some common causes of respiratory infection (e.g., rhinovirus, coronavirus) are rarely tested for in UK labs.

Table 8.4   Estimated Annual Contribution of Specific Pathogens to NHS Direct Calls About "Cough" and "Vomiting" (age 0-4 years) for England and Wales (October 2002– October 2004)

NHS Direct Syndrome	Goodness of Fit: R^2 Value	Significant Model Variables and Contribution from Other Causes	Estimated % Contribution to NHS Direct Syndromic Calls	Maximum % Weekly Estimated Contribution
NHS Direct cough calls (95,000 calls/yr)	0.91	Invasive *Streptococcus pneumoniae*	20	33
		Influenza	15	63
		RSV	12	49
		Rhinovirus	6	21
		Bank holidays	3	17
		Other causes	43	88
NHS Direct vomiting calls (age 0–4 years; 70,000 calls/yr)	0.80	Rotavirus	27	61
		Norovirus	15	39
		Other causes	58	92

This relatively straightforward modeling technique has provided estimates of the contribution of the proportions of NHS Direct calls attributable to specific microbio-

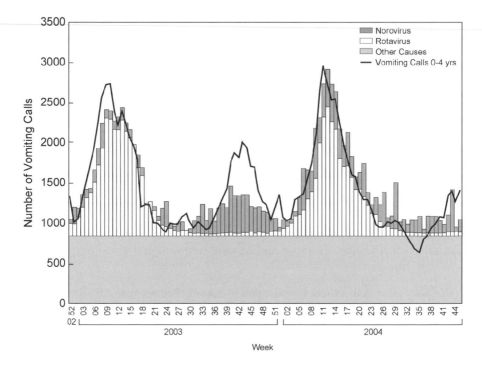

Fig. 8.11   Comparison of the observed weekly number of NHS Direct vomiting calls (age 0–4 years) (England and Wales) with the estimated numbers of weekly calls due to norovirus, rotavirus, and other causes (October 2002–October 2004).

logical causes. For example, most of the seasonal variation in NHS Direct respiratory calls is estimated to be caused by influenza, RSV, and invasive *pneumococcal* disease. Rotavirus and norovirus are estimated to be the main causes of NHS Direct gastrointestinal calls. The weekly estimates of the contribution of different pathogens to NHS Direct respiratory calls have provided greater confidence in the interpretation of sudden rises in syndromes reported to NHS Direct. Detailed estimates of the burden of specific respiratory diseases reported to NHS Direct have also fed into policy and planning documents [36].

8.5   CONCLUSIONS

8.5.1   Main Benefits of the System

Early warning. The main public health benefit of using NHS Direct tele-health data for syndromic surveillance in England and Wales is the early detection and tracking of rises in illness in the community at the national and regional levels. Use of timely and automated data has complemented existing surveillance systems, particularly for the surveillance of influenza-like illness and gastrointestinal disease. Experience has shown that the public may contact tele-health services about influenza symptoms before visiting family doctors or hospitals, demonstrating further the value of tele-health data for early warning and providing lead time for surveillance. A mechanism has also been developed by which tele-health callers can self-sample (e.g., for influenza and RSV), providing an alternative source of specimens for laboratory testing and a critical link between unspecific syndromic data and laboratory confirmation. NHS Direct data have also been used to monitor the environmental health effects of pollen, high temperatures [37], and poor air quality [38] and to characterize the areas and age groups affected for national and local public health teams.

Reassurance. Reassurance that a rise in illness is not occurring (during times of perceived higher risk) has been suggested as one of the main benefits of syndromic surveillance [39]. However, this reassurance is valid only if it has already been demonstrated (prospectively) that a surveillance system can detect similar rises in illness. Because NHS Direct data have been shown to exhibit a signal sufficient to alert a surveillance team to sudden and widespread rises in syndromic calls, these data can provide some reassurance that a widespread rise in disease has not occurred during times of increased perceived risk. Although the system detected a rise in respiratory illness around the time of a major oil depot explosion, mapping of these data demonstrated that the probable cause was a seasonal rise in respiratory disease rather than explosion-related. On two occasions (after traces of ricin were found in a London flat in January 2003 and after the London bombs of July 7, 2005), NHS Direct data provided reassurance that there was no suspicious rise in illness in the London area. Prompt reassurance was helped by the ability of the surveillance team to reduce the time interval of reporting (from every 24 hours to every 2 hours) and by mapping of NHS Direct calls.

Planning. The systematic collection of almost 5 years' worth of daily national tele-health call data with well-established statistical baselines means that the surveillance database is now a well-used resource, providing data extracts for emergency planning exercises and modeling work. Call data have been used for testing national contingency plans for pandemic influenza surveillance, for testing local resilience plans (using London as an example), and for modeling the potential impact and spread of a pandemic flu strain in the UK. Also, timely surveillance data have been fed back to NHS Direct to contribute to operational planning. For example, surveillance reports about rises in specific syndromes can be relayed to NHS Direct's online health information service and the NHS Direct responsive messaging service, used to inform callers of relevant topical information. The supporting clinical advice and rationales within the NHS CAS algorithms used by the nurses can be modified to reflect awareness of the prevailing respiratory infections (as highlighted by the linear regression modeling in Section 8.4.2).

Fostering multidisciplinary collaborative working. Syndromic data have provided a new source of information for ongoing routine surveillance, for monitoring health protection policy (e.g., providing estimates of the burden of specific diseases reported to NHS Direct), and for research (e.g., sociodemographic profiling of calls [15]). A diverse group of people — epidemiologists, medics, tele-health nurses, statisticians, and operational managers — have been brought together for various collaborative ventures. In turn, these collaborations have raised the profile of NHS Direct outside its core business, demonstrating its usefulness for public health and epidemiological purposes.

8.5.2   System Evaluation

The need for detailed evaluation of syndromic surveillance systems (in 2003, there were over 100 in the United States) led to the publication of the "Framework for evaluating public health surveillance systems for early detection of outbreaks" by the CDC in 2004 [40]. This framework was used for a preliminary evaluation of the HPA NHS Direct syndromic surveillance system in 2004, which concluded that the system was timely, representative, and useful [41]. The direct annual operating costs of the system — $280,000 per year — were considered to be low for a national surveillance system. This valuation did not include data costs, however, because the surveillance requirements of the system are embedded in the core operations of NHS Direct (the data provider). Plans for surveillance of calls to a private tele-health provider must consider data costs and variable costs associated with the investigation of surveillance signals (e.g., additional nonroutine tele-health data required, additional staff costs, cost of laboratory testing of samples from callers) may be prohibitive.

8.5.3   Cautionary Note for Future Work

The evaluation with the CDC framework also found that the system was more likely to detect large-scale events and generalized rises in syndromes than very localized outbreaks of communicable disease or disease caused by the deliberate release of a bioagent. Although there are clear benefits of the surveillance system (outlined in Section 8.5.1), to date it has not detected a succession of local disease outbreaks in advance of other surveillance systems. At present, total NHS Direct call rates are a fraction (approximately one-thirtieth) of total family doctor contacts in the UK. Therefore, even though almost 100% of the population has access to NHS Direct, the syndromic surveillance system captures only a fraction of illness reported in England and Wales. Opportunities to detect localized rises in illness (potential outbreaks) may increase as NHS Direct call rates rise over time, and the statistical methodology used to flag local data anomalies is refined (e.g., using integrated spatiotemporal analysis tools such as SaTScan [42]). In general, local outbreak detection via analysis of telephone triage data will be possible only in areas where phoning a telephone triage line is high on the population's list of health-seeking behaviors. For example, in a telephone survey of New York City residents with "flu-like-illness," calling a healthline was fifth on the list of health-seeking behaviors (4% of residents), behind pharmacy and physician-based services [43]. Therefore, to be confident of providing reassurance that local rises in disease are not occurring, more work is needed to define exactly which local events the HPA NHS Direct surveillance system will and will not detect given current call rates.

It is worth stressing that a pragmatic approach to surveillance has been taken. By necessity, routine syndromic data based on NHS Direct clinical algorithms have been used rather than the more specific case definitions usually associated with outbreak detection and laboratory-based surveillance systems. The influenza sampling study (Section 8.4.1) and regression modeling (Section 8.4.2) have provided additional confidence in interpreting nonspecific syndromic data. It may be possible, however, to improve the specificity of the surveillance system's case definitions through extraction of multiple symptoms from a single call record within the NHS Direct CAS relational database. The benefits of linking multiple symptoms to a single caller would have to be weighed against the additional workload associated with using other than routine data.

8.5.4   Integration with Other UK Primary Care Surveillance

Routine primary care data provide the means to systematically monitor a variety of syndromes that could provide early warning of health protection issues (microbiological and chemical). As well as NHS Direct data, two sentinel surveillance systems based on family doctor diagnoses currently operate in the UK: the Royal College of General Practitioners (RCGP) Weekly Returns Service [22] (established during the 1970s and covering 700,000 people) and the Q-Research [44]/Q-Flu [45] system (established in 2003 and covering 17 million people). It is possible, therefore, to use preprimary care (NHS Direct) and primary care data (family doctor diagnoses) to track illnesses that may not present to hospitals (e.g., chickenpox, conjunctivitis) or illnesses for which laboratory specimens are not routinely taken (e.g., influenza). The RCGP system has the benefits of long historical baseline data about an extensive list of medical conditions. The Q-Research/Q-Flu system has the advantage of being able to link diagnoses to socioeconomic risk factors and prescribing and vaccination details. The relative strengths and weaknesses of these three primary care surveillance systems and the HPA NHS Direct syndromic surveillance system complement each other to provide a timely picture of illness reported to primary care in the UK.

8.5.5   Recommendations

Twenty recommendations have been developed to aid the design, operation, and evaluation of a syndromic surveillance system based on tele-health triage data.

Design

1. Form a multidisciplinary, dedicated team of analysts and public health personnel.

2. Define and involve the stakeholders as early as possible.

3. Set expectations at an appropriate level by describing, if possible, the type of events the system will and will not detect.

4. Invest time and effort in developing investigation protocols that are integrated into the public health response.

5. Develop a clear link among data analysis, rapid evaluation of surveillance signals, and potential public health action.

6. Ensure that the data cover as wide a population and area as possible. Alternatively, define the system's representativeness.

7. Use as accurate a geographical identifier as is possible and legal.

8. Use tele-health data that are routinely available and automated.

9. If possible, link multiple symptoms, rather than single clinical algorithms, to individual callers.

Operation

1. Keep routine outputs clear, useful, and simple.

2. Analyze tele-health data alongside data from traditional surveillance systems (e.g., laboratory) to make epidemiological interpretation more confident and surveillance messages more persuasive.

3. Keep an open mind: there are benefits to the work where you least expect them.

4. Focus on areas where tele-health data can provide a unique picture of community morbidity and "added value" over existing surveillance.

5. Be prepared for software changes that may interrupt the flow of data and affect data coding and baselines.

6. Be prepared for resistance: the use of tele-health data for public health surveillance is a relatively new, innovative, and evolving field.

7. Engage those who are sceptical or critical of the work.

Evaluation

1. Incorporate into the surveillance system a method of evaluating the impact of syndromic surveillance signals and investigations on public health (the "so what" factor).

2. Calibrate the syndromic surveillance system against the CDC evaluation framework.

3. Try a variety of statistical aberration-detection methods (e.g., using simulation studies or retrospective analyses) to identify the method(s) that are most suitable for the data.

4. Publish as much as possible and share experience with other syndromic surveillance practitioners.

8.5.6 Final Remarks

Although syndromic surveillance systems based on data from regional telephone triage systems exist, the use of data from a national tele-health system (i.e., NHS Direct) is unique in the field of syndromic surveillance. The HPA NHS Direct syndromic surveillance system is also the only national daily surveillance system in the UK and provides a timely national snapshot of community morbidity. To date, no deliberate release of either a chemical or a biological agent has been detected. The main benefits of using NHS Direct telephone triage data for public health surveillance have been in providing early warning of rises in infectious disease and disease caused by environmental factors, tracking and verification of trends in community morbidity, and reassurance that widespread disease is *not* occurring when there is a perceived high public health risk. When the surveillance team took action, local or national agencies received surveillance reports within 24–48 hours of the time the NHS Direct calls were made. Secondary benefits of the system include the provision of data for monitoring public health policy, emergency planning exercises, and epidemic modeling. Future challenges for this system are the provision of surveillance data to a newly defined network of local primary care trusts in England and Wales, the integration of routine spatiotemporal analyses into the surveillance system, and a targeted evaluation of the usefulness of the surveillance outputs to public health practitioners.

8.6 STUDY QUESTIONS

8.1 Clinical decision-support software, used by nurses for telephone triage, may undergo regular software upgrades. The data providers should have detailed documentation of these upgrades. Upgrades may reduce or expand the list of syndromes available for surveillance and affect call classification (syndromic coding, outcome/disposition coding). *Q: What means of detecting these changes might you use? Once you have detected a change, how might you alter your syndromic surveillance system to maintain consistent data output and analyses?*

8.2 NHS Direct call centre data are noisy and subject to overdispersion (the variance of the data is greater than expected). *Q: What problems could this cause for signal detection? How would you overcome these problems?*

8.3 Many syndromic surveillance systems use hospital data (e.g., ED visits) or medical centre data (e.g., clinician visits) for early event detection. Telephone triage and nurse hotline data are less frequently used although these services may be the first point of contact for an unwell person. *Q: What are the main advantages of using telephone triage or nurse hotline data compared with the more common syndromic data sources?*

8.4 There is growing evidence that syndromic surveillance systems are particularly sensitive for detecting increases in acute viral disease (e.g., influenza, norovirus) and environmental health effects (e.g., atmospheric pollution). There are a wide variety of reasons, however, for calling a nurse hotline. *Q: Are there any other areas of health in which syndromic surveillance based on telephone triage data could be useful? What are they, and what syndromes could be useful for their surveillance?*

Acknowledgments

This work was funded by HPA and NHS Direct. The author wishes to thank NHS Direct for continuing support for the project and for supplying call data, the HPA/NHS Direct collaborative group for input into all aspects of the surveillance work, and NHS Direct colleagues Dr. Ewan Gerard and Frances Chinemana and Dr. Gillian Smith of the HPA for help with drafts of this chapter.

REFERENCES

1. The US Telemedicine Market. Jacksonville, OR: Feedback Research Services, 2000.

2. Schneider P. Telehealth core to WHO's missions. Healthcare Inf. July 1998:59-60.

3. Telehealth Ontario. Available at `http://www.health.gov.on.ca/english/public/program/telehealth/telehealth_mn.html`.

4. HealthDirect. Available at `http://www.health.wa.gov.au/services/detail.cfm?Unit_ID=799`.

5. NHS Direct Online. Available at `http://www.nhsdirect.nhs.uk/`. Accessed July 2006.

6. NHS 24. Available at `http://www.nhs24.com/html/content/default.asp`.

7. Healthline. Available at `http://www.moh.govt.nz/healthline`.

8. English Department of Health. Hospital episode statistics. Available at `http://www.performance.doh.gov.uk/hospitalactivity/index.htm`.

9. Rowlands S, Moser K. Consultation rates from the general practice research database. Br J Gen Pract. 2002;52:658-660.

10. Turner VF, Bentley PJ, Hodgson SA, et al. Telephone triage in Western Australia. Med J Aust. 2002;176(3):100-103.

11. Knowles E, Munro J, O'Cathain A, Nicholl J. Equity of access to health care. Evidence from NHS Direct in the UK. J Telemed Telecare. 2006;12(5):262-265.

12. Comptroller and Auditor General. NHS Direct in England. London: Stationery Office; 2002.

13. Ring F, Jones M. NHS Direct usage in a GP population of children under 5 years: is NHS Direct used by people with the greatest health need? Br J Gen Pract. 2004;54:211-213.

14. Burt J, Hooper R, Jessopp L. The relationship between the use of NHS Direct and deprivation in southeast London: an ecological analysis. J Publ Health Med. 2003;25:174-176.

15. Cooper DL, Arnold E, Smith GE, et al. The effect of deprivation, age and gender on NHS Direct call rates. Br J Gen Pract. 2005;5:287-291.

16. Cooper DL, Hollyoak V, O'Brien SJ, Vaughan M. Do socio-demographic factors affect calls to NHS Direct which are suggestive of infection? A geographical analysis of NHS Direct call data. In: Proceedings of the PHLS 27th Annual Scientific Conference, 2002:48.

17. Rodman JS, Frost F, Jakubowski W. Using nurse hotlines calls for disease surveillance. Emerg Infect Dis. April–June 1998; 4: 329-333.

18. Henry JV, Magruder S, Snyder M. Comparison of office visit and nurse advice hotline data for syndromic surveillance: Baltimore–Washington, DC, metropolitan area, 2002. MMWR. 2004; 53(suppl): 112-116.

19. Magruder SF, Henry J, Snyder M. Linked analysis for definition of nurse advice line syndrome groups, and comparison to encounters. MMWR. 2005;54(suppl):93-97.

20. Espino JU, Hogan WR, Wagner MM. Telephone triage: a timely data source for surveillance of influenza-like diseases. AMIA Annu Symp Proc. 2003:215-219.

21. Rolland E, Moore KM, Robinson VA, McGuinness D. Using Ontario's "Telehealth" health telephone helpline as an early-warning system: a study protocol. BMC Health Serv Res. February 2006;15(6):10.

22. Fleming DM. Weekly returns service of the Royal College of General Practitioners. Commun Dis Public Health. 1999;2:96-100.

23. Health Protection Agency, Chemical Hazards and Poisons Division. Public health surveillance of chemical incidents surveillance report, July 1 – September 30, 2005. Available at http://www.hpa.org.uk/chemicals/reports/incident_surv_q3_2005.pdf.

24. Armitage P, Berry G. Statistical Method in Medical Research 2nd ed. Blackwell Scientific; Oxford:1987.

25. Reis BY, Cooper DL, Smith GE, Gerard EM, Mandl KD. Data on the edge: detecting anomalies in evolving datasets. Presented at the National Syndromic Surveillance Conference, Seattle, WA; 2005.

26. Department of Health. The Caldicott Committee. Report on the review of patient-identifiable information. December 1997. Available at http://static.oxfordradcliffe.net/confidential/gems/caldrep.pdf.

27. Goddard NL, Joseph CA, Watson JM, Zambon M. Epidemiological features of a new strain of the influenza A virus: influenza A (H1N2) circulating in England and its public health implications. Virus Res. July 2004;103(1-2):53-54.

28. Cooke MK, Crofts JP, Joseph CA, et al. Influenza and other respiratory viruses surveillance in the United Kingdom: October 2003 to May 2004. CCR. 2005(suppl).

29. HPA Centre of Infections. Influenza/Respiratory Virus Team. National influenza season summary. May 2006. Available at http://www.hpa.org.uk/infections/topics_az/influenza/seasonal/activity0506/reports/Season_Summary0506.pdf. Accessed July 2006.

30. Bhalla PL, Swoboda I, Singh MB. Reduction in allergenicity of grass pollen by genetic engineering. Int Arch Allergy Immunol. 2001;124(1-3):51-54.

31. Buncefield Major Incident Investigation Board. Buncefield major incident investigation. Sudbury, UK: Health and Safety Executive;2006. Available at http://www.buncefieldinvestigation.gov.uk/reports/initialreport.pdf.

32. Health Protection Agency. Primary care surveillance. Available at http://www.hpa.org.uk/infections/topics_az/primary_care_surveillance/menu.htm.

33. Steiner-Sichew L, Geenko J, Hefferman R, Layton M, Weiss D. Field investigations of emergency department surveillance signals, New York City. In: Syndromic surveillance: reports from a national conference, New York, 2003. MMWR. 2004;53(suppl):184-189.

34. Muller-Pebody B, Edmunds WJ, Zambon MC, Gay NJ, Crowcroft NS. Contribution of RSV to bronchitis and pneumonia-associated hospitalizations in English children, April 1995–March 1998. Epidemiol Infect. 2002;129:99-106.

35. Melegaro A, Edmunds WJ, Pebody R, Miller E, George R. The current burden of pneumococcal disease in England and Wales. J Infect. 2006;52(1):37-48.

36. Health Protection Agency. Health protection in the 21st century: understanding the burden of disease; preparing for the future. 2005.

37. Leonardi G, Heat S, Covets RS, Smith GE, Cooper D, Gerard E. Syndromic surveillance use to detect the early effects of heat-waves: an analysis of NHS Direct data in England. Soc Preven Med. 2006;51(4).

38. Baker M, Smith GE, Cooper DL, et al. Early warning and NHS Direct: a role in community surveillance? J Public Health. 2003;25:362-368.

39. Sosin DM. Biosecure syndromic surveillance: the case for skillful investment. Bioterror. 2003;1(4):247-253.

40. Buehler JW, Hopkins RS, Overhage JM, Sosin DM, Tong V. CDC Working Group. Framework for evaluating public health surveillance systems for early detection of outbreaks: recommendations from the CDC Working Group. MMWR Recomm Rep. May 7, 2004;53(RR-5):1-11.

41. Doroshenko A, Cooper D, Smith GE, et al. Evaluation of syndromic surveillance based on NHS Direct derived data in England and Wales. MMWR. 2005;54(suppl):117-122.

42. Kulldorff M, Heffernan R, Hartman J, Assuncao R, Mostashari F. A space-time permutation scan statistic for disease outbreak detection. PLoS Med. March 2005;2(3):e59. Epub February 15, 2005.

43. Metzger KB, Hajat A, Crawford M, Mostashari F. How many illnesses does one emergency department visit represent? Using a population-based telephone survey to estimate the syndromic multiplier. MMWR. September 24, 2004; 53(suppl): 106-111.

44. Harcourt S, Smith GE, Hippisley-Cox J, et al. Report of the first year of a pilot, national, primary care surveillance project. In: Proceedings of the Health Protection Agency Annual Conference, 2005:119.

45. Hippisley-Cox J, Smith S, Smith G, et al. QFLU: new influenza monitoring in UK primary care to support pandemic influenza planning. Eur Surveill. June 22, 2006;11(6):E060622.4.

9 Surveillance for Emerging Infection Epidemics in Developing Countries: EWORS and Alerta DISAMAR

Jean-Paul Chretien, David Blazes, Cecilia Mundaca, Jonathan Glass, Sheri Happel Lewis, Joseph S. Lombardo, R. Loren Erickson

The previous three chapters presented examples of automated disease surveillance systems that have been implemented in the United States,Canada, and the United Kingdom. In these examples, the systems were developed either by local public health authorities or by academic institutions supporting local public health departments. This chapter presents surveillance systems that have been implemented in Indonesia and Peru through a collaboration between the U.S. military research laboratories and the public health authorities in their host countries. Examples are given of innovative approaches to capturing data from remote locations for surveillance and containment of infectious diseases.

In 2003, a highly pathogenic strain of avian influenza, A/H5N1, emerged in Vietnam. By early 2007, the strain had infected more than 250 people in Asia, the Middle East, and North Africa. More than half of these confirmed infections were fatal [1]. Although nearly all cases resulted from exposure to infected birds, the epidemic has generated serious international concern and resource commitments because influenza viruses undergo unpredictable genetic changes that influence pathogenicity and transmission characteristics. For example, an avian virus that acquired the ability to spread efficiently among humans probably caused the influenza pandemic of 1918–1919, in which around 50 million people died [2]. If genetic changes allow the H5N1 virus to spread efficiently from person to person (as seasonal influenza viruses do), the world would again face the possibility of a pandemic that could kill millions of people and devastate economies.

Avian influenza is an "emerging" infectious disease [3, 4], a category that includes diseases that have recently appeared (e.g., H5N1, which was first identified as a human pathogen in Hong Kong in 1997; acquired immunodeficiency syndrome [AIDS])

and ones that are known but changing in significant ways (e.g., malaria, which is spreading to new areas and returning to areas where it was previously eliminated; tuberculosis, which, like malaria, has developed resistance to many drugs). Effective public health response to emerging infections depends on surveillance systems to detect and characterize them and guide interventions [4, 5]. However, in much of the developing world, public health surveillance systems do not exist or are ineffective [5, 6]. Because many emerging infections, such as H5N1, spread easily beyond national borders, these deficiencies can have regional or global consequences. Heymann and Rodier of the World Health Organization (WHO) captured this interdependence in reflecting on the 2003 multicountry severe acute respiratory syndrome (SARS) epidemic: "Inadequate surveillance and response capacity in a single country can endanger national populations and the public health security of the entire world" [7].

This chapter explores strategies for implementing effective surveillance for emerging infection outbreaks in developing countries. After a general overview of challenges to effective surveillance in developing countries and possible solutions, it turns to two systems developed through host country–U.S. military collaboration. These case studies offer lessons that could be useful for developing countries, sponsoring agencies, and collaborators in developing and improving surveillance systems for emerging infections in resource-poor settings.

9.1 IMPROVING SURVEILLANCE IN RESOURCE-POOR SETTINGS

Developing countries face significant challenges in implementing effective public health surveillance systems. Some of these are similar in kind to, but of greater magnitude than, problems that developed countries encounter [8, 9]. For example, insufficient laboratory diagnostic capabilities [10, 11] and lack of personnel with necessary professional skills [12] limit surveillance effectiveness in developing countries, but affect wealthy nations as well.

More specific to poor countries are infrastructure constraints that can make even rudimentary surveillance functions difficult. For example, poor roads and lack of transportation can prevent public health staff from investigating outbreaks; computer-based information systems may be difficult to implement because electrical power is unreliable; and access to communication systems (such as the Internet) may be very limited by lack of or poor telecommunications lines [9]. The bureaucratic structure of the health sector may obscure lines of accountability for surveillance functions [13] and discordant data collection protocols by rival health agencies at the national and sub-national level may impair outbreak detection, reporting and response. When foreign assistance is provided to strengthen public health systems, well-intentioned donors may impose programmatic requirements that impede development of effective systems [9, 14].

Recent WHO efforts to strengthen global infectious disease surveillance depend on effective and coordinated national- and sub-national-level systems [15, 16]. For example, the International Health Regulations, revised in 2005 to address SARS and other emerging infections that can spread rapidly through a globalized world, place broader obligations on countries to build surveillance and response capacities [17] (the original International Health Regulations, instituted in 1969, focused on monitoring and control of three diseases capable of causing serious international epidemics: cholera, yellow fever, and plague). The Global Outbreak Alert and Response Network (GOARN), was established in 2000 to facilitate collaboration among existing institutions and surveillance networks in identifying, confirming, and responding to epidemics of international importance [18]. However, this network depends on effective national and sub-national surveillance systems to identify outbreaks in a timely manner.

Several innovative models have been developed for improving infectious disease surveillance in developing countries. A few successful, low-cost examples at the sub-national level include a community-based program in Cambodia that employs lay volunteers to identify outbreaks [19]; a hospital-based program in South Africa that trains infection-control nurses to identify syndromes that require immediate public health action [20]; and a public–private hospital network that monitors a range of infectious diseases in India [21]. The success of these and other effective approaches is due, in part, to detailed understanding of local public health system problems and capabilities.

9.2   U.S. MILITARY OVERSEAS PUBLIC HEALTH CAPACITY BUILDING

The U.S. military has long supported public health activities of foreign countries, but the formal capacity for surveillance of emerging infectious diseases was built within the U.S. Department of Defense (DoD) only relatively recently. A key DoD platform for public health capacity building abroad is a network of overseas medical research laboratories in Peru, Egypt, Kenya, Thailand, and Indonesia. DoD established these facilities between 1943 and 1983 to conduct tropical infectious disease research important to both host countries and the U.S. military. The U.S. military and host country staff work together to develop regional advanced laboratory capabilities, networks of field sites, and a spirit of collaboration and trust to produce medical advances of broad importance, including drugs for malaria and typhoid fever, fluid–electrolyte rehydration therapy for cholera, and vaccines for hepatitis A and Japanese encephalitis, among others [22, 23, 24, 25, 26, 27, 28, 29]. U.S. military scientists also supported host countries in responding to infectious disease outbreaks with laboratory diagnostics, epidemiologic field investigations, and training.

A seminal report by the U.S. Institute of Medicine in 1992 drew attention to emerging infectious diseases as a threat to global health and U.S. security [4]. The report called for greater U.S. engagement with emerging infections overseas, and identified the DoD overseas medical research laboratories as the most broadly based U.S. platforms for monitoring and responding to epidemics abroad. Building on this and subsequent reports, a 1996 presidential directive formally expanded the mission of DoD and its overseas medical research laboratories to include surveillance, outbreak response, host country personnel training, and research for emerging infectious diseases [30]. DoD established the Global Emerging Infections Surveillance and Response System (DoD-GEIS) to coordinate and support these efforts at the DoD overseas medical research laboratories and in the military health system.

Current DoD-GEIS supported surveillance networks include more than 50 countries in South America, the middle east, sub-Saharan Africa, and central and southeastern Asia [31]. A global, laboratory-based network monitors influenza [32], a top surveillance priority because of the ever-present pandemic threat. Other systems focus on malaria, dengue, diarrheal diseases, and sexually transmitted infections. All surveillance networks rely on close U.S. military–host country collaboration and must contend with the challenges described above to deliver accurate, timely information on emerging infections in resource-poor settings.

Sections 9.3 and 9.4 describe surveillance systems developed and sustained by a collaboration of host countries, DoD-GEIS, DoD overseas medical research laboratories, and other organizations. The purpose of both systems is to detect outbreaks of emerging infections early and to facilitate rapid public health intervention. The first, the early warning outbreak recognition system (EWORS), was developed by the U.S. Naval Medical Research Unit-2 (NAMRU-2; Jakarta) and deployed in collaboration with host country ministries of health in Indonesia, Lao PDR, Cambodia, and Vietnam. The U.S. Naval Medical Research Center Detachment (NMRCD; Lima) and the Peru Ministry of Health have also collaborated to implement a version of EWORS. The second case study focuses on Alerta DISAMAR, which was developed by NMRCD and the Voxiva corporation and deployed in collaboration with the Peruvian navy and army.

Several approaches to describing and evaluating public health surveillance systems have been proposed [33, 34, 35]. The case studies below draw on these approaches to present an overview of the systems and their operating environments, focusing especially on data acquisition, information flow, the critical connection between the surveillance systems and public health response, and features that facilitate effective surveillance in resource-poor environments. Rather than provide comprehensive evaluations of many system attributes (e.g., simplicity, flexibility, data quality, acceptability, sensitivity, specificity, timeliness, stability), the case studies explore a key attribute for surveillance systems designed for emerging infections — flexibility. The U.S. Centers for Disease Control and Prevention (CDC) describes *flexibility* this way: A flexible public health surveillance system can adapt to changing information needs or operating conditions with little additional time, personnel, or allocated funds. Flexible systems can accommodate, for example, new health-related events, changes in case definitions or technology, and variations in funding or reporting sources. In addition, systems that use standard data formats (e.g., in electronic data interchange) can easily be integrated with other systems and thus might be considered flexible [34].

Surveillance systems for emerging infectious disease outbreaks, such as EWORS and Alerta DISAMAR, must be flexible because clinical presentations of disease that could cause sever epidemics cannot be known in advance. Systems must be configured so that "unusual" events, such as syndromes not normally seen in an area or an increase in presentations of syndromes that are normally seen at lower rates, are identified and investigated. Ideally, systems should also allow for rapid implementation of new surveillance protocols: for example, after case definitions are established for a newly emerged disease, such as a pandemic influenza. Finally, all surveillance systems, but especially those in resource-poor settings, should be able to adapt to temporal and spatial variability across important operating environment parameters: for example, variation in communication and transportation infrastructure across a system's catchment area, turnover of system operators, and infusion of new resources from sponsors. These case studies illustrate different, important aspects of surveillance system flexibility.

9.3   CASE STUDY 1: EWORS (SOUTHEASTERN ASIA AND PERU)

Infectious diseases that cause localized epidemics across Indonesia and other Southeast Asian countries include malaria, dengue, and bacterial, parasitic, and viral diarrhea. Of global concern, influenza A/H5N1 was reported in humans in Indonesia in 1999 and re-emerged in 2003. During 2006, Indonesia reported more human cases ($N = 56$) and deaths ($N = 46$) than any other country, and the second highest cumulative number of cases ($N = 76$) after Vietnam and the most deaths ($N = 58$) since 2003 [1]. Most cases are thought to have had contact with infected poultry. However, a small number of cases have been identified in self-limited family clusters, and human-to-human transmission is strongly suspected [36].

NAMRU-2 and the Ministry of Health colleagues from Southeast Asia have responded to numerous infectious disease epidemics [37, 38, 39, 40, 41, 42, 43], but often found that the response was launched too late for effective intervention. In fact newspapers often carried the earliest warnings of epidemics. For example, an outbreak of influenza-like illness in the remote jungle on Irian Jaya in 1995–1996, which involved more than 4000 cases and 300 deaths, was noted first by local newspapers several months after the epidemic began [38]. This outbreak and other instances of delayed detection prompted NAMRU-2 to develop a more timely system for detecting and responding to epidemics capable of adapting to the resource scarcities and disparities in integration that impact the developing world; a system to empower both the national and sub-national users.

9.3.1   System Development, Configuration, and Operation

When development of what would become the Early Warning Outbreak Recognition System (EWORS) began in 1998, it was clear that implementing timely surveillance for disease-specific conditions would be difficult. Many clinics and hospitals lacked even basic laboratory diagnostic capabilities to make pathogen-specific diagnoses. The professional training and experience of clinical staff varied widely, with particular differences between urban and rural healthcare workers [44]. Skilled epidemiology resources also vary between urban and rural areas as well as between the national and sub-national levels. Remote or underdeveloped districts, often with low population densities, posed real challenges to establishing necessary rapid communication linkages and capturing rapidly spreading outbreaks. They generally do not use standard diagnostic coding and few acute care clinical databases can be accessed remotely.

To increase the likelihood of capturing a community outbreak and to minimize infrastructure investment requirements, the EWORS system is designed to be implemented in sentinel urban hospital centers — specifically, outpatient and acute care clinics (Fig. 9.1). The protocol relies on clinical identification of patients with suspected infectious diseases and manual data collection using a half-page, standardized questionnaire administered by nurses and physicians. The questionnaire collects demographic data as well as all of the patient's symptoms using medical terminology rather than a single diagnosis code or chief complaint.

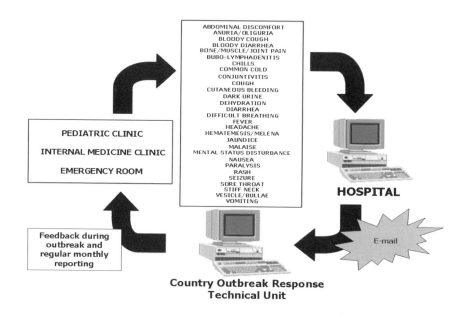

Fig. 9.1 Country outbreak response technical unit.

To collect and process that data, a simple, menu-driven software package that includes a database and data analysis capabilities was developed. This relies on on-site manual data entry of a clinical questionnaire and on-site and remote graphic-driven data analysis. Each participating hospital has a computer terminal where data is into the EWORS software. Data files are transmitted by email to the EWORS hub for additional analysis, ideally once per day. Medical staff and data entry personnel take approximately one minute each to complete each patient questionnaire. With a 56 Kbps modem, it takes approximately 10 minutes of internet connectivity to transmit the data file to the hub.

The software is designed to allow rapid, intuitive data interpretation by hospital-based operators with minimal epidemiologic training in addition to review by experienced epidemiologists. The user defines the syndrome to be analyzed; the definition may be based on WHO case definitions or local variants. Menus provide options for time series display based on surveillance sites, demographic groups, and syndromes (Figs. 9.2a–9.2c). Data are displayed in a line-chart format with observed case numbers by time, age group, or gender. Geographic information system (GIS) displays are easily generated for intuitive assessment of clustering over a period of time (Fig. 9.3). Analysis guidelines were developed without quantitative criteria. Instead, because the primary analytical tool was a time-series graphic, the analyst is advised to visually compare the case numbers with the previous month, the previous three months and the same time during the previous year. This is a crude method but simple to understand at the local level. The software also allows users to output raw data to statistical packages for more complex analysis.

Although NAMRU-2 maintains a central EWORS hub that provides software and clinical protocol enhancements, technical support, and training for all of the national EWORS networks in Southeast Asia, host countries have taken over responsibility for day-to-day operations, including formation of a national EWORS hub for outbreak identification and response. Thus, each country "owns" its EWORS data, and is not obligated to report to NAMRU-2. This has the benefit of building analysis and decision-making experience in-country, and satisfying national privacy concerns.

The software and the questionnaire have been developed in six languages, Indonesian, Lao, Khmer, Vietnamese, Korean and Spanish. The EWORS pilot implementation began in 1999 in Indonesia with large public hospitals in Jakarta (on the island of Java), Medan (Sumatra), Denpasar (Bali), Pontianak (Kalimantan), and Ujung Pandag (Sulawesi). In its first year, this first-generation network enrolled more than 10,000 cases. This network facilitated identification of a large cholera outbreak [44]. Since then, in collaboration with governments in Asia and South American, EWORS has expanded to include 11 sites on the five Indonesian islands (Fig. 9.4), 7 sites in Lao PDR, 10 sites Cambodia, and 9 sites Vietnam. Together, these Southeast Asia EWORS networks enrolled more than 5,000,000 cases. In 2005, NAMRU-2 and NMRCD collaborated to initiate EWORS in Peru. Though still in pilot stage, EWORS-Peru includes modifications based on the EWORS experience in Southeast Asia (discussed below).

9.3.2 Outbreak Detection and Response

At each national EWORS hub, up to two full-time analysts review daily reports from participating hospitals to identify increases in case counts for a particular syndrome that could signify an outbreak. Downloading, processing, and analyzing daily data from all sites usually requires approximately one day (two days may be required if there are data file errors). If a concerning increase in cases is identified, the analyst communicates with the affected site(s) to request additional clinical and epidemiologic information. If suspicion of an actual outbreak remains, the hub notifies the public

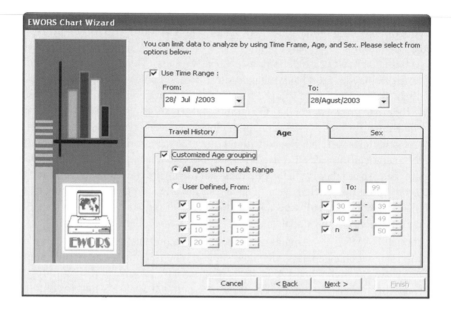

Fig. 9.2a   EWORS Chart wizard.

health authorities responsible for responding to outbreaks. In addition to outbreak alerts, the EWORS hub also sends a monthly report to each participating hospital summarizing surveillance data for that hospital. Provincial health departments also receive reports for EWORS hospitals in the province.

The process described has encountered three important challenges. First, linking EWORS-detected suspected outbreaks with outbreak response actions can require coordination of complex bureaucracies when agencies within ministries of health have compartmentalized roles and responsibilities. For example, in one EWORS country, the Ministry of Health must be invited or granted permission by the provincial authorities to assist in an outbreak response. There is bureaucratic complexity at national levels, too — within one Ministry of Health, three agencies must be involved to coordinate outbreak response. One has responsibility for public health surveillance and outbreak investigation, another for research and development, and the third for public hospital management. When the central government is stronger and the surveillance and response agencies better integrated, as in some EWORS countries, there is less delay in responding to suspected outbreaks. However, the scarcity of human and financial resources can impede investigations based on EWORS findings.

A second challenge has been standardizing procedures at the EWORS hub for identifying possible outbreaks. Early versions of EWORS software emphasized simplicity, but the decision of whether to issue an outbreak alert was based on suspicion, not validated statistical algorithms. With the lack of statistical thresholds to define a possible outbreak, EWORS staff — who themselves had variable epidemiological

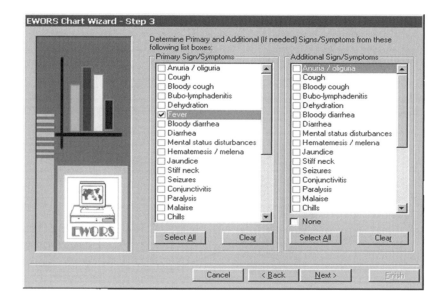

Fig. 9.2b   EWORS Chart wizard.

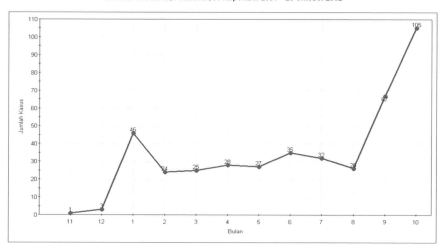

Fig. 9.2c   EWORS Line chart.

Distribusi kasus gejala #1: Demam, #2: Mual, Pendarahan kulit, Sakit kepala dan Sakit otot di Kalimantan Barat yang berobat ke RSUD Dr. Soedarso 01 Oktober 2002 -- 31 Oktober 2002

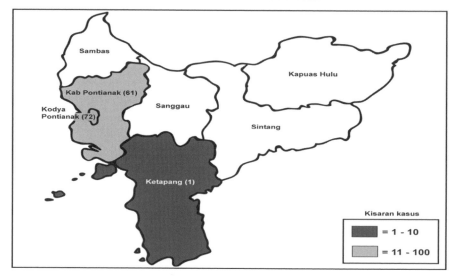

Fig. 9.3   Number of All Cases from Pirngadi Hospital, North Sumatra.

training — made decisions about abnormal signals based on subjective perception or ad hoc methods. For example, at one national hub, EWORS staff calculated historical means and standard deviations of case counts to define statistical thresholds for issuing alerts. Another national hub's process was to define an outbreak as a two-fold rise in cases over a two-week period. There was no validation performed as to how sensitive and specific such thresholds were. This lack of standardization brings an uncomfortable uncertainty to issuing outbreak alerts. In the context of scarce public health resources, therefore, committing those resources to subjective conclusions can be difficult for Ministries of Health.

To address this problem, NAMRU-2 and NMRCD have collaborated to incorporate automated statistical outbreak detection algorithms into EWORS software. The goal is to preserve the opportunity for intuitive, qualitative data assessment through graphical displays, and offer quantitative assessments and automatic "flags" using algorithms currently employed in syndromic surveillance systems in the United States.

The third challenge has been validating an outbreak detection system in a developing country with limited laboratory diagnostic capabilities (in fact, a primary purpose of EWORS is to fill a surveillance gap where there is no laboratory network) and scarce resources to investigate possible outbreaks. It is too costly to send outbreak investigations teams out on every EWORS alert. And, without constant surveillance from other systems, it is difficult to determine whether outbreaks are being missed.

In practice, EWORS in Southeast Asia has been useful less in generating the initial identification of an outbreak, and more in guiding the deployment of scarce

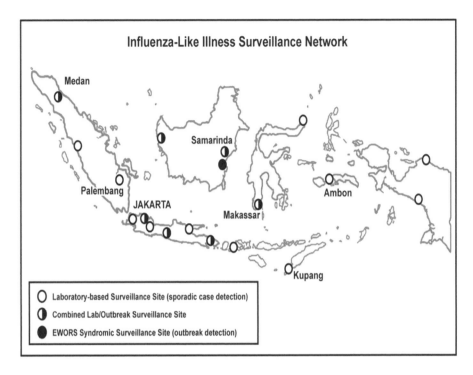

Fig. 9.4   Influenza-like illness surveillance network.

resources from central and provincial offices. Because up to three days may elapse between a patient presenting to a hospital with a syndrome under surveillance and analysis of the data at the EWORS hub, hospitals often have been aware that outbreaks are underway before an alert could be sent. Although hospital staff may know that an outbreak is underway, persuading provincial and central offices to provide epidemiologic or laboratory support can be difficult without convincing data — for example, the number of patients suspected of having the disease; the expected number of patients with similar presentations seen during a given timeframe; and patient clinical and demographic information. For hospitals that participate in EWORS, such data can be provided rapidly; in contrast, hospitals that do not routinely participate in EWORS or other surveillance systems can become too overwhelmed with patient care to produce such data during an outbreak. EWORS has been especially useful in demonstrating the geographic scope of outbreaks that have affected several hospitals and required mobilization of significant resources from provincial or central levels.

Although NMRCD implemented EWORS in Peru recently (2005), several features of that short experience are noteworthy. In Peru, the Ministry of Health's primary goal in supporting implementation of EWORS was improving the autonomy of the hospital and district level health authorities in infectious disease outbreak detection and response. For this reason, participating sites send surveillance data to the EWORS hub at NMRCD infrequently and are responsible for managing and interpreting their data.

This arrangement provided additional impetus to incorporate automated statistical detection algorithms into the software, and requires the EWORS hub to provide more training to participating sites that would be needed if data management and interpretation occurred centrally. An indirect benefit of this training, but one welcome by the Ministry of Health, has been improvement in outbreak preparedness in general — by learning the clinical, epidemiologic, and computer skills necessary to take an active role in EWORS, hospital staff have become better able to identify and investigate "unusual" events, whether or not they are reportable in EWORS.

In addition, the EWORS training program in Peru strengthens feelings of professional competence among hospital staff. This has been an important incentive for sites to participate in the system, especially because NMRCD staff made a strategic decision early in EWORS implementation not to provide financial or resource incentives to participating hospitals (e.g., salaries and computers) — a policy that has dissuaded some hospitals from participating, but ensured that ones that elect to participate are committed to the system and professional development, and not seeking ancillary benefits.

9.3.3   System Flexibility

NAMRU-2 and host countries developed EWORS to improve surveillance for a wide range of emerging infectious diseases. With concern growing for an influenza pandemic beginning in Asia, however, EWORS has been identified as a system that might provide an early warning capability critical for effective pandemic response. For example, the U.S. national strategy for pandemic influenza calls for continued support of EWORS as part of efforts to strengthen pandemic influenza surveillance overseas [45]. In the national influenza strategy of Lao PDR, EWORS is included as a major component of surveillance.

Computer simulation studies showing that rapid detection and public health intervention might contain an emerging pandemic suggest the utility of an early warning system [46, 47]. A draft WHO plan [48], based in part on such work, calls on countries to rapidly identify and report clusters of people with symptoms and exposures that could represent human-to-human transmission of a novel influenza virus–possibly the first indication of an emerging pandemic. WHO also has established large stockpiles of antiviral drugs to be deployed for pandemic containment, but only if the emerging pandemic is detected early enough for containment to be feasible [48].

Whether EWORS in its current forms could provide timely detection of an emerging influenza pandemic, or whether it is sufficiently flexible to accommodate modifications that would enhance early pandemic detection is unknown. To investigate these questions, DoD-GEIS, NAMRU-2, NMRCD, and The Johns Hopkins University/Applied Physics Laboratory (JHU/APL) initiated an "end-to-end" system evaluation in 2006. Because the success of pandemic containment is time dependent, with computer simulations providing guidance on how soon interventions must begin [46, 47], the evaluation team is using quantitative modeling approaches in addition to qualitative epidemiological assessments to understand how EWORS might perform in the face of an emerging pandemic. The system modeling framework will allow assessment of various EWORS modifications that could improve performance. One of the project's objectives is to guide future development of EWORS and other systems that countries may implement to improve early detection for pandemic influenza or other epidemic-prone respiratory viruses.

Although in the early stages, the EWORS evaluation has identified several features of EWORS and its operating environment that are likely to influence its effectiveness as an early warning system for an emerging influenza pandemic. For example, important system features could include the number and type of clinics at sentinel hospitals that participate in EWORS, the time lag between patient admission and data analysis, the background rate of syndromes for which an increase might indicate an outbreak of a viral respiratory illness such as influenza and many others. Approaches for evaluating syndromic surveillance systems in the United States [49, 50] will be adapted for evaluating such features in EWORS.

A realistic projection of EWORS performance for pandemic influenza, though, also requires analysis of factors that are external to the system. For example, local preferences for traditional medicine (which could reduce the effectiveness of a hospital-based surveillance system such as EWORS), referral patterns for patients with suspected avian influenza infection (which could direct such patients to or away from sentinel hospitals), population density (which could affect the rate of epidemic progression), location and type of laboratory testing capabilities (which could affect how rapidly a suspected outbreak is verified), and the administrative relationships between the EWORS surveillance hub and outbreak response offices are a few of the extra-system factors that a thorough evaluation should consider. Epidemiologic capabilities of the host country are also critical and will affect the number and skill of personnel available for surveillance activities.

A tool expected to result from this evaluation is a generic framework for establishing, enhancing, and evaluating surveillance activities in developing countries. When applied, a key consideration must be the ability of the system's host agency to sustain and validate recommended capabilities. While it is possible to suggest many enhancements to a system with limited existing capability, the host agency must be able to sustain the new features. If enhancements are accepted and sustained, they should be validated over time to continue improving the system and to assess the potential utility of such features for other systems.

9.3.4 Summary

A key lesson from several years of EWORS experience in Southeast Asia is the importance of the system's administrative context as a determinant of usefulness. In addition, providing actionable information using validated procedures is critical to developing confidence in a system that can trigger expenditures of human and financial resources. EWORS, in its present or in modified forms, may facilitate rapid detection and containment of pandemic influenza, but rigorous evaluation of the system and its operating environment is needed to define its role in pandemic influenza preparedness.

9.4   CASE STUDY 2: ALERTA DISAMAR (PERU)

The Peruvian Navy maintains dozens of training facilities, ports, and other bases across the country, from modern facilities in Lima to remote bases in border areas. Crowded living conditions and challenges to maintaining hygiene–which militaries in wealthy and developing countries alike may contend with–contribute to outbreaks of respiratory and diarrheal diseases among Peruvian naval personnel. The tropical, jungle environment poses additional risks of malaria, yellow fever, dengue, and other vector-borne diseases. Outbreaks of such diseases can render a large proportion of a base population ill and can significantly affect the Peruvian Navy's ability to execute missions.

Before 2002, the Peruvian Navy's public health surveillance system did not facilitate rapid detection, investigation, and control of infectious disease outbreaks among medical beneficiaries (approximately 25,000 active duty personnel and 100,000 family members in 2006). At each base, a medical officer recorded diseases targeted for surveillance by the Navy. Paper reports were mailed each month to the central naval medical office in Lima. Because of the long reporting interval and time required for mailed reports to reach Lima (especially for ones sent from remote border areas), surveillance data indicating infectious disease outbreaks often did not reach the central office until outbreaks were far along or over. Even if reports had reached the central office more rapidly, timely public health action might not have been taken because the Navy lacked an information system to support the small central staff in managing, analyzing, and interpreting the data. The cost of delayed outbreak response was great: the Peruvian Navy spent substantial amounts of money evacuating patients to the central hospital and treating patients with severe disease.

After a severe *Plasmodium falciparum* malaria outbreak at a base along the Colombian border in 2001, the Peruvian Navy acknowledged the need for more timely outbreak detection and response and committed to developing a more effective infectious disease surveillance system. For assistance, the Navy turned to NMRCD, which the Peruvian Navy had hosted at its national medical campus in Lima since 1983.

9.4.1   System Development, Configuration, and Operation

NMRCD and Peruvian Navy system planners recognized communications infrastructure as a key consideration in generating timely information. Developing a nationwide system that would cover all Navy facilities was an essential objective, but communication capabilities varied widely across the Navy. Some facilities had Internet access, whereas remote bases did not. Some of these even lacked telephones and used radio to communicate with higher level commands. After considering several possible solutions, system planners settled on an innovative, commercial technology that could integrate surveillance data across diverse communications platforms.

Developed by Voxiva, the system allows real-time data transmission by Internet or telephone [51]. Alerta DISAMAR was built around this information system in 2002, beginning with 11 reporting Navy facilities. The surveillance system has since expanded to 69 reporting units (including several Navy vessels) across the country, covering 97.5% of the Peruvian Navy medical beneficiary population (Fig. 9.5). Based on successful implementation in the Navy, the Peruvian Army has recently enrolled sites into the system, giving priority to posts in remote areas with endemic tropical diseases, such as the Amazon basin. The Air Force has also requested to be incorporated into the system.

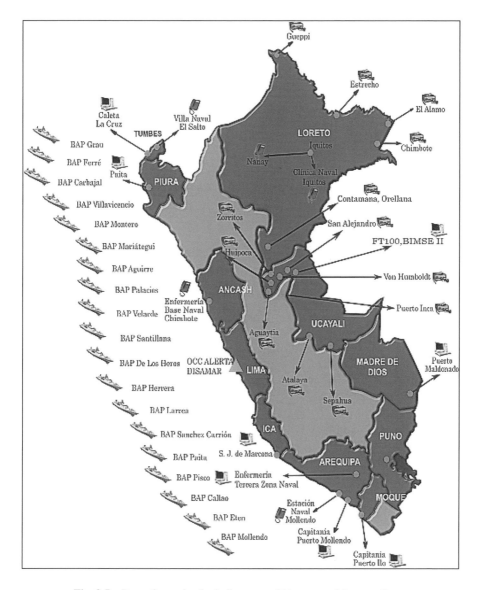

Fig. 9.5   Reporting units (including several Navy vessels) across Peru.

Figure 9.6 summarizes information flow through Alerta DISAMAR (the figure and the remainder of the case study focus on the more mature and extensive Navy network). At each site, a medical officer (physician or nurse) employed by the Peruvian Navy transmits data to the Alerta DISAMAR central hub at NMRCD by the most convenient means available: Internet or telephone (the call is toll-free from public land lines). Sites without access to either medium transmit reports by radio to regional hubs, where they are sent by Internet or telephone to the central hub.

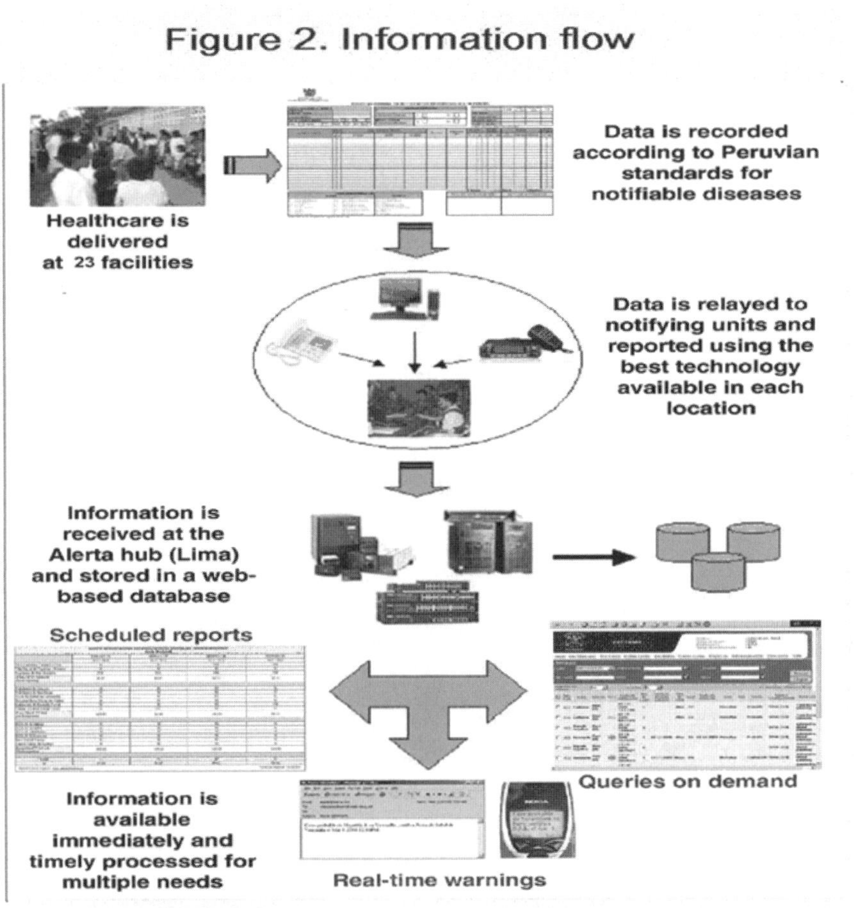

Figure 2. Information flow

Healthcare is delivered at 23 facilities

Data is recorded according to Peruvian standards for notifiable diseases

Data is relayed to notifying units and reported using the best technology available in each location

Information is received at the Alerta hub (Lima) and stored in a web-based database

Scheduled reports

Information is available immediately and timely processed for multiple needs

Real-time warnings

Queries on demand

Fig. 9.6   Information flow through Alerta DISAMAR.

Reports consist of demographic and clinical data for clinically suspected or laboratory-confirmed cases of diseases/syndromes identified as surveillance priorities by the Peruvian Ministry of Health or Navy (Fig. 9.7; approximately one-third of cases are laboratory-confirmed during routine surveillance, depending on on-site and nearby laboratory capabilities). Reporting frequency depends on the disease–some diseases require a daily report with demographic and clinical information on each case, while common syndromes (such as acute diarrhea or respiratory illness) are reported twice per week in batches to reduce data transmission time. All units must send a twice-per-week "zero report" if no reportable diseases are identified. The medical officer at each site devotes approximately 10-30 minutes per day to review medical records in preparation for reporting and approximately 2-3 minutes to transmit data on each case (or batch of cases for the twice-per-week report).

INDIVIDUAL REPORT		
ERUPTIVE BARTONELLOSIS	LEPTOSPIROSIS *	CONGENITAL SYPHILIS
SYSTEMIC BARTONELLOSIS	P. FALCIPARUM MALARIA	TETANUS
BRUCELLOSIS *	P. VIVAX MALARIA	NEONATAL TETANUS
ANTHRAX	MENINGOCOCIC MENINGITIS	EPIDEMIC TYPHUS
CHAGAS DISEASE	TB MENINGITIS	WHOOPING COUGH
DENGUE FEVER	MATERNAL DEATH	PULMONARY TB*
DHF	SNAKE BITES	HIV
DIPHTERIA	PLAGUE	TRAUMA
YELLOW FEVER	ACUTE FLACCID PARALYSIS	COLLECTIVE REPORT
TYPHOID FEVER *	RABIES	
HEPATITIS A *	RUBELLA	CHOLERA
HEPATITIS B	CONGENITAL RUBELLA	ADD (Acute diarrheal disease)
STD*	MEASLES	ARI (Acute respiratory infection)
CUTANEOUS LEISHMANIASIS	SARS	PNEUMONIA
MUCOCUTANEOUS LEISHMANIASIS	AIDS	ASTHMA

☐ Daily report   ■ Biweekly report

Fig. 9.7   Alerta DISAMAR diseases under surveillance, individual reports.

The Alerta DISAMAR hub staff includes one full-time physician employed by NMRCD and a senior noncommissioned officer and two part-time physicians assigned by the Peruvian Navy. The hub uses Voxiva software to convert data reported by different communication platforms into a common format to facilitate management and analysis. Quality assurance includes weekly manual review of automated procedures that track reporting timeliness (including "zero reporting"), completeness, and error rates (e.g., invalid diagnostic codes) by site (Figs. 9.8 and 9.9). All the data can be exported to Excel for further analysis. To identify excess cases rapidly, graphs are automatically generated in Excel with weekly counts of the most common diseases and expected counts based on historical averages by site within each Navy region (Fig. 9.10). The staff evaluates the graphs to assess whether additional follow-up is needed. Each week, reports summarizing epidemiologic data and quality assurance metrics for each site are generated automatically; these include counts of the most common diseases/syndromes and timely report rates (Fig. 9.11). Medical officers at reporting units and the central Peruvian Navy medical leadership can access these reports on a restricted, password-protected Internet site. Alerta DISAMAR personnel who lack Internet access may elect to receive compressed text reports by cellular telephone.

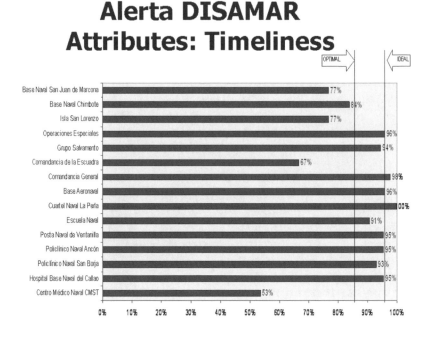

Fig. 9.8   Alerta DISAMAR attributes: timeliness.

9.4.2   Outbreak Detection and Response

When Alerta DISAMAR graphical displays of observed and usual case counts suggest that an outbreak may be underway, the central hub staff first checks the reports for obvious errors. The next step is to make contact with the reporting site's medical officer by telephone or radio, to verify the accuracy of the report, gather additional clinical information, and identify any additional cases not yet formally reported. Based on this assessment, the central hub team decides whether to launch an outbreak investigation. Frequently, discussion between central hub and field site staff results in a decision not to initiate an investigation — for example, if the etiology already is known, morbidity is not severe, and effective control measures are in place. Investigations launched as a result of Alerta DISAMAR have identified outbreaks of various infectious diseases, including malaria [52], dengue [53], and cyclosporiasis [54] (Fig. 9.12).

A critical element in this decision-making process is the Peruvian naval senior noncommissioned officer assigned to the Alerta DISAMAR central hub. This npers

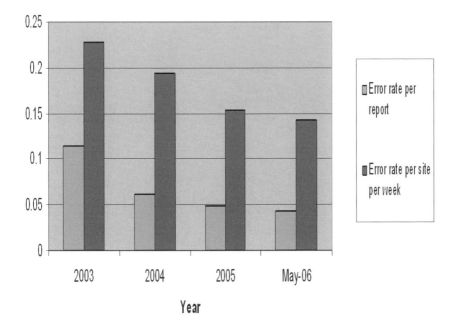

Fig. 9.9   Alerta DISAMAR attributes: sata quality.

maintains close contact with each site in the surveillance network (a full-time job) to provide feedback on reports, respond to requests for technical assistance, and assess whether an outbreak investigation is warranted. As a member of the naval service, his understanding of the surveillance sites facilitates communication with the sites and interpretation of surveillance data. The Peruvian Navy's decision to detail a senior noncommissioned officer to the Alerta DISAMAR central hub attests to its support for the system. Efforts are ongoing to persuade other Peruvian government agencies enrolling sites into Alerta DISAMAR to assign such a person to the central hub.

Once the central hub team reaches a decision to investigate a potential outbreak, it must obtain permission from the military installation commander or higher levels of command. The close relationship between NMRCD and Peruvian naval leadership facilitates this process as well. Rather than seek permission from installation commanders (who may not have the time or interest to host an outbreak investigation), the central hub team briefs the central naval medical leadership, which has authority to approve an investigation at any naval facility. The medical leadership has approved all requests for facility access to investigate outbreaks since Alerta DISAMAR was initiated. To facilitate collaboration with installation personnel, the investigation team, on arrival at the facility, briefs the facility commander on why the investigation is needed and how it will be executed.

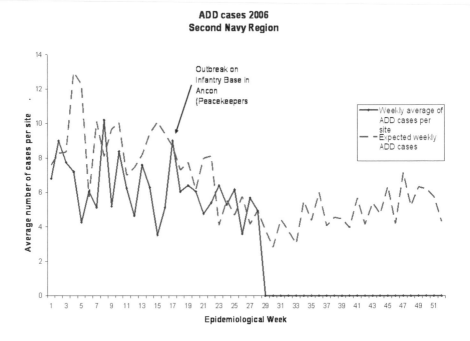

Fig. 9.10   ADD cases, 2006, Second Navy region.

Since outbreaks often are first identified as an increase in clinically suspected cases of an infectious disease, an early step in outbreak investigation is collection of specimens and their submission to a competent laboratory for confirmatory diagnosis; frequently, the medical staff at the affected site can take this action before the investigation team arrives. Most Peruvian naval medical facilities lack advanced diagnostic capabilities, so Alerta DISAMAR interfaces with national laboratory networks to identify outbreak etiology: public health laboratories operated by the Ministry of Health and a nationwide laboratory-based surveillance network operated by NMRCD in collaboration with the Ministry of Health.

This laboratory-based network, the Febrile Syndromic Surveillance System, enrolls patients presenting with febrile, respiratory, gastrointestinal, or hemorrhagic syndromes to 10 clinical sites across the country. Site staff collect demographic, historical, and clinical data and diagnostic specimens appropriate for the presenting syndrome. Data and specimens are sent at regular intervals to the central laboratory at NMRCD or an NMRCD field laboratory in Iquitos (northeastern Peru, in the Amazon basin), which use virological, serological, and polymerase chain reaction (PCR) methods to test for a wide range of likely pathogens. The transportation protocols established for this ongoing surveillance program facilitate transfer of specimens collected in an Alerta DISAMAR outbreak investigation to a competent laboratory,

Reporte de los daños mas frecuentes notificados en las cuatro últimas semanas epidemiológicas Alerta DISAMAR 2006

SE 2006 - 30		SE 2006 - 31		SE 2006 - 32		SE 2006 - 33	
Daño	Nro Casos	Daño	Nro Casos	Daño	Nro Casos	Daño	Nro Casos
IRA	435	IRA	729	IRA	598	IRA	687
EDA	128	EDA	144	EDA	102	EDA	142
Asma-SOB	3	Asma-SOB	8	Asma-SOB	4	Asma-SOB	6
Malaria Vivax	1	Malaria Vivax	2	Malaria Vivax	4	Malaria Vivax	3
Dengue Clasico	2	Dengue Clasico	3	Dengue Clasico	4	Dengue Clasico	3
Otros	0	Otros	2	Otros	1	Otros	2
Neumonia	0	Neumonia	0	Neumonia	0	Neumonia	2
Malaria Falciparum	0	Malaria Falciparum	0	Malaria Falciparum	0	Malaria Falciparum	1
TBC Pulmonar	0	TBC Pulmonar	1	TBC Pulmonar	2	TBC Pulmonar	1
Reporte Negativo *	28	Reporte Negativo *	25	Reporte Negativo *	26	Reporte Negativo *	30

Fig. 9.11   Example of report summarizing epidemiologic data and quality assurance for each site.

provided specimens can be directed to a Febrile Syndromic Surveillance System enrollment site.

On completion of the outbreak investigation, the Alerta DISAMAR central hub team prepares a report on its findings and recommendations for preventing or responding to future outbreaks to the central naval medical leadership, which may direct the affected facility (or others) to implement recommendations. Understanding and respecting such chain-of-command relationships has been critical for NMRCD's success in developing and expanding Alerta DISAMAR in the Peruvian Navy.

9.4.3   System Flexibility

Voxiva-developed Alerta DISAMAR software provides for system flexibility in key domains. As discussed earlier, the system's ability to integrate surveillance data from Internet and telephone is important because communication capabilities vary markedly across the Alerta DISAMAR network. The software also allows the central hub to define new reportable diseases and syndromes as the Peruvian Navy recognizes new health threats. This is an important capability for a system focused on emerging infectious diseases, which (by definition) are new or changing. However, experience in adding leptospirosis, sexually transmitted infections, and other diseases to the original list has shown that the process imposes significant requirements on the surveillance sites. Central software modification allows all sites to report new diagnostic codes,

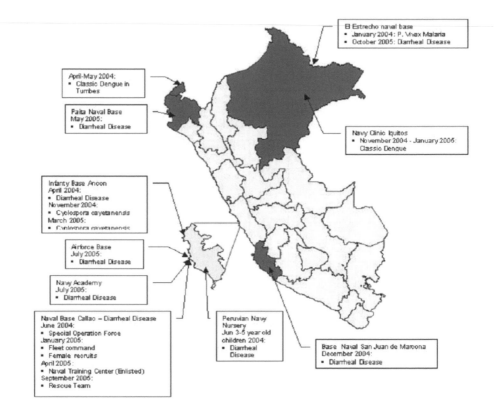

Fig. 9.12   Alerta DISAMAR usefulness: outbreaks detected.

but generating those new data requires busy medical staff to implement new clinical procedures (e.g., additional questions or physical examination components).

Voxiva and its software also have proven adaptable to the needs of the Peruvian Navy and central hub by incorporating new ways of entering and visualizing data. For example, the latest software upgrade allows staff at sites with intermittent Internet access to perform data entry offline on a PC, then upload the data to the central hub when an Internet connection is available. Reporting platforms are being expanded to include smart phones and PDAs. SMS/text messaging will provide another means of reporting to the central hub and communicating from the central hub to notify sites of new diseases to include in surveillance or of emergency procedures (e.g., if there is concern for SARS, pandemic influenza, or another novel, dangerous disease in the region).

The Web-based interface provides data visualization from anywhere with Internet access. Multiple "dashboards" have been created to customize data views for users with different needs (e.g., surveillance site staff versus central naval leadership). These Web-based interfaces display key information using indicators, graphs, alerts, and an interactive GIS map. Charts can be generated automatically that use standard epidemiologic formats or charts can be custom-made with user-specified data and formats. Data can be exported to standard statistical software packages for further analysis.

As a military surveillance system, an important challenge that Alerta DISAMAR contends with is personnel turnover. While most central hub staff members have worked there for several years, many medical officers at Navy surveillance sites are young physicians or nurses performing short, required national service duty. Although such frequent turnover demands frequent training, the central Peruvian naval command allocates time to Alerta DISAMAR training during initial medical officer training, a 2-day session in Lima before assignment to facilities across the country (an example of training material developed by the central hub is shown in Fig. 9.13). This arrangement allows the central hub to conduct one group basic training session each year for a new cohort of surveillance site medical officers, and is another example of how high system acceptability by the major stakeholder, the Peruvian Navy, contributes to efficiency and effectiveness.

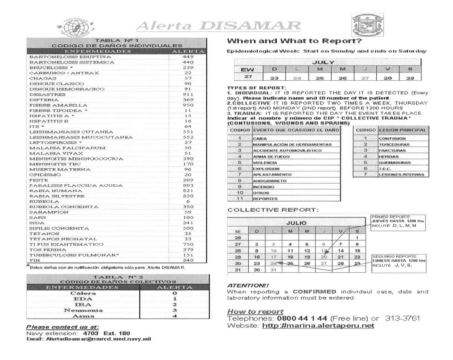

Fig. 9.13   Alerta DISAMAR training material.

Finally, broadly based training of surveillance site staff allows them to respond appropriately to possible outbreaks, even if modification of usual system procedures is required. In one recent example, the medical officer on a naval ship noticed an increase in diarrhea cases during a 2-day period over that considered normal on the ship. Because diarrhea is not uncommon in the population, and Alerta DISAMAR reporting draws staff away from other important clinical duties, system procedures call for reporting of diarrhea cases twice per week. However, the medical officer, who had completed an NMRCD outbreak response course as part of Alerta DISAMAR training, recognized the increase as a possible outbreak requiring immediate reporting. She contacted the Peruvian naval representative at the central hub, who quickly verified that other ships in the area that had shared a training environment were experiencing excess diarrhea cases as well.

9.4.4 Summary

The Peruvian Navy and NMRCD have found Alerta DISAMAR to be useful for timely detection of emerging infectious disease outbreaks [55]. Key factors that contribute to the system's effectiveness are software that integrates surveillance data across diverse communication platforms, thus extending surveillance to remote facilities with minimal communication capabilities; broadly based training of system operators, which prepares them to respond appropriately to situations that require modification of usual system procedures; and, perhaps most important, strong stakeholder support, which facilitates communication with surveillance sites, addition of new sites to the network, physical access to sites for outbreak investigation, and centralized training of surveillance site medical officers. As with many infectious disease surveillance systems in developing countries, Alerta DISAMAR often reports clinically suspected rather than laboratory-confirmed diagnoses. In outbreak scenarios, though, integration with laboratory-based networks can provide diagnostic confirmation.

9.5 CONCLUSIONS

The two short case studies presented in this chapter illustrate a few common themes: the importance of gaining visible endorsement for the surveillance system from offices whose authority is recognized by clinical and public health personnel participating in the system; the utility of broadly based training for system operators, which prepares them to address new situations not covered by the system's standard operating procedures; and the need for integrating laboratory-based and syndromic surveillance. Although the case studies covered surveillance systems in developing countries, these points apply to systems in wealthy countries as well.

It would be wrong to assume, however, that evaluations of and experience with surveillance systems in wealthy countries provides sufficient guidance for implementing systems in resource-poor settings. While challenges and solutions may appear similar at a high level of abstraction, the brief treatment of EWORS and Alerta DISAMAR here shows that some features of the developing country environment call for technological or administrative strategies that might not be needed in, for example, a county health department in the United States. There are significant challenges in developing countries that money alone cannot solve: for example, lack of skilled personnel to operate surveillance systems, and issues of legal authority in outbreak investigations or the implementation of new systems.

The need for surveillance system evaluations in developing countries is greater than ever, as concern for an influenza pandemic has driven wealthy countries to provide substantial resources for improvement of public health capacity in developing countries. Fundamentally, there is a need to identify the advantages, disadvantages, and appropriate applications of various sponsorship and support models. For example, how useful is direct aid in developing public health capacity in poor countries? How does this experience compare with that of overseas platforms like NAMRU-2, NM-RCD, and other broadly based laboratories? What models not yet implemented might work best? Analyses that answer such questions could prove very useful in guiding efficient, effective investment in the public health systems of developing countries.

9.6 STUDY QUESTIONS

9.1 Incentives can be a useful tool in enrolling and maintaining sites in a surveillance system. But they can increase system sustainment cost and possibly affect data validity (for example, if incentives are based on number of events reported). *Q: Besides financial and equipment incentives, what are some ways that busy hospitals or clinics in developing countries could be persuaded to participate in a surveillance system?*

9.2 In many developing countries, people may seek care at hospitals only after pursuing other options (e.g., treatment at home or a traditional healer or pharmacist). *Q: In such places, how could surveillance systems be designed to capture timely and accurate information?*

9.3 This chapter described one system (Alerta DISAMAR) that uses the Internet and telephones to communicate surveillance data from remote locations. *Q: What are some other methods of communicating surveillance data that could be implemented in resource-poor settings?*

9.4 Developing country ministries of health usually have small budgets for investigating outbreaks. Even if a surveillance system is in place and provides convincing evidence that an outbreak is under way, decision makers may elect not to expend precious resources on a response. *Q: What data could a surveillance system in a developing country collect to help authorities decide whether to launch an investigation?*

9.5 Several approaches to evaluating surveillance systems have been proposed. Some have been informed primarily by experience in high-income countries. *Q: What are some features of surveillance systems (or their operating environments) in developing countries that might require special attention in an evaluation?*

Disclaimer. The views expressed here are the private views of the authors and are not intended to be construed as official, or as reflecting the true views of the U.S. Department of the Army, U.S. Department of the Navy, or U.S. Department of Defense.

REFERENCES

1. World Health Organization. Cumulative number of confirmed human cases of avian influenza A/(H5N1) reported to WHO. July 20, 2006. Available at http://www.who.int/csr/disease/avian_influenza/country/cases_table_2006_07_20/en/index.html.

2. Taubenberger JK, Reid AH, Lourens RM, Wang R, Jin G, Fanning TG. Characterization of the 1918 influenza virus polymerase genes. Nature. 2005; 437(7060): 889-893.

3. Morens DM, Folkers GK, Fauci AS. The challenge of emerging and re-emerging infectious diseases. Nature. 2004; 430(6996): 242-249.

4. Institute of Medicine. Emerging Infections. Microbial Threats to Health in the United States. Washington, DC: National Academies Press; 1992.

5. Institute of Medicine. Microbial Threats to Health. Emergence, Detection, and Response. Washington, DC: The National Academies Press; 1998.

6. Cooper RS, Osotimehin B, Kaufman JS, Forrester T. Disease burden in sub-Saharan Africa: what should we conclude in the absence of data? Lancet. 1998;351 (9097):208-210.

7. Heymann DL, Rodier G. Global surveillance, national surveillance, and SARS. Emerg Infect Dis. 2004; 10(2): 173-175.

8. Nsubuga P, White ME, Thacker SB, et al. Public health surveillance: a tool for targeting and monitoring interventions. In: Jamison DT, Breman JG, Measham AR, et al., eds. Disease Control Priorities in Developing Countries. 2nd ed. New York: Oxford University Press; 2006: 997-1016.

9. White ME, McDonnell SM. Public health surveillance in low- and middle-income countries. In: Teutsch SM, Churchill RE, eds. Principles and Practice of Public Health Surveillance. New York: Oxford University Press; 2000: 287-315.

10. Berkelman R, Cassell G, Specter S, Hamburg M, Klugman K. The "Achilles Heel" of global efforts to combat infectious diseases. Clin Infect Dis. 2006; 42(10): 1503-1504.

11. Petti CA, Polage CR, Quinn TC, Ronald AR, Sande MA. Laboratory medicine in Africa: a barrier to effective health care. Clin Infect Dis. 2006; 42(3): 377-382.

12. Williams T. Building health information systems in the context of national strategies for the development of statistics. Bull World Health Organ. 2005; 83(8): 564.

13. Hotchkiss DR, Eisele TP, Djibuti M, Silvestre EA, Rukhadze N. Health system barriers to strengthening vaccine-preventable disease surveillance and response in the context of decentralization: evidence from Georgia. BMC Public Health. 2006; 6(1): 175.

14. AbouZahr C, Boerma T. Health information systems: the foundations of public health. Bull World Health Organ. 2005; 83(8): 578-583.

15. Public-health preparedness requires more than surveillance. Lancet. 2004; 364(9446): 1639-1640.

16. Durrheim DN, Speare R. Communicable disease surveillance and management in a globalised world. Lancet. 2004; 363(9418): 1339-1340.

17. World Health Organization. International Health Regulations. Geneva, Switzerland, WHO; 2005.

18. Heymann DL, Rodier GR. Hot spots in a wired world: WHO surveillance of emerging and re-emerging infectious diseases. Lancet Infect Dis. 2001; 1(5): 345-353.

19. Oum S, Chandramohan D, Cairncross S. Community-based surveillance: a pilot study from rural Cambodia. Trop Med Int Health. 2005; 10(7): 689-697.

20. Durrheim DN, Harris BN, Speare R, Billinghurst K. The use of hospital-based nurses for the surveillance of potential disease outbreaks. Bull World Health Organ. 2001; 79(1): 22-27.

21. John TJ, Samuel R, Balraj V, John R. Disease surveillance at district level: a model for developing countries. Lancet. 1998; 352(9121): 58-61.

22. Artenstein AW, Opal JM, Opal SM, Tramont EC, Peter G, Russell PK. History of U.S. military contributions to the study of vaccines against infectious diseases. Mil Med. 2005; 170(4 suppl): 3-11.

23. Bavaro MF, Kelly DJ, Dasch GA, Hale BR, Olson P. History of U.S. military contributions to the study of rickettsial diseases. Mil Med. 2005; 170(4 suppl): 49-60.

24. Endy TP, Thomas SJ, Lawler JV. History of U.S. military contributions to the study of viral hemorrhagic fevers. Mil Med. 2005; 170(4 suppl): 77-91.

25. Gambel JM, Hibbs RG Jr. U.S. military overseas medical research laboratories. Mil Med. 1996; 161(11): 638-645.

26. Hoke CH Jr. History of U.S. military contributions to the study of viral encephalitis. Mil Med. 2005; 170(4 suppl): 92-105.

27. Lim ML, Murphy GS, Calloway M, Tribble D. History of U.S. military contributions to the study of diarrheal diseases. Mil Med. 2005; 170(4 suppl): 30-38.

28. Ockenhouse CF, Magill A, Smith D, Milhous W. History of U.S. military contributions to the study of malaria. Mil Med. 2005; 170(4 suppl): 12-16.

29. Crum NF, Aronson NE, Lederman ER, Rusnak JM, Cross JH. History of U.S. military contributions to the study of parasitic diseases. Mil Med. 2005; 170(4 suppl): 17-29.

30. Presidential Decision Directive NSTC-7. 1996.

31. Chretien JP, Gaydos JC, Malone JL, Blazes DL. Global network could avert pandemics. Nature. 2006; 440(7080): 25-26.

32. Canas LC, Lohman K, Pavlin JA, er al. The Department of Defense laboratory-based global influenza surveillance system. Mil Med. 2000; 165(7 sSuppl 2): 52-56.

33. Buehler JW, Hopkins RS, Overhage JM, Sosin DM, Tong V. Framework for evaluating public health surveillance systems for early detection of outbreaks: recommendations from the CDC Working Group. MMWR Recomm Rep. 2004; 53(RR-5): 1-11.

34. German RR, Lee LM, Horan JM, Milstein RL, Pertowski CA, Waller MN. Updated guidelines for evaluating public health surveillance systems: recommendations from the Guidelines Working Group. MMWR Recomm Rep. 2001; 50(RR-13): i-35.

35. Romaguera RA, German RR, Klaucke DN. Public health surveillance in low- and middle-income countries. In: Teutsch SM, Churchill RE, eds. Principles and Practice of Public Health Surveillance. New York: Oxford University Press; 2000: 176-193.

36. Kandun IN, Wibisono H, Sedyaningsih ER, Yusharmen, Hadisoedarsuno W, Purba W, Santoso H, Septiawiti C, Tresnaningsih E, Heriyanto B, Yuwono D, Harun S, Soeroso S, Giriputra S, Blair PJ, Jeremijenko A, Kosasih H, Putnam SD, Samaan G, Silitonga M, Chan KH, Poon LL, Lim W, Kilmov A, Lindstrom S, Guan Y, Donis R, Katz J, Cox N, Peiris M, Uyeki TM. Three Indonesian clusters of H5N1 virus infection in 2005, N Engl J Med 2006;355:2186-94.

37. Corwin AL, Larasati RP, Bangs MJ, et al. Epidemic dengue transmission in southern Sumatra, Indonesia. Trans R Soc Trop Med Hyg. 2001; 95(3): 257-265.

38. Corwin AL, Simanjuntak CH, Ingkokusumo G, et al. Impact of epidemic influenza A-like acute respiratory illness in a remote jungle highland population in Irian Jaya, Indonesia. Clin Infect Dis. 1998; 26(4): 880-888.

39. Corwin AL, Subekti D, Sukri NC, Willy RJ, Master J, Priyanto E, Laras K. A large outbreak of probable rotavirus in Nusa Tenggara Timur, Indonesia. Am J Trop Med Hyg, 2005; 72(4): 488-494.

40. Laras K, Sukri NC, Larasati RP, et al. Tracking the re-emergence of epidemic chikungunya virus in Indonesia. Trans R Soc Trop Med Hyg. 2005; 99(2): 128-141.

41. Richards AL, Bagus R, Baso SM, et al. The first reported outbreak of dengue hemorrhagic fever in Irian Jaya, Indonesia. Am J Trop Med Hyg. 1997; 57(1): 49-55.

42. Sukri NC, Laras K, Wandra T, et al. Transmission of epidemic dengue hemorrhagic fever in easternmost Indonesia. Am J Trop Med Hy. 2003; 68(5): 529-535.

43. Simanjuntak CH, Larasati W, Arjoso S, et al. Cholera in Indonesia in 1993–1999. Am J Trop Med Hyg. 2001; 65(6): 788-797.

44. Corwin AL, McCarthy M, Larasati RP, et al. Developing regional outbreak response capabilities: Early Warning Outbreak Recognition System (EWORS). Navy Med. September–October 2000: 1-5.

45. Homeland Security Council. National strategy for pandemic influenza. Implementation plan. 2006.

46. Longini IM Jr, Nizam A, Xu S, et al. Containing pandemic influenza at the source. Science. 2005; 309(5737): 1083-1087.

47. Ferguson NM, Cummings DA, Cauchemez S, et al. Strategies for containing an emerging influenza pandemic in Southeast Asia. Nature. 2005; 437(7056): 209-214.

48. World Health Organization. WHO pandemic influenza draft protocol for rapid response and containment. 2006.

49. Buckeridge DL, Burkom H, Moore A, Pavlin J, Cutchis P, Hogan W. Evaluation of syndromic surveillance systems: design of an epidemic simulation model. MMWR. 2004; 53(suppl): 137-143.

50. Lombardo JS, Burkom H, Pavlin J. ESSENCE II and the framework for evaluating syndromic surveillance systems. MMWR. 2004; 53(suppl): 159-165.

51. Mundaca CM, Araujo RV, Moran M, et al. Use of an electronic disease surveillance system in a remote, resource limited setting: Alerta DISAMAR in Peru. Presented at the American Society of Tropical Medicine and Hygiene 54th Annual Meeting, December 11-15, 2005; Washington, DC.

52. Araujo-Castillo R, Mundaca CM, Moran M, Ortiz M, Blazes DL. Malaria surveillance using an electronic reporting system in Navy personnel in Loreto, Peru.

Presented at the American Society of Tropical Medicine and Hygiene 54th Annual Meeting, December 11-15, 2005; Washington, DC.

53. Araujo-Castillo RV, Mundaca CM, Moran M, er al. Use of an electronic surveillance system (Alerta) to detect a dengue outbreak among a Peruvian Navy population in Iquitos, Peru. Presented at the American Society of Tropical Medicine and Hygiene 54th Annual Meeting, December 11-15, 2005; Washington, DC.

54. Mundaca CM, Torres PA, Moran M, et al. Use of PCR in an outbreak of cyclosporiasis at a Naval base in Ancon, Lima, Peru. American Society of Tropical Medicine and Hygiene 54th Annual Meeting; 2005 December 11-15; Washington, D.C.

55. Mundaca CM, Araujo RV, Moran M, et al. Self-evaluation of an electronic disease surveillance system in a resource limited under-surveilled setting: Alerta DISAMAR in Peru. Presented at the American Society of Tropical Medicine and Hygiene 54th Annual Meeting, December 11-15, 2005; Washington, DC.

Part III: Evaluation, Education, and the Future

10 Evaluating Automated Surveillance Systems

David L. Buckeridge, Michael W. Thompson, Steven Babin, Marvin L. Sikes

Part II of this book presented several examples of automated disease surveillance systems. Chapter 6 considered systems used locally and nationally in the United States and Chapters 7–9 examined systems used in Canada, the United Kingdom, Southeastern Asia and South America. Each of the systems examined provides surveillance solutions that take advantage of locally available resources for conducting disease surveillance.

Part III of this book examines issues in evaluation, training, and research as they relate to automated disease surveillance systems. Chapter 10 presents methods for evaluating disease surveillance system considering the context in which evaluations are performed, the components of the evaluation process and approaches to measuring system performance.

10.1 THE CONTEXT OF EVALUATION

10.1.1 Why? — The Need to Evaluate

Automated syndromic surveillance is a novel public health tool characterized by real-time data capture and the use of prediagnostic data. These characteristics produce systems with low operating costs [1], the ability to detect outbreaks rapidly and the capacity to enhance "situational awareness". The ease of system implementation, coupled with concerns over bioterrorism, have prompted public health agencies to implement hundreds of automated surveillance systems in the United States and around the world [2, 3] at a cost of millions of dollars [4].

While the rapid growth in automated surveillance systems is seen by many in public health as an exciting and important development, this growth has also prompted questions about the need for and the effectiveness of syndromic surveillance within a limited public health budget [4, 5, 6]. One concern relates to the practical role of syndromic surveillance in the day-to-day operations of a public health department [5]. Another concern is whether syndromic surveillance works for outbreak detection [6]. These appropriate and important questions, which remain unanswered to a large extent, are due to the limited evaluation of syndromic surveillance. As discussed in this chapter, evaluation should identify not only if syndromic surveillance works, but rather the benefits of using syndromic surveillance for defined outcomes in defined contexts. In some cases, it may be difficult to quantify the benefit of syndromic surveillance for applications such as ruling-out outbreaks and providing situational awareness. Evaluation is, nevertheless, essential to ensure the appropriate use of syndromic surveillance within an evolving public health infrastructure.

Early evaluations of syndromic surveillance were limited in number [7], but the number of published evaluation studies has increased in recent years [8]. This increasing interest in the evaluation of syndromic surveillance is well placed because many questions about syndromic surveillance remain unanswered. As more data sources become available electronically in real time in the future, the increased availability will lower the barrier to implementing syndromic surveillance. Only when the benefits of automated syndromic surveillance are defined clearly will it be possible to answer questions about the cost effectiveness of adding automated surveillance to the public health toolkit.

10.1.2   What? — The Focus of Evaluation

An evaluation study should be driven by a clear question, which may be motivated by an issue important to a single location or of more general interest. In posing the question and defining the scope of the evaluation, it is helpful to start from an evaluation framework.

A few evaluation frameworks are relevant to automated syndromic surveillance systems. A working group established by the CDC adapted existing guidelines for evaluating surveillance systems [9] to the evaluation of automated surveillance systems focused on rapid outbreak detection [10]. The CDC evaluation framework includes system description, evaluation of outbreak detection, and assessment of system experience. Other, more general, evaluation frameworks are also relevant to syndromic surveillance systems. The DeLone and McLean (D&M) model of information system success, originally published in 1992 [11] and updated recently [12], contains constructs for information quality, system quality, service quality, intention to use, use, user satisfaction, and net benefits. The Public Health Informatics Institute has developed a logic model framework based on the D&M model for evaluating public health information systems [13].

In general, frameworks identify potential evaluation foci as (1) the quality of the system, (2) the quality of the information used in the system, (3) user experiences interacting with the system, and (4) the benefits of the system (Table 10.1). As stated earlier, two potential benefits of syndromic surveillance are rapid outbreak detection and enhanced situational awareness. This chapter focuses on the evaluation

Table 10.1   Potential Foci Identified by Frameworks for Evaluation of an Automated Surveillance System. Source: Buehler et al. [2], Delone and McLean [11], PHII [13]

Evaluation Focus	Examples
Information quality	Validity of diagnostic codes, frequency of missing values
System quality	Stability of software and hardware, security
User experience	Ease of use, time to perform tasks
System benefits	Accuracy and timeliness of outbreak detection, infections averted, cost-effectiveness

of outbreak detection and considers evaluation of both the human response to statistical aberrations in the data and aberration detection itself.

10.1.3   How? — The Methods of Evaluation

The steps in an evaluation process are (1) define the evaluation, (2) identify or create the evaluation data, (3) apply detection algorithms and response protocols to the evaluation data, and (4) measure performance. In the remainder of this chapter, each of these four steps is discussed in turn.

10.2   DEFINING THE EVALUATION

At the outset of an evaluation, the initial tasks are to clarify the evaluation question, identify the configuration of the surveillance system, define the outbreak scenario, and describe the overall evaluation plan.

10.2.1   Question and Scope

The question to be answered through evaluation may have a specific focus in a practical setting. For example, an analyst may be interested in the magnitude of a signal that a specific surveillance system will detect or the optimal threshold for an algorithm in the context of a specific type of signal. Alternatively, the question may be more general or may be related to how results from the system are used in practice. For example, a public health department may be interested in how much time it takes to rule out false alarms, how analysts tend to interpret alarm signals, or how well their personnel work with other agencies in an outbreak situation. The specific question should help to determine the appropriate system configuration and outbreak scenario. For evaluations aimed at response protocols, the U.S. Federal Emergency Management

Agency (FEMA) has developed a process to assist planners in ensuring that their objectives are clear and accurate [14].

10.2.2   System Configuration

The surveillance system may be a real system or a model of an operating system. A model of a system may be preferable for evaluation studies where performance will be examined across many outbreaks because it is generally more efficient to conduct multiple tests in a model than an operational system. Multiple tests — thousands to tens of thousands — are usually required for evaluations of outbreak detection that use simulated outbreaks. Conversely, if the evaluation is aimed at human response protocols to statistical alarms, it may be preferable to use a real system in situ to ensure that the exercise is realistic.

10.2.3   Outbreak Scenario

The outbreak scenario may range from a simple "increase in incidence" with few additional details to a complex scenario involving the release of infectious agents at multiple locations with a spatially mobile population [15]. While the outbreak scenario should have complexity sufficient for answering the question, the scenario should, at the same time, not be overly complex. A practical test of complexity is whether the scenario will provide data that are sufficiently complex for the outbreak detection algorithms that will be used in the evaluation or the response protocol that will be evaluated. For example, if a space-time statistical method is being used without adjustment for covariates, the scenario must specify the spatial characteristics of the scenario, but details about age groups are not necessary unless this information is required by a simulation model that will be used to generate outbreak signals. Details beyond those required by the statistical detection algorithms are also needed in an evaluation aimed at response protocols, where analysts may need to view individual records as a first step in investigating a statistical aberration. The story line of events must also be credible and, if possible, based on real-world events [16]. At a minimum, the scenario must be supported by realistic threats and data.

10.2.4   Evaluation Plan

The evaluation plan describes the steps that will be taken to conduct the evaluation, ide-ally in sufficient detail to repeat the evaluation, if desired. For a quantitative evaluation focused on outbreak detection or other aspects of detection algorithm performance, the evaluation plan may be similar to a protocol for a research study and include such factors as the specific data streams and date ranges to be used, the algorithm thresholds at which performance will be evaluated, and the number of simulations that will be performed. For an evaluation focused on response protocols, considerable resources and planning may be required. Accurate planning for the logistical requirements is essential for a successful exercise involving many personnel. Planning may include reservation of conference facilities and classrooms, establishment of necessary telephone and computer network access, security, and administrative support. Once the question is stated clearly, the configuration of the surveillance system is determined, the outbreak scenario is described, and the overall evaluation plan is in place, the next step is to identify or create the evaluation data.

10.3 IDENTIFYING OR CREATING EVALUATION DATA

10.3.1 Data for Evaluation

Data for evaluation must contain outbreaks, ideally with known characteristics. Evaluators use authentic data (i.e., real data, usually taken from historical data in an operating surveillance system) or simulated data, alone or in combination, to create the data needed for an evaluation. The following combinations are used most commonly in evaluations of outbreak detection and response protocols, and each approach has distinct advantages and disadvantages [17, 18, 19]:

1. Authentic background data with authentic disease outbreaks

2. Authentic background data with simulated disease outbreaks

3. Simulated background data with simulated disease outbreaks

Although using authentic background data with authentic disease outbreaks may seem initially to be the best option, this approach has a number of drawbacks. First, it is often difficult to identify with certainty authentic outbreaks in evaluation data. Small, sporadic outbreaks may be missed altogether, and when outbreaks are identified, it can be difficult be to determine their onset precisely and to identify which cases are attributable to the outbreak and which belong to the endemic background. In other words, the characteristics of the outbreak signal cannot be derived without error from inspection of the data alone. Investigation of individual cases and other coincident data sources may help, but this type of validation can be prohibitively expensive. An additional problem with using all-authentic data is that few historical time series are available containing verified disease outbreaks, and even fewer are available containing outbreaks associated with bioterrorism or emerging infectious diseases.

For these reasons, algorithm detection performance is often measured using the *semisynthetic approach*, where simulated disease outbreaks are injected into authentic background data [18, 19, 20]. This approach enables evaluation of an alerting algorithm using many outbreak signals with as much variation as desired. Figure 10.1 is an example of a simulated outbreak injected into authentic data. Because the outbreaks are simulated, their signal characteristics, including onset and magnitude, are known with certainty; and because the outbreaks are injected, tests can be repeated with and without the outbreaks present, as well as with random variation in the outbreak signals, to obtain precise estimates of key performance statistics, such as sensitivity, specificity, and timeliness of detection. One drawback to this approach is that it cannot be proven that the background data do not contain any undocumented outbreaks. Another drawback is that simulated outbreak signals might not adequately represent the authentic outbreaks encountered by the surveillance system. This question is addressed in Section 10.3.3, where approaches to simulating outbreak signals are considered.

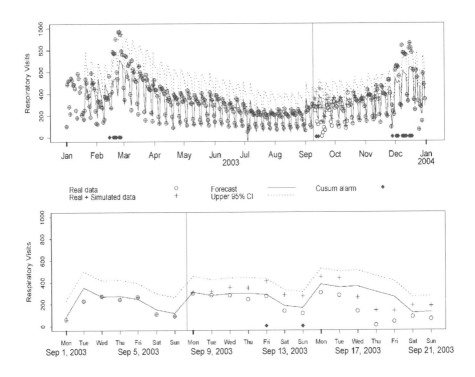

Fig. 10.1   Example of a simulated outbreak injected into authentic background data. The top panel shows a year of data, and the bottom panel shows data around the onset of the inject. The vertical line indicates the timing of exposure to inhalational anthrax for a simulated population.

A third possibility is to inject simulated disease outbreaks into simulated background data. With this approach, the evaluator has complete control over the test data. The characteristics of the background data are known with certainty, the background data contain no hidden outbreaks, and both background and signal can be varied to produce an even wider variety of test cases. As with the semisynthetic method, effects of typical data problems are easily added to the data to evaluate algorithm robustness. Furthermore, tests can be repeated with some random variation in both the background data and the outbreak signals to study the temporal variation of key performance statistics, such as sensitivity and specificity. Drawbacks to this approach are the difficulty of modeling the background data and the possibility that simulated data might not adequately represent the authentic data encountered by the surveillance system. Sections 10.3.2 through 10.3.4 discuss methods for and issues associated with using authentic outbreaks, simulated outbreaks, and simulated background.

10.3.2 Authentic Outbreaks

Authentic outbreaks tend to be used in evaluations with qualitative outcomes for several reasons: authentic outbreaks are generally small in number, it can be difficult to distinguish between background and outbreak cases, and it can be difficult to establish when an outbreak begins. Evaluations using authentic outbreaks have tended to focus on explaining false positive and false negative detections [1, 21]. Because the data are real, evaluators can identify the impact on outbreak detection of factors such as population sampling and health care utilization patterns. Despite the difficulty of gathering enough data on a number of authentic outbreaks for a quantitative evaluation, some researcher have conducted quantitative evaluations using authentic data [22, 23]. In these situations, the onset of the outbreaks were determined through expert review of the authentic data or use of another external gold standard. The results from such evaluations are useful, but the reliance on an external and imperfect standard to define outbreaks and the constraint of using only outbreaks that have occurred limit the accuracy and usefulness of results from this type of evaluation.

10.3.3 Simulated Outbreaks

Simulated outbreaks are useful for quantitative evaluation of outbreak detection and response protocols, but they do not allow the type of careful qualitative analysis of detection performance that is possible with authentic outbreak data. The methods used to simulate outbreaks vary in complexity. As with the definition of the outbreak scenario, the selection of the simulation method should be tied to the evaluation question, and data produced should be of sufficient but not excessive complexity. The main approaches to simulating outbreaks entail the use of mathematical functions, empirical outbreak distributions, and "mechanistic" models.

10.3.3.1 Mathematical Functions Outbreaks simulated using mathematical functions are used frequently in evaluations involving time-series data. Mathematical (e.g., step, linear) or probability (e.g., exponential, lognormal) functions are used to generate the incidence of the variable under surveillance over time. This is a simple approach to simulating outbreaks that requires few resources and produces an outbreak signal of complexity sufficient for many questions and scenarios of interest [6, 24]. In particular, the lognormal function is a good model of the time to onset of symptoms for many infectious diseases [25].

The limitations on using mathematical functions to generate outbreak signals are the limited complexity of the signals produced by these functions, their limited ability to incorporate information, and the difficulty of relating these abstract shapes to specific outbreak scenarios. Although mathematical functions can generate outbreak time series in a straightforward manner, they cannot generate realistic space-time series or individual records with multiple attributes. In addition, if an evaluator is interested in the impact of increased virulence on outbreak detection, for example, it is not clear how to adjust a mathematical function to mimic a change in virulence. Finally, while some functions, such as lognormal probability distribution functions, may generate realistic symptom-onset epidemic curves, these abstract shapes are still difficult to relate to a specific scenario of public health interest. For this reason, the results from evaluation studies using mathematical functions to simulate outbreaks may be difficult to apply in practice.

10.3.3.2 *Empirical Density Functions*   Empirical density functions [26] estimated from authentic outbreaks can be used to generate simulated outbreaks (Fig. 10.2). As with mathematical functions, these functions are best suited to producing time series, although it is possible to estimate space-time empirical density functions. The function can be taken directly from an observed outbreak, or the empirical density function may be altered by smoothing or scaling. The signals produced are more authentic than the signals generated by a mathematical function, but the drawback is that the signal will also represent faithfully peculiarities of the original scenario that may not be relevant to the evaluation scenario. So, while the signal may be "authentic" for a particular location where the outbreak occurred, it may not be the signal that would be seen if the same outbreak occurred in another location. General-purpose software, such as the GenKern package for the R statistical software, can be used to estimate a function from historical data [27]. Specialized software is also available to facilitate the use of empirical density functions to evaluate outbreak detection [28].

10.3.3.3 *Mechanistic Models*   Mechanistic simulation models generate outbreak signals with enough complexity for evaluating many types of outbreak detection algorithms, for staging realistic response scenarios, and for comparing surveillance to other approaches to outbreak detection. These models are called *mechanistic* because they describe the mechanisms underlying an outbreak, including disease, infection, and health care utilization. People are modeled in either an agent or a network-based framework [29] or as independent stochastic processes [17, 18, 20]. The agent-based model extends naturally to communicable diseases (i.e., an infectious disease that can be spread from person to person), but these models have many parameters and they require extensive computing resources, especially if multiple simulation runs are required.

Modeling people as independent stochastic processes works well for noncommunicable diseases and in scenarios where only primary disease cases are of interest: for example, following a large aerosol release of a bioagent or a large common-source exposure to a foodborne disease. An example of a model used to simulate an outbreak following an aerosol release of anthrax spores is shown in Fig. 10.3. This approach to modeling tends to have fewer parameters than agent-based models because independence is assumed between persons. This simplifying assumption limits the number of parameters in the simulation model and decreases the computational requirements of

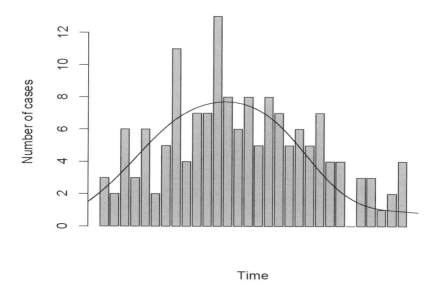

Fig. 10.2 Simulated outbreak generated by an empirical density function. The bars represent the frequency of symptom onset over time, and the line demonstrates an empirical density function [26] fit to the simulated counts.

the model relative to agent-based approaches. To model communicable diseases, this type of model could be linked to the output of a deterministic or stochastic epidemic compartment model.

Both types of models have many parameters, and the influence of parameter value selection on the results may be profound. Evaluations using these types of models should therefore assess the sensitivity of results to parameter value choices. This assessment can be accomplished through univariate sensitivity analysis [18] or a Latin Hypercube Sampling (LHS) design in which all parameter values are varied simultaneously over their prior distributions [30]. LHS is an approach to sampling parameter values from a high-dimensional parameter space to obtain estimates of output variables that are more efficient and precise than would be obtained with simple random sampling [31]. The LHS approach is also attractive because in a study using LHS, the evaluation results integrate uncertainty in parameter values with random variation. When a simulation model is specified, there are K parameters. A given run of the simulation model requires a value for each parameter, or a set of parameter values $\mathbf{X} = \{X_1, \ldots, X_K\}$. Each parameter has a space of possible values $\mathbf{S} = \{S_1, \ldots, S_K\}$. In LHS, the space for each parameter is partitioned into N intervals of probability size $1/N$. The Cartesian product of these intervals partitions

S into N^K cells, which form a hypercube. Obtaining **X** for a simulation run requires random sampling of a partition for each parameter and then sampling a parameter value from within that partition, assuming that values are uniformly distributed within a partition. Figure 10.4 shows an example of the parameter values sampled for the disease model shown in Fig. 10.3.

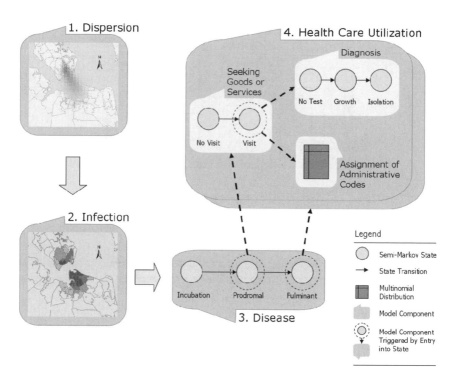

Fig. 10.3 Overview of the components in a mechanistic simulation model using inhalational anthrax as an example. The dispersion component (1) models the release of an agent into the environment and the dose to which a person is exposed at locations throughout the simulation region. The infection component (2) determines the probability of infection given a person's home location. The disease component (3) models the progression over time of infected persons through distinct disease states: incubation, prodromal, and fulminant. Finally, a health care utilization component (4) is associated with a state in the disease component. In this example, the model associated with the prodromal disease state is shown in detail. Upon entering a disease state, a person may seek health care goods or services (i.e., "Visit"). If care is sought, the person may be assigned an administrative code (the subject of syndromic surveillance). In addition, once care is sought, diagnostic tests may be ordered (blood culture, in this example), which may ultimately lead to detection of an outbreak through clinical case findings. A separate health care utilization component may be associated with different states in the disease component.

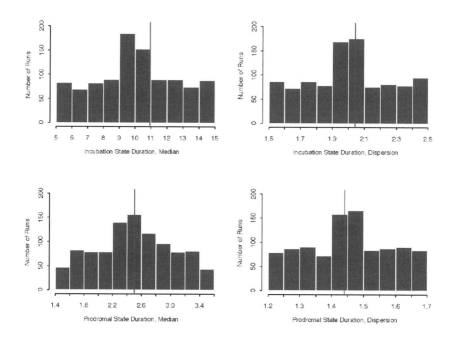

Fig. 10.4   Distribution of sampled values for parameters in the disease component. The vertical lines indicate the best estimate of the value.

10.3.4   Simulated Background

If authentic background data are not available, it is possible to simulate the background. Most healthcare utilization data have regular patterns, such as seasonal and day-of-week patterns, and the background simulated must contain a similar structure.

To generate simulated background data, a time series can first be constructed that represents the time-varying expected value $\mu(t)$ of the data stream. Seasonal fluctuations are added by including an oscillatory term:

$$\mu(t) = \mu_0(1 + A\cos[2\pi(t - t_0)/T]) \qquad (10.1)$$

where μ_0 is the long-term time-series mean, $A \leq 1$ is the relative peak amplitude of the seasonal fluctuations, t is time, t_0 is a time value corresponding to one of the peaks of the fluctuations, and T is the period of the fluctuations.

To produce random variability in this time series, a random draw is taken from the appropriate statistical distribution for each element of the series. The particular distribution used is determined by the expected value $\mu(t)$ and the desired variance-to-mean ratio of the data stream, $k = \sigma^2(t)/\mu(t)$, which should be a constant. If $k = 1$, the appropriate distribution is Poisson with a mean equal to $\mu(t)$. If $k < 1$, the appropriate distribution is binomial with the number of independent trials equal to **round**$[\mu(t)/(1-k)]$ and the probability of success in any given trial equal to $1-k$. If $k > 1$, the appropriate distribution is negative binomial with the number of successes observed equal to $\mu(t)/(k-1)$ and the probability of success in any given trial equal to $1/k$. The resultant time series is adjusted for day-of-week and holiday variability by shifting cases among the elements of the series.

Some statistical software also has packages that are useful for simulating background data. The surveillance package created for the R statistical software is one example [27].

10.4   APPLYING DETECTION ALGORITHMS AND RESPONSE PROTOCOLS

10.4.1   Combining Background and Outbreak Data

If authentic background and outbreak data are used, there is no need to combine data. Otherwise, the outbreak data must be injected into or superimposed onto the background data, which is usually done by adding the outbreak data beginning on randomly selected days in the background data. If desired, a stratified random sample of days can be used to oversample the types of days of interest (e.g., season or day of week). When simulated outbreak data are combined with authentic background data, the usual approach is to combine many different outbreaks in turn with the same series of background data. For data that are entirely simulated, multiple baseline and outbreak series are generated and combined.

10.4.2   Applying Outbreak Detection Algorithms

If the evaluation is using a small number of outbreak series, or if the aim of the exercise is to evaluate the response of analysts to aberration detection, it is preferable to use a real system. The realism will enhance the face validity of the results and will allow analysts to respond naturally during large-scale exercises. On the other hand, if many outbreak series will be used, a model of a real system may be preferable for reasons of efficiency. Operational surveillance systems often contain many features that are not necessary in an evaluation study and that take time to perform. In addition, when large numbers of analyses are performed — usually thousands of runs — vast amounts of data are generated, and mechanisms must be established for storing and indexing the generated data.

10.4.3   Applying Response Protocols

The steps taken to apply response protocols within an evaluation will depend on the type of exercise and the focus of the evaluation (Table 10.2). In most cases, activities will include introductions and orientation; an opportunity to interact with the

Table 10.2   Types of Exercises Conducted to Evaluate the Response to Alarms and System Information in Public Health Settings

Exercise Type	Focus and Purpose
Orientation seminar	Training and familiarization. Provides participants with an overview of concepts, protocols, resources, and expectations.
Tabletop	Training and problem solving. Provides senior staff and planners with an opportunity to discuss response protocols that guide action in a specific scenario.
Drill	Testing and evaluation. Performed to test response times, equipment, personnel readiness, and communication.
Functional	Testing and evaluation. Conducted to test and evaluate capabilities, functions, and activities of the response system.
Full scale	Testing and evaluation. Conducted to test and evaluate a major area or the entire emergency response system.

surveillance system and other resources in an unstructured or semistructured manner; the exercise itself, including data collection; and a postexercise meeting. In the case of multiagency or multijurisdictional exercises, the users can respond and communicate with one another as different people evaluate the data from their regional or agency perspectives. In these cases, an exercise control room is often used with people who can direct the exercise and can simulate responses from different groups (e.g., police, fire, hospital, labs) to inquiries from public health users. A method should be used, such as audio recording or participant observers, to capture key events, decisions, and outcomes throughout each phase of the exercise.

10.5   MEASURING PERFORMANCE

Performance measurement is the step in the overall evaluation where the results from the outbreak detection algorithms or the results of applying the response protocols are analyzed to answer the questions posed at the outset of the evaluation. Several methods are available for evaluating the detection performance and robustness of alerting algorithms used in public health surveillance. These include receiver operating characteristics (ROC) and activity monitoring operating characteristics (AMOC) curves, time-varying ensemble statistics, and summary statistics. The performance metrics should be chosen early in the design of the evaluation.

10.5.1 Outbreak Detection

Sensitivity and specificity are two basic metrics for assessing outbreak detection. A ROC curve allows sensitivity and specificity to be compared over a range of algorithm decision thresholds. Timeliness measures the speed with which an outbreak is detected and can be plotted against specificity in an AMOC curve [32] or against both specificity and sensitivity in a timeliness receiver operating characteristics (TROC) surface [33].

In addition to these measures of accuracy and timeliness, time-varying ensemble statistics allow assessment of detection performance over time, and summary statistics enable characterization of algorithm robustness. These metrics are discussed in more detail in Sections 10.5.1.1 through 10.5.1.6. The discussions use the concept of the alarm value A for an algorithm at a given threshold h for each interval (e.g., day) analyzed j. The alarm value is a binary measure, or

$$A(h)_j = \quad 1 \quad \text{if } S(h, j) > h \qquad (10.2)$$
$$= \quad 0 \quad \text{otherwise}$$

where $S(h, j)$ is a value returned from the algorithm after analysis of the interval j with threshold h.

10.5.1.1 *Specificity*   Specificity is the probability of no alarm when there is no outbreak:

$$\text{specificity} = P(\overline{A}|\overline{O}) = \frac{n(\overline{A}, \overline{O})}{n(\overline{O})} \qquad (10.3)$$

where $n(\overline{O})$ is the number of intervals (e.g., days) in the background data, and $n(\overline{A}, \overline{O})$ is the number of alarms when the algorithm is applied to the background data without any superimposed outbreaks. Specificity is calculated at a decision threshold h as:

$$\text{Sp}(h) = \frac{1}{m} \sum_{j=1}^{m} A(h)_j \qquad (10.4)$$

where there are m analysis intervals in the background data. Note that specificity is calculated using only non-outbreak, or background, data. To determine specificity, an algorithm is applied at a given threshold to the background data. An assumption implicit in this approach to calculating specificity is that any alarm in the background data is a false alarm. This assumption is reasonable if one is interested in detecting only outbreaks due to the specific agent being modeled, but it may lead to conservative estimates of specificity if one is interested in detecting other types of outbreaks as well.

Specificity is calculated per analysis interval and can be converted to an alarm rate per unit time by multiplication by the number of analyses per time interval. People may find it easier to interpret the alarm rate per unit time than specificity.

10.5.1.2 Sensitivity Sensitivity is the probability of an alarm given an outbreak:

$$\text{sensitivity} = P(A|O) = \frac{n(A, O)}{n(O)} \tag{10.5}$$

where $n(O)$ is the number of outbreaks and $n(A, O)$ is the number of outbreaks during which an alarm was sounded. Sensitivity is calculated at a decision threshold h over some number n of evaluation data sets i as:

$$\text{Se}(h) = \frac{1}{n} \sum_{i=1}^{n} \min(1, \sum_{j=1}^{m_i} A(h)_{ij}) \tag{10.6}$$

where there are m_i analysis intervals in data set i. Note that sensitivity measures only whether an alarm occurred at any point during an outbreak; it does not measure the timing of an alarm within an outbreak interval. (This formulation assumes that only one outbreak exists in each evaluation data set.)

Sensitivity is calculated only from the algorithm results during outbreak intervals. The drawback of calculating sensitivity per outbreak is that sensitivity and specificity are not calculated on the same scale, which complicates direct comparison of the two metrics see Section 10.5.1.3). Also, the calculation of sensitivity depends on the definition of outbreak intervals. The outbreak interval can be defined to include the time between the initial infection and the peak day of the outbreak, the entire outbreak period, or some other interval of interest.

10.5.1.3 Accuracy The ROC curve is a means of comparing specificity and sensitivity graphically over a range of algorithm thresholds. Figure 10.5 shows an example ROC curve that quantifies the trade-off between sensitivity and specificity.

In addition, the area under the ROC curve (AUC) is a summary measure of accuracy. It is important to note, however, that the standard approach to calculating the AUC weighs each point on the curve equally, when in reality, points farther to the left (i.e., with higher sensitivity and specificity) are usually of greater interest because this is the range in which it is usually practical to operate a surveillance system. A simple solution to this problem is to plot the ROC and calculate the AUC over a subset of the specificity range, as is done in Figure 10.5. Another note of caution relates to the concept of "random" performance, which is usually a diagonal line on the ROC plot. When sensitivity is calculated per outbreak and specificity is calculated per analysis interval, however, the random line is not necessarily diagonal.

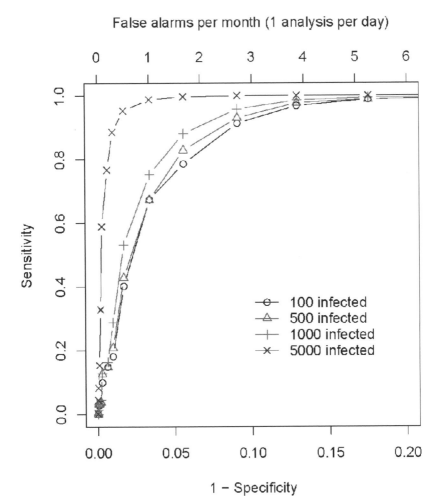

Fig. 10.5 ROC curves for outbreak detection with different numbers of people infected. Note that more outbreaks are detected (i.e., the sensitivity improves) at a given alarm rate as the number infected increases.

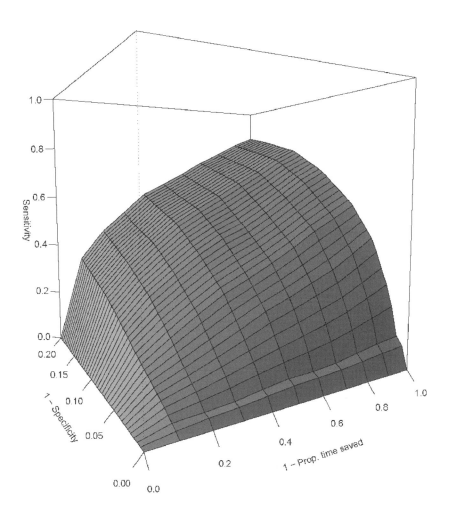

Fig. 10.6 Example timeliness ROC surface. The surface shows, at different alarm rates (FP), the frequency (TP) with which a proportion of time was saved through surveillance compared with outbreak detection through clinical case finding. See Buckeridge et al. [30] for details of the model to estimate the time to detection through clinical case finding. The top-right corner demonstrates, for example, that some time was saved (i.e., 1 – proportion of time saved was ≤ 1.0) in over 80% of outbreaks when 1 – specificity (or FP) rose to 0.2. See Fig. 10.7 for two-dimensional slices through the surface at different alarm rates.

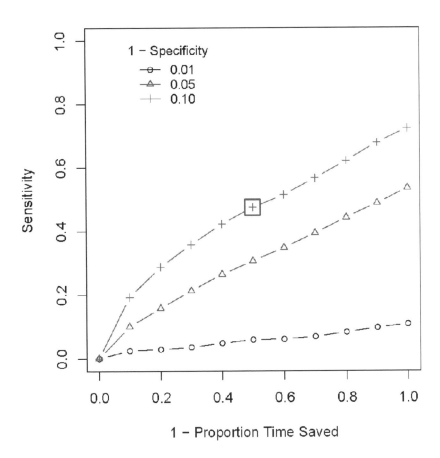

Fig. 10.7   Two-dimensional slices through the TROC surface shown in Fig. 10.6.   These two-dimensional slices demonstrate the proportion of outbreaks (sensitivity) for which a given amount of time was saved through syndromic surveillance relative to clinical case finding (1-proportion of time saved) at three alarm rates.   The point in the box indicates that when the system was operated at an alarm rate of 0.10, surveillance saved at least 50% of the time (i.e., 1-proportion of time saved, on the horizontal axis) in nearly half of the simulated outbreaks (i.e., sensitivity, on the vertical axis).

10.5.1.4 Timeliness   Timeliness of outbreak detection can be measured relative to the onset of the outbreak or relative to the time of detection through another method. In both cases, timeliness can be expressed as units of time or the proportion of time saved. Timeliness is calculated relative to the onset of an outbreak for a single simulated outbreak as:

$$T(h, i) = \min_{j}(j : A(h)_{ij} = 1) \qquad (10.7)$$

where there are m_i intervals i, and timeliness is not defined if $\sum_{j=1}^{m_i} A(h)_{ij} = 0$. It is possible to plot timeliness against specificity, to generate an AMOC curve [32]. Timeliness is undefined when the outbreak is not detected, however, so AMOC curves must be interpreted in the context of the corresponding sensitivity across the range of specificity. One solution is to plot ROC and AMOC curves together, allowing both to be inspected simultaneously. Another solution is to plot the three-dimensional surface formed by specificity, sensitivity, and timeliness, as shown in Fig. 10.6. The volume under this TROCS surface provides a summary measure of accuracy-weighted timeliness, analogous to the AUC for the ROC [33]. This surface plot, however, presents a considerable amount of information and may be difficult to interpret. An alternative is to plot two-dimensional cuts through the surface, as shown in Fig. 10.7.

10.5.1.5 Time-Varying Ensemble Statistics   Although ROC curves, AMOC curves, and TROC surfaces are useful for characterizing overall detection performance, they are less useful for describing how detection performance varies with respect to time in a given data stream, information that is helpful for characterizing algorithm robustness. One method of investigating this behavior is simply to plot the individual time series associated with a number of key statistics, such as the daily count values predicted by the alerting algorithm and the corresponding test statistics.

However, if fully simulated data are being used, a much more powerful analysis can be conducted. First, multiple random realizations of the data stream are generated for the test case of interest. Each of these realizations is processed individually by the algorithm being evaluated, and the ensemble statistics of interest are then calculated and plotted as functions of time element by element across all realizations of the series. Some potentially useful statistics that can be plotted in this manner include the median values and confidence intervals of the observed count, the expected count, the threshold count (which is the minimum count needed to trigger an alert), the standardized alert threshold (defined in the next paragraph), the test statistic, the sensitivity to a sudden spike, and the specificity. If multiple levels of alerts are used, the multinomial distribution of alert types can also be plotted as a function of time. A typical presentation of some time-varying ensemble statistics is shown in Fig. 10.8.

An especially useful statistic for quantifying algorithm robustness is the *standardized alert threshold*. This statistic, which is expressed in multiples of the standard deviation of the data stream expected on a given day, can be obtained by dividing the difference between the threshold count and the observed count by the expected time-varying standard deviation $\sigma(t) = \sqrt{k\mu(t)}$. Whenever the value of this statistic

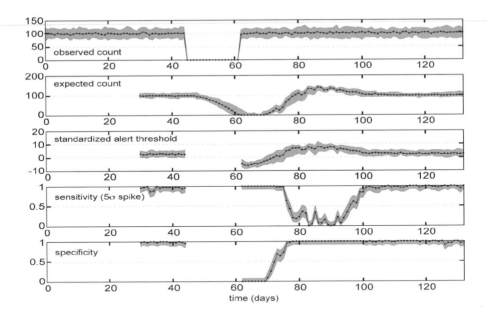

Fig. 10.8 Examples of time-varying ensemble statistics for evaluating the variation in detection performance as a function of time of a data stream.

is zero or negative, an alert is produced. Whenever the value is positive, an alert would have been produced by a sudden spike with a magnitude greater than or equal to that number of standard deviations above the observed count. With this statistic, algorithm robustness may be understood in terms of the time variation of algorithm sensitivity and specificity.

A useful statistic for quantifying detection sensitivity and timeliness is the *detection log-likelihood ratio*. First, a time series is calculated representing the running probability of obtaining at least one alert after the beginning of an upsurge. A reference series is calculated similarly, but without the upsurge. The detection log-likelihood ratio is then obtained by dividing the probability with the upsurge present by the probability with the upsurge absent and taking the base 10 logarithm. When the value of this statistic is positive, the alerting algorithm has a larger than random likelihood of detecting the upsurge, while a negative value means a smaller than random likelihood. The more rapid the rise of this statistic after the beginning of the upsurge, the more timely the detection.

10.5.1.6 Summary Statistics   Although curves such as those discussed can be useful for characterizing algorithm performance in great detail, it is often helpful to distill the key information to a few summary values, especially for characterizing algorithm robustness. Calculation of the average values of certain statistics during a fixed time interval following a transient event (e.g., the sensitivity and specificity during the

Test Case	Detector 1		Detector 2		Detector 3		Detector 4	
	ST	DOR	ST	DOR	ST	DOR	ST	DOR
Startup	8	7	8	3	31	30	15	14
Startup: Leading Zeros	8	7	8	3	NaN	NaN	16	15
DOW: Civilian Office Visits	29	7	29	3	31	30	15	14
DOW: Military Office Visits	6	5	5	4	31	30	15	14
DOW: School Absenteeism	22	11	9	2	31	30	35	23
Post-Upsurge	13	12	13	12	1	0	1	0
Post-Outlier	31	26	31	26	1	0	1	0
Post-Dropout	31	2	1	0	1	0	1	0
Post-Step: Up	11	10	11	10	26	12	27	11
Post-Step: Down	31	30	31	30	17	16	17	16

Fig. 10.9 Examples of summary statistics for evaluating the robustness of detection performance. ST refers to settle time, DOR to days out of range and DOW to day of the week.

7 days after the resumption of data following a drop-out), usually allows algorithm robustness to be characterized quite effectively with respect to that event.

In addition to the time-averaged sensitivity and specificity, two other summary statistics that can be useful for characterizing algorithm robustness are the *settle time* (ST) and the *days out of range* (DOR). ST is defined as the number of days required for the standardized alert threshold to settle within some acceptable range following a transient event. DOR is defined as the number of days on which the standardized alert threshold does not lie within the acceptable range during the settling period.

Two summary statistics that can be useful for characterizing detection sensitivity and timeliness are the *maximum detection log-likelihood ratio* (MDLLR) and the *detection time* (DT). MDLLR is defined as the peak value of the detection log-likelihood ratio curve. DT is defined as the number of days required from the beginning of the upsurge to achieve that peak value.

To evaluate the detection performance and robustness of an alerting algorithm quickly or to compare the performance of multiple algorithms, it can be useful to display the summary statistics in a series of tables. A separate table can be prepared for each group of related statistics (e.g., specificity and sensitivity, ST and DOR, MDLLR and DT). Within each table, the results for each test case can be listed in separate rows, the values of each summary statistic can be listed in minor columns, and the results for each algorithm can be grouped into major columns. Cell shading can be used to indicate whether these values are acceptable, unacceptable, or indeterminate. An example of such a table is shown in Fig. 10.9.

10.5.2 Response Protocols

The approach to measuring performance by the application of response protocols is linked to the type of exercise performed (see Section 10.4.3). The kinds of questions that might be considered include:

- How do the actions taken by participants compare to the actions described in the response protocol?

- What are the differences between the actions and the protocol, and what is the likely impact of these differences?

- What system or protocol changes, or training, may be needed to address the differences observed?

Evaluation of response protocol performance may be quantitative, but it is more likely to be qualitative. For example, if a participant observer collected notes during the application of the response protocols, the dominant themes may be identified and summarized for discussion in a focus group. A similar approach could be taken by transcribing audio recordings of the exercise and using qualitative data analysis to identify important issues. Surveys or interviews of participants may also provide useful information.

10.6 SUMMARY

As interest and investment in automated syndromic surveillance increases, evaluation is required to ensure that the method is used effectively by public health agencies. An evaluation that examines many components of a surveillance system from many different perspectives is needed. For some types of evaluations, such as those that evaluate system quality, information quality, and user experiences, suitable methods exist and should be applied [34]. Evaluation of outbreak detection and human response to system alarms, however, requires novel methods.

This chapter presents the steps to evaluate outbreak detection and alarm protocols, and examines in some detail recently developed methods for these types of evaluations. In particular, the focus is on methods for simulating disease outbreaks and for measuring outbreak detection performance. The number of evaluations of automated syndromic surveillance is increasing and more attention is being given to the methods used in these evaluations. This development and application of evaluation methods is important, and it is expected that the understanding of the effectiveness and benefit of automated syndromic surveillance in defined settings for defined tasks will increase as this evaluation work continues.

10.7   STUDY QUESTIONS

10.1 This chapter focuses on evaluation of outbreak detection and response protocols. As discussed in Section 10.1.2, however, there are other aspects of a surveillance system that could be the focus of an evaluation. *Q: Describe the steps that you would take to evaluate system quality and information quality.*

10.2 The use of mathematical functions to simulate disease outbreaks was discussed in Section 10.3.3. These functions are convenient to use but may not reflect the temporal dynamics of a real outbreak. *Q: If you assume that a real outbreak will have a shape like a lognormal distribution, what might be the effect on sensitivity and timeliness of using an exponential or linear function to simulate outbreaks for use in an evaluation?*

10.3 In an evaluation of response protocols, extensive resources may be required to conduct an exercise where public health personnel respond to a simulated outbreak scenario. *Q: Describe the resources that would be required for an exercise involving only a small surveillance team within a public health department. How would the required resources change if other agencies, such as police and health care institutions, were to be included in the exercise?*

10.4 In measuring timeliness, equal weight can be given to time at the outset of an outbreak and time later in an outbreak. For example, outbreak detection on day 2 of an outbreak lasting 4 days will save 2 days, and outbreak detection on day 10 of an outbreak lasting 12 days will also save 2 days. Intuitively, however, the first example seems more useful. *Q: How can you take this type of scenario into account when calculating timeliness?*

REFERENCES

1. Heffernan R, Mostashari F, Das D, Karpati A, Kulldorf M, Weiss D. Syndromic surveillance in public health practice, New York City. Emerg Infect Dis. 2004;10(5):858-64.

2. Buehler JW, Berkelman RL, Hartley DM, Peters CJ. Syndromic surveillance and bioterrorism-related epidemics. Emerg Infect Dis. 2003; 9(10): 1197-1204.

3. Sosin M, DeThomasis J. Evaluation challenges for syndromic surveillance: making incremental progress. MMWR. 2004; 53(suppl): 125-129.

4. Becker J. High-tech health watch draws cash, questions. The Washington Post, November 23, 2003;A17.

5. Reingold A. If syndromic surveillance is the answer, what is the question? Biosecurity Bioterrorism. 2003;1(2):77-81.

6. Stoto MA, Schonlau M, Mariano LT. Syndromic surveillance: is it worth the effort? Chance. 2004; 17(1): 19-24.

7. Bravata DM, McDonald KM, Smith WM, et al. Systematic review: surveillance systems for early detection of bioterrorism-related diseases. Ann Intern Med. 2004; 140(11): 910-922.

8. Buckeridge DL. Outbreak detection through automated surveillance: a review of determinants of detection. J Biomed Inf. 2007; submitted.

9. Centers for Disease Control and Prevention. Updated guidelines for evaluating public health surveillance sytems: recommendations from the Guidelines Working Group. MMWR 2001; 50(RR-13).

10. Buehler JW, Hopkins RS, Overhage JM, Sosin DM, Tong V. Framework for evaluating public health surveillance systems for early detection of outbreaks: recommendations from the CDC working group. MMWR Recomm Rep. 2004; 53(RR-5): 1-11.

11. DeLone WH, McLean ER. Information systems success: the quest for the dependent variable. Inform Sys Res. 1992;3(1):60-95.

12. DeLone WH, McLean ER. The DeLone and McLean model of information systems success: a ten-year update. J Manage Inf Sys. 2003;19(4):9-30.

13. Public Health Informatics Institute. Towards measuring value: an evaluation framework for public health information systems. PHII Technical Report. April 2005.

14. US Department of Homeland Security; Office of Domestic Preparedness. Homeland security exercise and evaluation program, Vol I: Overview and doctrine. Technical Report. 2003.

15. Happel Lewis SL, Cutchis PN, Babin SM, Burkom HS. Simulated release of plague in Montgomery County, Maryland. Johns Hopkins APL Tech Dig. 2003; 24(4): 354-359.

16. Association of State and Territorial Health Officials. Guide to preparedness evaluation using drills and table top exercises. Technical Report. 2002.

17. Buckeridge DL, Burkom HS, Moore A, Pavlin J, Cutchis PN, Hogan W. Evaluation of syndromic surveillance systems: design of an epidemic simulation model. MMWR. 2004; 53(suppl): 137-143.

18. Buckeridge DL, Switzer P, Owens D, Siegrist D, Pavlin J, Musen M. An evaluation model for syndromic surveillance: assessing the performance of a temporal algorithm. MMWR. 2005;54(suppl):109-115.

19. Mandl KD, Reis B, Cassa C. Measuring outbreak-detection performance by using controlled feature set simulations. MMWR. 2004; 53(suppl): 130-136.

20. Kleinman KP, Abrams A, Mandl K, Platt R. Simulation for assessing statistical methods of biologic terrorism surveillance. MMWR. 2005; 54(suppl): 101-108.

21. Balter S, Weiss D, Hanson H, Reddy V, Das D, Heffernan R. Three years of emergency department gastrointestinal syndromic surveillance in New York City: what have we found? MMWR. 2005; 54(suppl): 175-180.

22. Siegrist D, Pavlin J. Bio-Alert biosurveillance detection algorithm evaluation. MMWR. 2004; 53(suppl): 152-158.

23. Hogan WR, Tsui FC, Ivanov O, et al. Detection of pediatric respiratory and diarrheal outbreaks from sales of over-the-counter electrolyte products. J Am Med Inf Assoc. 2003;10(6):555-562.

24. Reis BY, Pagano M, Mandl KD. Using temporal context to improve biosurveillance. Proc Natl Acad Sci USA. 2003; 100(4): 1961-1965.

25. Sartwell PE. The distribution of incubation periods of infectious diseases. J Hyg. 1950; 51: 310-318.

26. Gentle JE, ed. Elements of Computational Statistics. New York:Springer-Verlag; 2002.

27. R Development Core Team. R: A Language and Environment for Statistical Computing. Vienna, Austria; R Foundation for Statistical Computing; 2006.

28. Wallstrom GL, Wagner M, Hogan W. High-fidelity injection detectability experiments: a tool for evaluating syndromic surveillance systems. MMWR. 2005; 54(suppl): 85-91.

29. Eubank S. Network based models of infectious disease spread. Jpn J Infect Dis. 2005;58(6):S9-S13.

30. Buckeridge DL, Owens DK, Switzer P, Frank J, Musen MA. Evaluating detection of an inhalational anthrax outbreak. Emerg Infect Dis. 2006; 12(12).

31. McKay MD, Beckman RJ, Conover WJ. A comparison of three methods for selecting values of input variables in the analysis of output from a computer code. Technometrics. 1979;21:239-245.

32. Fawcett T, Provost F. Activity monitoring: noticing interesting changes in behavior. Presented at the 5th International Conference on Knowledge Discovery and Data Mining; 1999.

33. Kleinman K, Abrams A. Metrics for assessing the performance of spatial surveillance. Stat Methods Med Res. 2006;15(5).

34. Friedman CP, Wyatt JC, eds. Evaluation Methods in Biomedical Informatics. 2nd ed. New York:Springer; 2006.

11 Educating the Workforce: Public Health Informatics Training

Harold Lehmann

The "workforce" in public health comprises many professions, ranging from office clerks to national directors, from direct providers of health care to formulators of health policy. Since the publication of the Institute of Medicine's (IOM) seminal position statement [1], the American public health community has researched the state of that workforce, has formulated the educational needs, and has worked at fulfilling those needs. Disease surveillance ranks as a core competency in the IOM-based framework, under the guise of "monitoring health status," and different educational approaches meet its needs to a varying degree [2]. This chapter reviews the educational framework for training in surveillance as currently practiced, including distance-education-based opportunities and reports on the state of public health informatics training, a novel approach to meeting these educational needs.

11.1 COMPETENCIES FOR DISEASE SURVEILLANCE

Curriculum developers increasingly structure teaching around the concept of *competencies* [3], measurable behaviors that a person needs to demonstrate [4]. *Competence*, on the other hand, tends to refer to the (minimum) standards that those behaviors ought to achieve [5]. A core competency takes the role that functional specifications do in information system design, providing specifications for teaching (learning) objectives and providing the basis for evaluating students and programs.

In public health, the Council on Linkages Between Academia and Public Health Practice and the Public Health Foundation, both of whose agendas concern implementation of the IOM framework, put core competencies at the focus of their efforts. They define core competencies as "the individual skills desirable for the delivery of Essential Public Health Services" [6]. The two relevant services for our purposes are (1) to monitor health status to identify community health problems, and (2) to diagnose and investigate health problems and health hazards in the community (see Table 11.1). A focus on competencies is the recommendation of a recent policy article as well [3], a follow-up on these authors' 2004 article [7]. In bioterrorism self-assessment, surveillance was not raised as an important skill [8]. However, the strategy Healthy People 2010, which defines the U.S. government's public health approach, raises surveillance as an important function of the public health infrastructure [9].

Table 11.1   Essential Health Services in Public Health (From Office of Disease Prevention and Health Promotion [54]).

1.	Monitor health status to identify community health problems
2.	Diagnose and investigate health problems and health hazards in the community
3.	Inform, educate, and empower people about health issues
4.	Mobilize community partnerships to identify and solve health problems
5.	Develop policies and plans that support individual and community health efforts
6.	Enforce laws and regulations that protect health and ensure safety
7.	Link people to needed personal health services and assure the provision of health care when otherwise unavailable
8.	Assure a competent public health and personal health care workforce
9.	Evaluate effectiveness, accessibility, and quality of personnel and population-based health services
10.	Research for new insights and innovative solutions to health problems

Within the Council on Linkage's definition of core competency, intended levels of mastery, and therefore learning objectives for workers within each competency, will differ depending on their backgrounds and job duties [6]. Educators must specify core competencies further, based on the skill goal of their students. The Council on Linkages specifies three levels of job categories — front-line staff, senior-level staff, and supervisory and management staff — and three levels of skill:

- *Aware:* basic level of mastery of the competency. Individuals may be able to identify the concept or skill but have limited ability to perform the skill.

- *Knowledgeable:* intermediate level of mastery of the competency. Individuals are able to apply and describe the skill.

- *Advanced:* advanced level of mastery of the competency. Individuals are able to synthesize, critique or teach the skill. (Formerly used *proficient*). [6]

The current chapter will address these three skill levels.

To help in defining teaching objectives within the core competencies, Tables 11.2a-11.2h lay out the skill classes needed within the two primary essential services. The tables show the large amount of overlap in the two services, with few skills unique to either one. These tables and the Case Studies in (Chapters 6 to 10) make clear the relevance for surveillance of skills beyond the technical expertise in outlier detection.

Table 11.2a   Core Competencies for Essential Services 1 (Monitor Health Status) and 2 (Diagnose & Investigate Health Problems and Health Hazards in the Community), continued. *Source*: **Public Health Foundation [55].**

Policy Development/ Program Planning Skills	*Essential Service # 1*	*Essential Service # 2*
Collects, summarizes, & interprets information relevant to an issue	√	√
States policy options & writes clear & concise policy statements		√
Articulates the health, fiscal, administrative, legal, social, & political implications of each policy option		√
States the feasibility & expected outcomes of each policy option		√
Decides on the appropriate course of action	√	√
Develops mechanisms to monitor & evaluate programs for their effectiveness & quality		√

The September 11 terrorist attacks, the anthrax attacks, and the worldwide increase in terrorism have promoted public health preparedness as a vital function. Rather than define preparedness as an essential service, public health leaders have mapped the needs of preparedness to the existing services [10] and have turned those competencies into curricula [11]. Although the World Health Organization (WHO) publishes many guidances for training in areas of public health, surveillance does not get specific treatment in the WHO library.

From the informatics perspective, competencies have been defined by the Education Working Group of the International Medical Informatics Association for informatics training that does refer to public health, but the competencies listed are not really specific to public health, and certainly not to surveillance [12].

Table 11.2b   Core Competencies for Essential Services 1 (Monitor Health Status) and 2 (Diagnose & Investigate Health Problems and Health Hazards in the Community). *Source*: **Public Health Foundation [55].**

Analytic/Assessment Skills	Essential Service #1	Essential Service #2
Defines a problem	√	√
Determines appropriate uses & limitations of both quantitative & qualitative data	√	√
Selects and defines variables relevant to defined public health systems	√	√
Identifies relevant & appropriate data & information sources	√	√
Evaluates the integrity & comparability of data & identifies gaps in data sources	√	√
Applies ethical principles to the collection, maintenance, use, & dissemination of data & information	√	√
Partners with communities to attach meaning to collected quantitative & qualitative data		√
Makes relevant inferences from quantitative & qualitative data	√	√
Obtains & interprets information regarding risks & benefits to the community	√	√
Applies data collection processes, information technology applications, & computer systems storage/ retrieval strategies	√	
Recognizes how the data illuminate ethical, political, scientific, economic, & overall public health issues	√	√

Table 11.2c   Core Competencies for Essential Services 1 (Monitor Health Status) and 2 (Diagnose & Investigate Health Problems and Health Hazards in the Community), continued. *Source*: **Public Health Foundation [55].**

Communication Skills	*Essential Service # 1*	*Essential Service & 2*
Communicates effectively both in writing & orally, or in other ways	√	√
Solicits input from individuals & organizations	√	
Advocates for public health programs & resources	√	
Leads & participates in groups to address specific issues	√	√
Uses the media, advanced technologies, & community networks to communicate information	√	√
Effectively presents accurate demographic statistical, programmatic, & scientific information for professional & lay audiences	√	√
Listens to others in an unbiased manner, respects points of view of others, & promotes the expression of diverse opinions & perspectives (attitude)	√	√

Table 11.2d   Core Competencies for Essential Services 1 (Monitor Health Status) and 2 (Diagnose & Investigate Health Problems and Health Hazards in the Community), continued. *Source*: **Public Health Foundation [55].**

Cultural Competency Skills	*Essential Service # 1*	*Essential Service # 2*
Utilizes appropriate methods for interacting sensitively, effectively, & professionally with persons from diverse cultural, socioeconomic, educational, racial, ethnic & professional backgrounds, & persons of all ages & lifestyle preferences	√	√
Understands the dynamic forces contributing contributing to cultural diversity (attitude)	√	√

Table 11.2e **Core Competencies for Essential Services 1 (Monitor Health Status) and 2 (Diagnose & Investigate Health Problems and Health Hazards in the Community), continued.** *Source*: **Public Health Foundation [55].**

Community Dimensions of Practice Skills	Essential Service # 1	Essential Service # 2
Develops, implements, and evaluates a community public health assessment	√	√
Accomplishes effective community engagements		√
Identifies community assets & available resources		√

Table 11.2f **Core Competencies for Essential Services 1 (Monitor Health Status) and 2 (Diagnose & Investigate Health Problems and Health Hazards in the Community), continued.** *Source*: **Public Health Foundation [55].**

Basic Public Health Sciences Skills	Essential Service # 1	Essential Service # 2
Defines, assesses, & understands the health status of populations, determinants of health & illness, factors contributing to health promotion & disease prevention, & factors influencing the use of health services	√	√
Identifies & applies basic research methods used in public health		√
Applies the basic public health sciences including behavioral and social sciences, biostatistics, epidemiology, environmental public health, & prevention of chronic & infectious diseases & injuries	√	√

Table 11.2g   Core Competencies for Essential Services 1 (Monitor Health Status) and 2 (Diagnose & Investigate Health Problems and Health Hazards in the Community), continued. *Source*: **Public Health Foundation [55].**

Financial Planning & Management Skills	Essential Service # 1	Essential Service # 2
Develops & presents a budget	√	√
Manages program within budget constraints	√	√
Applies budget processes	√	√
Develops strategies for determining budget priorities	√	√
Monitors program performance	√	√
Prepares proposals for funding from external sources	√	√
Applies basic human relations skills to the management of organizations, motivation of personnel, & resolution of conflicts	√	√
Manages information systems for collection, retrieval, & use of data for decision-making	√	√

Table 11.2h   Core Competencies for Essential Services 1 (Monitor Health Status) and 2 (Diagnose & Investigate Health Problems and Health Hazards in the Community), continued. *Source*: **Public Health Foundation [55].**

Leadership and Systems Thinking Skills	Essential Service # 1	Essential Service # 2
Creates a culture of ethical standards within organizations & communities	√	√
Identifies internal & external issues that may impact delivery of essential public health services (i.e., strategic planning)	√	√

11.2   PROFESSIONS OF DISEASE SURVEILLANCE

The WHO defines *surveillance* as "ongoing systematic collection, collation, analysis and interpretation of data and the dissemination of information to those who need to know in order that action may be taken" [13, 14], while CDC uses the definition, "the ongoing systematic collection, analysis, and interpretation of outcome-specific data for use in the planning, implementation and evaluation of public health practice" [15]. *Screening*, a component of surveillance, is "the use of simple tests across a healthy population in order to identify individuals who have disease, but do not yet have symptoms" [16]. The workforce in public health comprises many professions: ranging from office clerks to national directors; from direct providers of health care to formulators of health policy. Literature searches in PubMed and EMBASE focused specifically on surveillance and workforce education and training yield no references. Several surveys over the past few years have assessed the size, activity profile, and educational needs of each contributing profession for the more general essential services. The most recent was in 2005, commissioned by the Health Resources and Services Administration (HRSA) and examined six states — New Mexico, Montana, Georgia, California, Texas, and New York — representing different formulas for the relationship between the state and local public health agencies [17]. An earlier assessment was published in 2000 [18]. These surveys did not examine the performance or needs of managed care organizations as deliverers of population health. The following paragraphs summarize the 2005 report, filtered through the concerns of disease surveillance and reinforced by cognate research in North Carolina [19], further research in Texas [20], and rural UK [21]. Surveillance or screening per se is not addressed in these last three reports.

The HRSA report [17] acknowledges the range of public health professions, at a proportion of 60 to 95 per 100,000 population: general, nurse, physician, oral health, nutrition, social work, health education, epidemiologist, and so on. The researchers found a uniform need for health practitioners to improve their knowledge of bioterrorism and disaster preparedness, core public health principles, and epidemiology. Scientific/investigative work comprised 3 to 20% of the workforce; epidemiologists were 1 to 5% of the practitioners. All expressed a need for more education, especially training that bridged the academic and practice communities. However, there was a "substantial opportunity costs for individuals who sought MPH training," indicating a need either for true release time or for novel approaches to training, especially for senior staff.

11.3   TRAINING OPPORTUNITIES IN PUBLIC HEALTH EDUCATION

To match the demonstrated needs of the workforce for traditional and novel methods of learning, the public health community has assembled a range of options for students and practitioners. This section will address surveillance training provided in the context of public health education; the next section will address surveillance training in the context of informatics training.

The Council on Education for Public Health [22] defines the accreditation criteria for schools and programs. The most recent amendment (June 2005) contains neither surveillance, screening, nor informatics criteria. The Master's Degree in Public Health Core Competency Development Project of the Association of Schools of Public Health lists screening in its epidemiology competencies but has not yet incorporated informatics formally [23], although researchers in the workforce see that coming soon [3]. Public health surveillance, as a topic, can garner continuing education credits.

Despite the lack of current formal stipulations, many schools and training centers currently offer students and professionals the opportunities called for by analyses of the workforce. HRSA established under Section 766 of the Public Health Service Act, as amended by Public Law 105-392 in November 1998 a national network of 14 public health training centers [24]. The centers focus on providing courses, over half of them distance-based. Few courses relate directly to surveillance. For instance, the Mid-America Public Health Training Center provides a course on surveillance in rural counties [25], and the Northwest Center for Public Health Practice offers a course on public health surveillance and hot topics in preparedness [26].

The Centers for Disease Control and Prevention (CDC) manages educational programs of its own. For practitioners around the country, they publish lecture and learning material of a host of topics, including over 100 lectures on surveillance topics alone. For professionals wanting more formal training, they offer several epidemiology-related programs [27]. None is focused specifically on surveillance.

Partners in Information Access for the Public Health Workforce [28] provides a comprehensive list of training opportunities throughout the workforce, including many distance-education opportunities. The Association of Schools of Public Health maintains a list of distance-education opportunities, indexed by the essential services (see the association's website for further information) [24].

11.4 INFORMATICS TRAINING

The need for informatics in public health and for informatics training in public health predates the recent upsurge of interest in disease surveillance, but the promise of real-time biosurveillance has heightened the awareness of the relationship between informatics and biosurveillance [29]. Certainly, public health researchers and practitioners were involved in public health informatics even before this discipline had a name. Self-identified programs in public health informatics training date at least back to the mid-1990s, when the CDC began its informatics course for public health managers [30] and began its informatics training fellowship. The need for workforce training in informatics was recognized at the seminal spring meeting of the American Medical Informatics Association in 2001 [31], where 16 recommendations were offered. The Northwest Center for Public Health Practice took one of those recommendations to heart and formed a working group to assemble public health informatics competencies [32]. Bryant Karras, under a contract with the CDC, is currently working on updating those competencies (personal communication).

The International Medical Informatics Association (IMIA) recommendations for health informatics training divide informatics students into two groups: information technology (IT) users and health and medical informatics professionals [12]. The 2002 public health informatics competencies divide the users into those who require effective use of information, effective use of information technology, and effective management of information technology projects [32]. Covvey and colleagues in their exemplary document on health informatics training objectives divide the informatics field into applied, research and development, and clinician [33]. Lehmann extended these further into two axes (see Fig. 11.1): professional role [34] and informatics role [35]. These axes implicitly define 25 sets of competencies (one at each intersection box), where many specific competencies overlap.

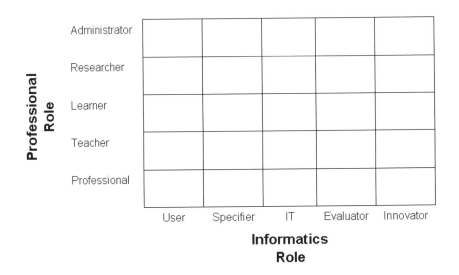

Fig. 11.1 Proposed space for educational interventions in public health informatics. *Professional role:* A single person may have these multiple roles: public health professional (epidemiologist, policymaker, etc.), teacher (to clients, colleagues), learner (continuously), researcher (at the least, describing his or her own performance across cases), and administrator. *Informatics role:* Users (use information via information technology for decision making and other aspects of their job), specifier (domain professional who defines the specifications of an information system), IT (ranging from tech support to system developer), evaluator (confirming that a system meets its specifications but also whether the system as intervention has achieved its goals), and innovator (informatics researcher or novel policymaker).

The needs for surveillance professionals mirror those of informatics. In the professional-role axis, public health practitioners must make judgments regarding diseases for which they screen and perform surveillance; they must teach and explain to their supervisors and to the public the implications of their results; they must continually learn and update their knowledge about the specific diseases as well as surveillance methods; they must either perform research as part of their practice or simply review their performance across instances of surveillance; and they must administer the surveillance program. From the informatics perspective, each professional level must use information, may specify the system that collects and manages the information, must develop and manage the system, may evaluate the system, or may innovate to create new systems, from either the technical or policy perspectives.

11.4.1 Training Opportunities in Public Health Informatics

Training opportunities in public health informatics range from certificates, based on a small number of courses, through degree programs. The University of Pittsburgh offers a five-course certificate in biosurveillance [36], and Loma Linda, in geoinformatics [37]. The University of Maryland [38] and University of Texas [39] offer a certificate program in the more general public health informatics. The program at the University of Illinois–Chicago can be taken online, for either a master's degree or a certificate [40]. Emory also offers both levels of programs [41].

The CDC has provided training in public health informatics for several years [42] where public health-trained professionals gain experience in developing public health information systems. The Robert Wood Johnson Foundation, partly to implement the training recommendation of the 2001 AMIA Spring Conference [31], initiated in 2004 a fellowship training program in public health "as a strategy to catalyze the development of the field and create a sustainable pipeline of future leaders in public health informatics" [43]. Partnering with the National Library of Medicine, extra fellowship slots were added to existing informatics-training programs at Columbia University [44], Johns Hopkins [45], the University of Utah [46], and the University of Washington [47].

Programs outside the United States include Lancashire's distance certificate program in public health informatics [48], the MPH in public health informatics at the University of Essex [49], the new certificate program at Curtin University of Technology in Perth [50], and the more general health informatics program at the School of Public Health at the University of New South Wales [51].

With the recent attention to national health care information infrastructure and networking, it is clear that many informatics specialists will be needed to see these efforts through. Although the Office of the National Coordinator for Healthcare Information Technology did not place informatics training in their framework [52], the American Medical Informatics Association is committed to training "10,000 informatics specialists by 2010" in their "10 × 10" program [53]. Although public health informatics is not an offering at the time of this writing, it probably will be by the time of publication or shortly thereafter. The need for the 10 x 10 program is evident from the various national efforts for a national health care information network that will require informatics expertise, although training of informatics specialists was not part of the initial national framework

11.5   CONCLUSIONS

Education and training in public health, surveillance, and informatics is achieving greater professionalization and organization. There are no outcomes data regarding the effectiveness of the new programs, either to advance individual careers or to improve the public's health. However, these recent efforts show great promise to apply the results of informatics results to the practice of public health and to improve the health of the nation and the world.

11.6   STUDY QUESTIONS

11.1 *Q: Assemble a list of competencies from the prior chapters. Next to each, check off the level you would like to attain: aware, knowledgeable, advanced. Has this book satisfied the "aware" and "knowledgeable" columns?*

11.2 *Q: To what extent do you feel that it is adequate to leave surveillance spread across the other essential services? Is it important enough to stand alone?*

11.3 *Q: The skills listed in Table 11.1 are relatively generic. How would you make them more specific for surveillance?*

11.4 Educational competency is often expressed in terms of "Knows that" and "Knows how." *Q: How would you construct a study to evaluate the effectiveness of general public health training in satisfying the "Knows how" set of competencies?*

11.5 Looking at yourself as a public health practitioner, peruse the public health training centers' educational offerings. *Q: What impresses you? What is missing?*

11.6 Locate yourself in as many boxes as is relevant in the grid in Fig. 11.1. *Q: Rate how confident you are with your knowledge and skills in each of those locations. What experiences (educational, practical) do you need to raise each box to its highest level? Are those experiences available?*

Acknowledgments

Thanks to our informatics fellows, Gregory Butchy, Paulina Sockolow, Patricia Abbot, Naima Carter-Monroe, Yakubo Owolabi, and Katherine Ball, for vetting the model in Figure 11.1.

Thanks to Nancy Roderer for reviewing an earlier draft of this chapter. Dr. Lehmann's educational activities are supported by T15 LM007452.

REFERENCES

1. Institute of Medicine, Committee for the Study of the Future of Public Health. The Future of Public Health. Washington, DC: National Academies Press; 1988.

2. Gebbie K, Rosenstock L, Hernandez LM, eds, Committee on Educating Public Health Professionals for the 21st Century. Who Will Keep the Public Healthy? Educating Public Health Professionals for the 21st Century. Washington, DC: National Academies Press; 2003.

3. Gebbie KM, Turnock BJ. The public health workforce, 2006: new challenges. Health Aff (Millwood). July–Aug 2006;25(4):923–933.

4. Strebler M, Robinson D, Heron P. Getting the Best Out of Your Competencies. Brighton, UK: Institute for Employment Studies; 1997.

5. Hoffman T. The meanings of competency. J Eur Ind Train. 1999;23(6):275–285.

6. Council on Linkages Between Academia and Public Health Practice. Prologue to the core competencies for public health. Washington, DC: Public Health Foundation. August 2005. Available at http://www.phf.org/Link/prologue.htm. Accessed September 22, 2006.

7. Gebbie K, Merrill J, Hwang I, Gebbie EN, Gupta M. The public health workforce in the year 2000. J Public Health Manage Pract. 2003;9(1):79–86.

8. Kerby DS, Brand MW, Johnson DL, Ghouri FS. Self-assessment in the measurement of public health workforce preparedness for bioterrorism or other public health disasters. Public Health Rep. March–April 2005;120(2):186–191.

9. US Department of Health and Human Services. Public health infrastructure. In: Healthy People 2010. 2nd ed. Washington, DC: US Government Printing Office; November 2000. Chap 23. Available at http://www.healthypeople.gov/document/HTML/Volume2/23PHI.htm. Accessed September 22, 2006.

10. Centers for Disease Control and Prevention. Bioterrorism and emergency readiness: competencies for all public health workers. Report TS 0740. Atlanta, GA: CDC; 2002.

11. University of North Carolina School of Public Health. Preparedness Center Training Site. Available at http://www2.sph.unc.edu/nccphp/training/. Accessed September 22, 2006.

12. Recommendations of the International Medical Informatics Association (IMIA) on education in health and medical informatics. Methods Inf Med. 2000;39(3):267–277.

13. Integrated Disease Surveillance and Response. Geneva, Switzerland: World Health Organization; 2006. Available at http://www.who.int/countries/eth/areas/surveillance/en/index.html. Accessed September 22, 2006.

14. Integrated Disease Surveillance Programme. Geneva, Switzerland: World Health Organization; Available at http://www.who.int/csr/labepidemiology/projects/surveillance/en/index.html. Accessed September 22, 2006.

15. Thacker SB, Berkelman RL. Public health surveillance in the United States. Epidemiol Rev. 1988;10:164–190.

16. Screening and Early Detection of Cancer. Geneva, Switzerland: World Health Organization; 2006. Available at http://www.who.int/cancer/detection/en/. Accessed September 22, 2006.

17. Public Health Functions Project. The Public Health Workforce: An Agenda for the 21st Century. Rockville, MD: National Center for Health Workforce Analysis; 2005.

18. Potter M, Pistella C, Fertman C, Dato V. Needs assessment and a model agenda for training the public health workforce. Am J Public Health. Aug 2000;90(8):1294–1296.

19. Harrison LM, Davis MV, MacDonald PD, et al. Development and implementation of a public health workforce training needs assessment survey in North Carolina. Public Health Rep. 2005;120 (suppl 1):28–34.

20. Borders S, Blakely C, Quiram B, McLeroy K. Considerations for increasing the competences and capacities of the public health workforce: assessing the training needs of public health workers in Texas. Hum Resour Health. July 26, 2006;4(1):18.

21. Brown JS, Learmonth A. Mind the gap: developing the PH workforce in the North East and Yorkshire and Humber regions: a scoping stakeholder study. Public Health. January 2005;119(1):32–38.

22. Council on Education for Public Health. Accreditation Criteria for Public Health Programs. Amended June 2005. Washington, DC: Council on Education for Public Health; 2005.

23. Association of Schools of Public Health. Final MPH Core Competency, Version 2.3. January 2006. Available at http://www.asph.org/. Accessed September 22, 2006.

24. Association of Schools of Public Health. Public health training centers: preparing public health professionals in a changing world. 2006. Available at

http://www.asph.org/document.cfm?page=780. Accessed September 22, 2006.

25. Course RH-SEC7: Surveillance in rural counties. 2006. Available at http://maphtc.uic.edu/Public/Catalog/. Accessed September 22, 2006.

26. Northwest Center for Public Health Practice at the University of Washington School of Public Health and Community Medicine. Courses and exercises. 2006. Available at http://www.nwcphp.org/training/courses-exercises/index.html. Accessed September 22, 2006.

27. CDC Public Health Training Opportunities: Epidemiology. Atlanta, GA: Centers for Disease Control and Prevention. Available at http://www.cdc.gov/phtrain/epidemiology.html. Accessed September 22, 2006.

28. Partners in Information Access for the Public Health Workforce. Education and training. August 23, 2006. Available at http://phpartners.org/educ.html. Accessed September 22, 2006.

29. Wagner MM, Moore AW, Aryel RM, eds. Handbook of Biosurveillance. Amsterdam, Netherlands: Elsevier Academic Press; 2006.

30. O'Carroll P, Yasnoff W, Wilhoite W. In: Public Health Informatics: A CDC Course for Public Health Program Managers, 1998. Philadelphia, PA: Hanley & Belfus; 1998:472–476.

31. Yasnoff W, Overhage J, Humphreys B, LaVenture M. A national agenda for public health informatics: summarized recommendations from the 2001 AMIA spring congress. J Am Med Inf Assoc. 2001;8(6):535–545.

32. Public Health Informatics Competencies. Seattle, WA: Northwest Center for Public Health Practice; August 2002. Available at http://nwcphp.org/resources/phicomps.v1. Accessed September 22, 2006.

33. Covvey HD, Zitner D, Bernstein RM, eds. Pointing the Way: Competencies and Curricula in Health Informatics. Edmonton, Alberta, Canada: Healthcare Information Management and Communication; 2001.

34. Lehmann HP. Medical informatics, educational technology, and the new curriculum, In: DeAngelis CD, ed. The Johns Hopkins University School of Medicine Curriculum for the Twenty-First Century. Baltimore: Johns Hopkins University Press; 1999:128–169.

35. Lehmann HP. Informatics in the health sciences. In: Armitage P, Colton T, eds. Encyclopedia of Biostatistics. 2nd ed. Chichester, UK: Wiley; 2005:2552–2554.

36. Biomedical informatics training certificate program. Pittsburgh, PA: University of Pittsburgh; August 15, 2006. Available at http://www.cbmi.pitt.edu/trainingprogram/certificate.htm. Accessed September 22, 2006.

37. Certificate in health geoinformatics (CHG): 2006 Summer Institute. Loma Linda, CA: Loma Linda University. Available at http://www.llu.edu/llu/sph/geoinformatics/chg06.html. Accessed September 22, 2006.

38. Graduate certificate program. College Park, MD: University of Maryland. Available at http://www.professionalstudies.umd.edu/phi/. Accessed September 22, 2006.

39. Certificate program overview. Houston, TX: University of Texas. August 3, 2006. Available at http://www.shis.uth.tmc.edu/education/certificate-program. Accessed September 22, 2006.

40. Public health informatics. Chicago: University of Illinois. Available at http://www.uic.edu/sph/phi/.

41. MSPH in Public Health Informatics. Atlanta, GA: Emory University. April 8, 2005. Available at http://www.sph.emory.edu/bios/phi.php. Accessed September 22, 2006.

42. Public health informatics fellowship program. Atlanta, GA: Centers for Disease Control and Prevention; January 3, 2006. Available at http://www2.cdc.gov/epo/dphsi/faq.asp. Accessed September 22, 2006.

43. Public health informatics fellows training program. Princeton, NJ: Robert Wood Johnson Foundation. Available at http://www.rwjf.org/applications/solicited/solicitedgrants.jhtml. Accessed September 22, 2006.

44. Education and training. New York: Columbia University. Available at http://www.dbmi.columbia.edu/publichealth/docs/et.html. Accessed September 24, 2006.

45. Masters of science candidates, 2007. Baltimore, MD: Johns Hopkins University; July 1, 2006. Available at http://dhsi.med.jhmi.edu/content/admissions.html. Accessed September 24, 2006.

46. Training track: public health informatics. Salt Lake City, UT: University of Utah; 2006. Available at http://uuhsc.utah.edu/medinfo/index.cfm?Content=DBcontent&mcid=1148. Accessed September 24, 2006.

47. Public health informatics group. Seattle, WA: University of Washington; 2006. Available at http://phig.washington.edu/. Accessed September 24, 2006.

48. University certificate public health informatics. Preston, UK: University of Central Lancashire. Available at http://www.uclan.ac.uk/courses/factsheets/health/lpsofmh/4752.pdf. Accessed September 24, 2006.

49. Masters in public health (MPH) postgraduate diploma in public health. Colchester, UK: University of Essex. Available at

http://www.sx.ac.uk/hhs/pg/pgt/msc_ph.htm. Accessed September 24, 2006.

50. Courses. Perth, Australia: Curtin University of Technology; February 16, 2006. Available at http://www.publichealth.curtin.edu.au/html/areasofstudy_courses.htm. Accessed September 24, 2006.

51. Health informatics programs additional information. Sydney, Australia: University of New South Wales. May 3, 2006. Available at http://www.sphcm.med.unsw.edu.au/SPHCMWeb.nsf/page/HI. Accessed September 24, 2006.

52. Thompson TG, Brailer DJ. The decade of health information technology: Delivering consumer-centric and information-rich health care framework for strategic action. Rockville, MD: US Department of Health and Human Services; 2004.

53. AMIA 10 x 10: 10,000 trained by 2010. Bethesda, MD: American Medical Informatics Association; August 30, 2006. Available at http://www.amia.org/10x10/. Accessed September 24, 2006.

54. Public health in America. Rockville, MD: Office of Disease Prevention and Health Promotion; January 1, 2000. Available at http://www.health.gov/phfunctions/public.htm. Accessed September 24, 2006.

55. Core competencies for public health professionals. Public Health Foundation; August 3, 2006. Available at http://www.phf.org/competencies.htm. Accessed September 24, 2006.

12 The Road Ahead: The Expanding Role of Informatics in Disease Surveillance

Joseph S. Lombardo

The previous chapters in this book presented the components of automated disease surveillance systems as well as case studies of systems that have found practical use within the public health community. Automated surveillance systems present a considerable advance over manual approaches, but the field of automated disease surveillance will continue to advance as operational experience and technology improvements are incorporated within new or existing surveillance tools. This final chapter surveys a few areas where significant progress is currently being made and where advances will probably be available within the next few years.

12.1 INTRODUCTION

Advances in information technology are having a major impact on the way that health departments conduct the business of disease surveillance. Currently, most major health departments use some form of computer application to conduct disease surveillance. Many of these applications are first-generation systems that were developed rapidly with funding related to bioterrorist threats to enable early disease recognition. The terrorist attacks of September 11, 2001, and the use of the U.S. Postal Service to transmit *Bacillus anthracis* caused federal and local health officials to recognize the urgent need for improvements to their disease surveillance processes. Many health departments enhanced their surveillance activities by requiring hospital emergency departments to fax them their patient encounter logs. These records were processed manually to look for abnormal trends in disease [1]. However, it quickly became evident that manual collection and processing of hospital records i.e. "active" reporting was a time-consuming and labor-intensive process that was taking a toll on health department personnel and funds.

The introduction of automated disease surveillance applications, developed by commercial, federal, and academic groups, provided an alternative to manual surveillance for public health departments. In many cases, however, these applications were not designed to take into account unique characteristics of specific jurisdictions, so many health departments elected to develop their own surveillance applications. Even these custom-built systems were implemented when limited knowledge existed about how best to use the data that were being acquired. As a result of this rush to implement first-generation systems, the potential for major improvements in existing surveillance applications is profound, especially as increased knowledge is obtained through the operation and analysis of current processes.

Several areas exist where improvements in automated public health surveillance are likely in the near future.

1. The enhancement of the interoperability among systems so that national, regional, and local disease surveillance networks can be assembled to collect and share data and information.

2. The adoption of a stable set of standards for the collection, sharing, and visualization of data and information among agencies responsible for disease surveillance.

3. The leveraging of enhancements in the electronic patient record, community and regional health information networks, and electronic laboratory reporting.

4. The streamlining of disease surveillance operations by leveraging public health informatics.

The remainder of this chapter addresses medical and public health informatics activities that could lead to major improvements in disease surveillance.

12.2   INTEGRATION OF DISEASE SURVEILLANCE SYSTEMS

One of the important functions of any public health informatics application is interoperability. Most public health organizations have, over time, developed and operated several applications. Many of these applications address some specific objective in surveillance or response. Examples from the local health departments include archiving and monitoring the occurrences of reportable diseases, cancer registries, medical examiners' reports, and the monitoring of hospital emergency departments and overall bed capacity in support of emergency medical systems response.

At the federal level, the Centers for Disease Control and Prevention (CDC) developed many different informatics applications in support of disease surveillance. Examples include the Early Warning Infectious Disease Surveillance program focused at states bordering Canada and Mexico, the 121 Cities Mortality Reporting System, the 8-City Enhanced BioTerrorism Surveillance Project, the Influenza Sentinel Physician Program, the Medical Examiner and Coroner Information Sharing

Program, the National Electronic Disease Surveillance System (NEDSS), the Health Alert Network (HAN), and BioSense. Information sharing among these programs should allow public health personnel to better understand disease trends that may be difficult to interpret from examination of one system alone. The ability to fuse data and information collected across many different systems is made possible through interoperable data sharing using standard representation of data elements and standard formats for transmission of data elements among systems.

Another example of interoperability enhancements in disease surveillance is the exchange of data and information among local, regional, and federal partners sharing resources in a secure, controlled environment. Some data sources, such as local emergency departments, may be acquired more easily by local health departments, where as, other such as over-the-counter medications sales, may be acquired more easily nationally by federal agencies. Public Health partners may use disease surveillance system of their own design or may use a common system. A surveillance network could include the distribution of responsibilities among participants for capturing, sharing, and analyzing surveillance data as well as supporting follow-up activities for investigating abnormal disease events. Sharing responsibilies among several partners could reduce the overall cost of surveillance while pooling knowledge from each of the partners.

12.2.1 Data Privacy and Public Health Networks

The Health Insurance Portability Accountability Act (HIPAA) Privacy Rule recognizes the legitimate need for public health authorities and others responsible for ensuring public health and safety to have access to protected health information to carry out their public health mission. The rule also recognizes that public health reports made by covered entities are an important means of identifying threats to the health and safety of the public at large as well as to individuals. Accordingly, the rule permits covered entities to disclose protected health information without authorization for specified public health purposes [2]. More specific information regarding the HIPAA rules is presented in Chapter 3.

In the past, most health departments have taken a relatively conservative approach to maximizing privacy when acquiring data for surveillance use. These health departments minimize the collection and use of personal identifiers to live within the spirit of HIPAA even though such information can be acquired legally and used by public health departments for surveillance. More recently, some states have passed laws mandating the collection of hospital emergency department data [3]. For example, in March 2004, the state of Indiana passed a law requiring the state health department to collect data related to symptoms and health syndromes that may be a threat to public health. This same law required schools to report to the local health departments the percentages of students absent above a set threshold. Similar laws have enabled health departments to acquire data from covered entities that may have previously taken a conservative approach to sharing surveillance data.

However, it may sometimes be difficult for local surveillance systems to share data because agreements with local data providers typically do not permit data transfer to third parties. Many data-sharing agreements restrict health departments from sharing even portions of their data over a surveillance network outside their local boundaries. Because infectious diseases do not honor jurisdictional boundaries, public health agencies will need to find solutions for sharing information and performing surveillance among neighboring jurisdictions.

12.2.2   Standards for Information Sharing

In September 2005, the U.S. Department of Health and Human Services (DHHS) chartered the American Health Information Community (AHIC) to provide input and recommendations to DHHS on how to make health records digital, interoperable, private, and secure. AHIC consists of 17 members from both the federal government and private industry. AHIC adopted three priority issues: increasing biosurveillance capabilities, adopting standards for electronic health records, and defining data fields and algorithms for care quality measures. In support of AHIC, the Healthcare Information Technology Standards Panel (HITSP) was formed to recommend a set of standards to enable interoperability among software applications for local, regional, and national networks. Within HITSP, three committees have been formed: biosurveillance, consumer empowerment, and electronic health records.

The biosurveillance committee is chartered with providing recommendations for acquiring emergency department data for conducting disease surveillance. In September 2006, an initial draft of recommendations of the biosurveillance committee was submitted [4]. The overall scope of activities for the biosurveillance committee recommendations are described in the following six areas:

1. Populate biosurveillance information systems (BIS) with data from emergency departments.

2. Support detection of public health threats with the data provided.

3. Support ongoing monitoring of an event with a continuing receipt of data.

4. Support rapid response management of an event using information received.

5. Evaluate the BIS performance.

6. Improve the BIS performance as needed.

The Public Health Information Network (PHIN) is a CDC initiative to define a set of standards and business practices that support interoperability among public health applications [5]. The process of identifying appropriate standards for public health informatics applications has been slow and laborious. The process is complicated because technology is advancing much faster than standards can be established. Many health departments that developed applications based on one set of standards, found that by the time their applications became operational, the interoperability standards had changed and the interpretation of the standard used when development began was no longer valid. This confusion resulted in developers implementing applications with communication solutions that were not able to communicate. AHIC and the HITSP will expedite the PHIN standardization process to help prevent this type of occurrence in the future.

12.2.3   Regional and National Networks

Regional health information organizations (RHIOs), are regional- or state-supported projects to assist in the development of privacy and business rules for health information exchange. There are currently over 100 regional projects funded by the federal government and many more are supported by private industry or state legislatures. A good example of such an initiative is the California Regional Health Information Organization (CalRHIO), whose objectives are to construct a secure network for the exchange of health information across the state [6].

Two projects initiated by CalRHIO that benefit disease surveillance are emergency department linking and personal health records. The emergency department linkage project will provide information needed for point-of-care decisions, but because the project is to link all of the state's 350 hospitals, the data could also be used for disease surveillance by capturing disease trends across the state. The personal health record initiative will provide a longitudinal record of a person's health. This record could be used to increase the specificity of the information used in surveillance. Use of standard vocabularies and communications protocols are the key for the success of the CalRHIO projects. Figure 12.1 provides a roadmap for the implementation of these standards by CalRHIO.

Regional networks have been formed specifically for the purpose of conducting surveillance across jurisdictional boundaries. Within the National Capital Region (NCR), the state and local health departments surrounding Washington, DC, have formed an enhanced surveillance operating group to share surveillance data and analysis protocols across the region. Each member of the group provides data into an aggregated surveillance system that is used by each member health department in the region. This initiative has worked very well because each stakeholder has a vested interest in making the network succeed. Details of this network are presented in Chapter 6.

Also as mentioned in Chapter 6, the CDC is establishing a national network to acquire data for the BioSense system. The results of analyses conducted at CDC with data collected locally are made available to local health departments. The intent of BioSense is to share unprocessed data received locally with local health departments using the standards proposed in BioSense. If this goal is accomplished, a two-way linkage will be established between the local health departments and the CDC. The next step will be to create linkages within the network so that local health departments can share data and information within a defined region.

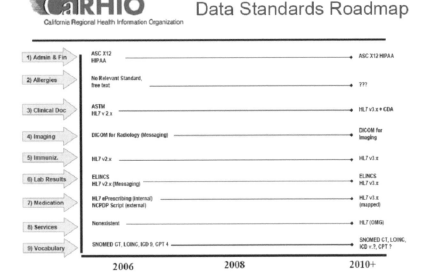

Fig. 12.1   CalRHIO road map for the implementation of standards in California.

12.3   SURVEILLANCE SYSTEM ENHANCEMENTS

12.3.1   Better Health Indicators

Current initiatives in standardization for electronic medical records, interoperability and communications, and the development of regional and national networks have the potential to increase the timeliness and specificity of disease surveillance (biosurveillance) systems.

12.3.1.1   Electronic Medical Record   The electronic medical record (EMR) contains electronic documents as well as functions including [7]:

- Patient demographics

- Medical history, examination, and progress reports

- Medicine and allergy lists and immunization status

- Scheduling, retrieval, and archiving of laboratory and other tests

- Graphic image display of x-rays, MRIs, and other medical imaging studies

- Medication ordering, including patient safety functions to minimize interactions or side effects

- Evidence-based recommendations for specific medical conditions, termed *clinical practice guidelines*

- Appointment scheduling

- Claims and payment processing

- Patient reminders of follow-up appointments, test completion, and preventive health practices

Many institutions are developing EMRs. However, because of this institutional perspective, EMRs permit viewing only by caregivers who perform their duties within a medical institution or medical group. Most EMRs do not permit patients or caregivers who work outside the group to view their data.

The term *electronic health record* (EHR) has been used to refer to a record that can be accessed by any caregiver providing care to a patient. Ideally, the EHR can be accessed for point-of-care service within a physician's office, emergency department, or outpatient clinic. This type of record requires one or more archives or repositories to be accessed securely, with information merged and presented to those seeking the information.

One component of the EHR is the continuity of care record (CCR), which is a historical record of a single patient's encounters and treatments for every health care provider supporting the care of the patient. The CCR provides summaries of patients' historical and present health status for primary care physicians and specialists supporting the care of the patient. The CCR plays an important role in making decisions on how to treat and support a patient with a history of illness.

Both the U.S. Department of Defense Tri-Service Healthcare System, known as TriCare, and the Veterans' Health Administration (VHA) have made much progress in the development and implementation of the EHR. Health maintenance organizations (HMOs) have also developed components of the EMR, EHR, and CCR for the care of their enrollees. These successes have occurred because the records remain within the local networks for organizations holding data. Challenges remain regarding information exchange among different organizations competing for health insurance revenues from large employers.

Once again, standards are key to the interoperability of EMRs and EHRs. The following list includes standards relevant to EMRs [7]. This list will be replaced when the HITSP biosurveillance committee completes its mission.

1. *ASTM (CCR):* a patient health summary standard based on XML, the CCR can be created, read, and interpreted by various EHR or EMR systems, allowing easy interoperability between otherwise disparate entities.

2. *ANSI X12 (EDI):* a set of transaction protocols used to transmit virtually any aspect of patient data. This has become popular in the United States for transmitting billing information because several of the transactions are required by the

Health Insurance Portability and Accountability Act (HIPAA) for transmitting data to Medicare.

3. *CEN-EHRcom:* EN13606, the European standard for the communication of information from EHR systems.

4. *DICOM:* a frequently used standard for representing and communicating radiology images and reporting.

5. *HL7:* HL7 messages are used for interchange between hospital and physician record systems and between EMR systems and practice management systems; HL7 Clinical Document Architecture (CDA) documents are used to communicate documents such as physician notes and other material.

6. *ISO:* ISO TC215 has defined the EHR and produced a technical specification, ISO 18308, describing the requirements for EHR architectures.

7. *openEHR:* next-generation public specifications and implementations for EHR systems and communication, based on a complete separation of software and clinical models.

8. Electronic laboratory reporting.

In response to the antiterrorism policies outlined in Presidential Decision Directive 39 [8], the CDC established the Laboratory Response Network (LRN) [9]. The objective of this project is to increase the capacity of state and local laboratories to support analysis of samples from acts of bioterrorism. The network is also being used to analyze environmental samples collected under the Department of Homeland Security's (DHS) BioWatch Program [10]. The LRN provides a unique asset linking state and local public health laboratories with the CDC. Similar networks are needed to link hospital and private clinical laboratories in support of early warning for public health surveillance.

For several years there have been initiatives to improve the laboratory reporting of reportable diseases to state health departments. These initiatives are collectively designated *electronic laboratory reporting* [11]. These initiatives also require the acceptance of standards to permit interoperability among the local laboratories and health departments to which they report. Once the implementation issues are resolved, the data will be invaluable to health departments for their surveillance mission because the laboratory data provide needed specificity that is missing in most of the other health care indicators being used for early alerting. Consideration has been given to the use of laboratory requests as an early indicator of specific diseases for surveillance at both the national and local levels [12].

12.3.2   Biostatistics

Developing analytic processes for the early identification of abnormal disease trends is challenging for several reasons. Algorithms are typically designed and evaluated against a data characteristic from a specific data source. Because of the wealth of possible sources of data that could be used as health indicators, it is unlikely that any single algorithm will perform on all data sources. Different time lags exist between creation of the data element and the time those data are received by the disease surveillance system. Not all data can be received in real time, and the algorithms must take into account lags among the data sources.

The time when an abnormal disease indication may first be evident also varies in different data sources and is a function of several parameters, including availability of insurance coverage, socioeconomic class, and disease. One might expect self-medication to occur early in the stage of a disease compared to an emergency department encounter when the symptoms are more acute. Using over-the-counter (OTC) medications as an early indicator would not be very effective for socioeconomic classes who do not have the ability to purchase these medications. At the other end of the socioeconomic spectrum, an early indication would not be expected for those who have the resources to stock up with medications frequently used to relieve symptoms of common ailments.

Many modern disease surveillance systems process only homogeneous data sources because the differences in characteristics vary widely among data sources. For example, many systems only use chief complaint data from emergency departments. To fully exploit the data available for surveillance, analytical techniques will need to be able to fuse all data types that provide value for early recognition of a health event. The set of analytics will vary for diseases with different signs and symptoms. Time-stepped data fusion techniques are needed to take into account the sequence of health- seeking behaviors occurring in different indicators.

Many algorithms currently exist for the identification of changing conditions. Process control techniques used in manufacturing have been found useful in detecting health events. Many of the current data mining techniques used to link data from several sources could be applied if privacy laws didn't restrict the use of data elements that could be used for linking. Much work is needed to adapt these techniques to achieve high values of sensitivity and specificity for early detection of public health events.

12.3.3 Information Technology

As more data sources become available for use in disease surveillance systems, additional techniques will be needed to capture data for use in surveillance processes as well as for viewing the vast amount of information collected. The most successful systems have relied on capturing data from existing systems. Manual collection of data specifically for disease surveillance has proven to be too labor intensive to be sustainable over long time periods. New technologies that automate the process of data entry are needed.

Surveillance systems have an enhanced value if they permit the user to see not only the outputs of analytical processes, but also the basic data elements. Many users of surveillance systems rely on their knowledge of the data sources to resolve false alarms that occur as a result of a variety of factors. As more items become available for possible viewing, newer techniques will be needed for digesting large amounts of data by the user. Data viewed in a specific format may provide insights for some events and not for others, so a wide variety of formats may be needed to obtain optimal use of the data.

12.3.4   Health Department Business Processes

As health departments expand their use of informatics applications, traditional business processes must be modified or expanded. Automated disease surveillance systems provide the time-saving benefits of capturing, archiving, and processing large amounts of data, but most health departments do not have the personnel and financial resources to follow up on alerts that are not true health events. Fortunately, more experienced surveillance system users have learned to recognize alerts that can easily be explained away or are interesting, but of little significance, as opposed to a public health event requiring intervention.

Disease surveillance systems must have the flexibility to adapt to the ever-changing challenges facing health departments. System users must be able to add new data sources and define or modify case definitions, syndrome groupings, or analytic processes without having to go back to the system developers or health department IT staff. The enhancements mentioned above have the potential for increasing the performance of modern disease surveillance systems while also increasing their value to support the management of public health events.

12.4   STUDY QUESTIONS

12.1   Interoperability — the ability to share data and information using a common format among different surveillance systems developed by different organizations — is a critical improvement. Agreement on a set of standards to make systems interoperable is making significant progress. These standards will permit the formation of networks at state, local, regional, and national levels. Disease surveillance networks require not only interoperability at the application level, but also require the ability to share data and information covered by current privacy laws. *Q: How would you propose to resolve the legal and ethical data-sharing issues across public health surveillance networks?*

12.2   Soon, many more sources of data will become available for use in public health surveillance systems. Because these data will not have common characteristics, automated processing will result in more false alerts, requiring more data to be viewed by public health monitors of surveillance systems. *Q: Given the time constraints of public health employees, suggest business processes to monitor large quantities of data, information, and algorithm outputs more efficiently.*

12.3 Most automated disease surveillance systems rely on acquiring data that have been collected for other purposes. A good example is billing using ICD-9 disease codes. Many other sources of data could also be useful for surveillance if the labor needed to collect the data was minimal. One example is the monitoring of animals that might be good sentinels for acts of terrorism. Currently, no automated data collection systems exist to monitor the animals that are most sensitive to diseases resulting from acts of bioterrorism. *Q: Describe mechanisms that could be used to acquire surveillance data automatically from sources that are currently very manually intensive.*

REFERENCES

1. Begier EM, Sockwell D, Branch LM, et al. The National Capitol Region's emergency department syndromic surveillance system: Do chief complaint and discharge diagnosis yield different results? Emerg Infect Dis. 2003;9(3):393–396.

2. US Department of Health and Human Services, Office for Civil Rights–HIPAA. Medical privacy: national standards to protect the privacy of personal health information. 2003. Available at `http://www.hhs.gov/ocr/hipaa/privacy.html`. Accessed September 13, 2006.

3. Indiana House Enrolled Act 1202. An act to amend the Indiana Code concerning health. Second Regular Session 113th General Assembly. Source: IC 16-19-10-8. 2004. Available at `http://www.in.gov/legislative/bills/2004/HE/HE1202.1.html`. Accessed September 13, 2006.

4. US Department of Health and Human Services, Office of the National Coordinator for Health Information Technology. Healthcare Information Technology Standards Panel (HITSP), Use Case 1, Biosurveillance: providing emergency room and lab result data, Version 1.0, via ANSI Public Document Library. 2006. Available at `http://public.ansi.org/ansionline/Documents/`. Accessed September 13, 2006.

5. US Department of Health and Human Services, Centers for Disease Control and Prevention. Public Health Information Network. Available at `http://www.cdc.gov/phin/`. Accessed September 13, 2006.

6. California Regional Health Information Organization. Available at `http://www.calrhio.org/`. Accessed September 13, 2006.

7. Wikipedia. Electronic medical record. Available at `http://en.wikipedia.org/wiki/Electronic_medical_record`. Accessed September 13, 2006.

8. The White House. 1995. U.S. policy on counterterrorism. Presidential Decision Directive 39. Available at `http://www.fas.org/irp/offdocs/pdd39.htm`. Accessed September 13, 2006.

9. US Department of Health and Human Services, Centers for Disease Control and Prevention. The Laboratory Response Network Partners in Preparedness. 2005. Available at `http://www.bt.cdc.gov/lrn/`. Accessed September 13, 2006.

10. Shen DA, Lister SA. The BioWatch Program: detection of bioterrorism. Congressional Research Services Report RL 32152. 2003. Available at `http://www.fas.org/sgp/crs/terror/RL32152.html`. Accessed September 13, 2006.

11. Jernigan DB. Electronic laboratory-based reporting: opportunities and challenges for surveillance, Emerg Infect Dis. 2001;7(3) (suppl): 538.

12. Haobo Ma, Rolka H, et al. Implementation of laboratory order data in BioSense early event detection and situational awareness. MMWR Suppl. 2005;54:27–30.

Index